Examination
Intensive Care
Medicine

2nd edition

Examination Intensive Care Medicine

2nd edition

Carole Foot
MBBS (Hons), FACEM, FCICM, MSc International Health Management

Liz Steel
BMedSci, MBChB (Hons), MRCP, FCICM

Kim Vidhani
MBChB, FRCA, FCICM, FANZCA

Bruce Lister
MBBS, FANZCA, FCICM, MBA

Matthew Mac Partlin
LRCP&SI, MB, BCh, BAO, MRCPI, FACEM, FCICM

Nikki Blackwell
MBBS, BSc, FRCP, FRACP, FAChPM, FJFICM, DTMH, PSM

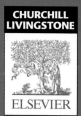

CHURCHILL LIVINGSTONE

ELSEVIER

Sydney   Edinburgh   London   New York   Philadelphia   St Louis   Toronto

Churchill Livingstone
is an imprint of Elsevier

Elsevier Australia. ACN 001 002 357
(a division of Reed International Books Australia Pty Ltd)
Tower 1, 475 Victoria Avenue, Chatswood, NSW 2067

ELSEVIER

This edition © 2012 Elsevier Australia

National Library of Australia Cataloguing-in-Publication Data

Title: Examination intensive care medicine / Carole Foot … [et al.].

Edition: 2nd ed.

ISBN: 9780729539623 (pbk.)

Notes: Includes index.

Subjects: Joint Faculty of Intensive Care Medicine
          (Australasia)--Examinations.
          Critical care medicine--Australia--Textbooks.
          Anesthesia--Australia--Textbooks.

Other Authors/Contributors: Foot, Carole.

Dewey Number: 616.028

Publisher: Sophie Kaliniecki
Developmental Editor: Neli Bryant
Publishing Services Manager: Helena Klijn
Project Coordinator: Geraldine Minto
Edited by Margaret Trudgeon
Proofread by Kerry Brown
Illustrations by Shaun Jury
Cover and adaptation of internal design by Lamond Art & Design
Index by Cynthia Swanson
Typeset by TNQ Books and Journals
Printed by China Translation and Printing Services Ltd

Dedication

To   Tom Czarniecki [CF]

Daniel, Katie and Rocky Steel [LS]

Leo and family; Tania, Pat and family [KV]

Tui Phantomlobo [BL]

La, Fiona, Ciara, Kevin and Nora Mac Partlin [MMacP]

Jeremy Hayllar and Paget [NB]

In memory of Lynne Dowd (1959–2011), wife, mother, doctor.

Her warmth and ability to listen, combined with enthusiasm for a challenge and life in general, will be missed by her family, friends and patients.

Text contents

DVD Contents   xiii
About the DVD   xv
Foreword   xvii
Preface   xix
About the authors   xxi
Acknowledgements   xxiii
DVD Acknowledgements   xxv

Chapter 1 Training in intensive care medicine in Europe and
           Australasia   1
           European Diploma of Intensive Care Medicine (EDIC)   1
               EDIC Part 1: Multiple choice question (MCQ) paper 2
               EDIC Part 2: Clinical and oral examination   3
           UK Intercollegiate Diploma in Intensive Care Medicine (DICM) 4
               Dissertation   5
               Expanded case summaries   6
               Exam format   6
           Fellowship of the College of Intensive Care
           Medicine (FCICM) training requirements   6
               Core knowledge and resources   6
               CICM Primary examination   7
               CICM Fellowship examination   9

Chapter 2 Strategies for success   12
           Timing   12
           Preparation courses   12
               EDIC/DICM   12
               FCICM   13
           Textbooks, journals and online resources   14
           Study notes   15
           Looking after yourself   17
           Study groups   18
           Clinical cases   20
           Vivas   20
           Creating the right impression   21
           Travel considerations   21
           On the day   21
           Coping with failure   22

Chapter 3 Basic sciences for intensive care medicine   24
           Introduction   24
           Physiology   25
               Respiratory system   26
               Cardiovascular system   33
               Renal system   39
               Neurological system   44
               Gastrointestinal system   46
               Thermoregulation   48
               Musculoskeletal system   48

Immunology and host defence 49
Haematological system 49
Obstetrics 50
Endocrine and nutrition 52
Pharmacology 52
Diagrams and graphs 52
Tables 55
Lists 58
Applying concepts to consolidate learning 60
Mind maps 60
Facts cards 61
Past papers 61
Making your own questions 64
Exam templates 66
Quizzes 66

Chapter 4   Equipment 68
Equipment overview 68
Arrangement of the equipment library 70
Physics and clinical measurement 75

Chapter 5   Practical and procedural skills 77
Overview 77
Classification of assessment types 77
Actor stations 77
Part task trainers 78
Full body manikins 78
Hybrids 78
Advice for approaching procedural skill assessments 78
Examples of scenarios 80
Actor stations 80
Part task trainers 82
Anatomy 85
Full body manikins 91
Questions examining practical and procedural
skills in the various exams 92
Demonstration of brainstem death clinical tests 92
High peak airway pressures in a ventilated patient 96
Hybrids 99

Chapter 6   Data interpretation for intensive care medicine 101
Overview of data interpretation 101
Imaging studies 102
Chest X-rays 103
CT scans – chest and neck 117
Abdominal X-rays 121
Abdominal ultrasound 126
CT scans – abdomen 127
CT scans – head 131
Skeletal and soft tissue imaging 136
Other imaging modalities 146
Electrocardiographs 147
Haemodynamic monitoring 151

Central venous pressure waveforms 151
Mixed venous oxygen saturation (SvO_2) and central
venous oxygen saturation ($ScvO_2$) 152
Arterial waveforms 152
Intra-aortic balloon pump waveforms 153
Pulmonary artery catheters 155
Newer haemodynamic measurement devices 158
Echocardiography 159
Respiratory function tests 167
Spirometry 167
DLCO 167
Flow–volume loops 168
Pressure–volume loops 170
Ventilator waveforms 171
Indirect calorimetry 174
Capnography 174
Biochemistry tests 175
Arterial blood gas analysis 175
Biochemistry data sets 179
Autoimmune markers 184
Short Synacthen test 185
Thyroid function tests 186
Iron studies 186
Tumour markers 186
Miscellaneous other tests 186
Haematology 187
Blood counts 187
Coagulation studies 190
Haematologic datasets 193
Analysis of body fluids 195

Chapter 7 Vivas 201
Generic advice 201
Format 203
Viva topics for the EDIC, DICM and CICM Fellowship
examinations 203
Possible viva topics 204
Vivas for the Primary examination of the CICM 208

Chapter 8 Clinical cases in the ICU 209
Introduction 209
A generic approach to the clinical case 210
Environmental clues 211
Systematic clinical examination 213
Presenting to the examiners 214
Diagnostic problems 217
1. Why does this patient have severe respiratory failure? 217
2. Why is this patient failing to wean from ventilation? 219
3. Can you extubate this patient? 221
4. Why is this patient shocked? 223
5. Why is this patient not passing urine? 225
6. Why is this patient jaundiced? 226
7. Why is this patient not waking up? 228

8. Why is this patient weak?   229
9. Is this patient brain dead?   231
10. Why is this patient febrile?   233
11. What injuries has this multiple trauma patient
 sustained?   235
12. How is this patient with multi-organ failure
 progressing?   238
Specific patient groups   238
1. The patient with chronic obstructive
 pulmonary disease   238
2. The cardiac arrest survivor   240
3. The post-cardiac surgical patient   242
4. The patient with a subarachnoid
 haemorrhage   245
5. The patient with a head injury   246
6. The patient with a spinal injury   249
7. The patient with an intra-abdominal catastrophe   251
8. The patient who has had an abdominal
 aortic aneurysm repair   253
9. The obstetric patient   254
10. The transplant patient   256
11. The oncology patient   258
12. The patient with burns   261
13. The patient receiving extracorporeal life support   263
14. The bariatric patient   265
15. The long-stay patient   267

Chapter 9 Critical care literature   269
Introduction to the reference library   269
Statistics   271
Data   272
Inferential statistics – which test to use and when   272
Trials   274
Factors involved in study design   275
Meta-analysis   275
Diagnostic tests   276
Looking at papers   277

Chapter 10 Paediatric intensive care   279
Introduction   279
Key paediatric facts   280
The paediatric component of the FCICM   283
Training in Paediatric Intensive Care Medicine
in Australasia   283
Training requirements   283
Strategies for success   284
Blueprint for the PIC Fellowship examination   284
The clinical component of the FCICM   291
Clinical cases   291
1. Is this child suitable for extubation?   291
2. The post-cardiac surgical paediatric case   292
3. The child on extracorporeal life support (ECLS)   295
4. The child post-transplant   297

5. The child with a head injury   299
6. The child with acute kidney injury   301
Paediatric critical care literature   304
   Brain death and organ donation   304
   Burns   304
   Cardiovascular medicine   305
   Endocrine   309
   Fluids and electrolytes   309
   Haematology   310
   Neurology   310
   Nutrition   312
   Renal medicine   313
   Resuscitation   313
   Respiratory medicine   314
   Sedation and analgesia   316
   Sepsis   316

List of abbreviations   319
Index   327

DVD contents

Introduction

Chapter supplements

    Equipment
        Cardiovascular
        Respiratory
        Renal
        Gastroenterology
        Neurology
        Infection control
        Other

    Practical & procedural skills
        Central venous line insertion
        Arterial line insertion
        Pulmonary artery catheter insertion
        Intra-aortic balloon pump insertion
        Defibrillation/Electrical Cardioversion
        Transcutaneous pacing
        Temporary transvenous pacing wire insertion
        Pericardiocentesis
        Intra-osseous needle insertion
        Standard intubation via the oral route
        Laryngeal mask insertion
        Cricothyroidotomy
        Percutaneous tracheostomy
        Emergency thoracocentesis
        Chest drain insertion
        Small bore catheter insertion
        Diagnostic bronchoscopy
        Nasogastric tube insertion
        Minnesota tube insertion
        Lumbar puncture

    Data interpretation
        Microbiology
        Transcranial doppler studies
        Electroencephalography
        Intracranial pressure monitoring
        Cardiotocography

    Critical care literature
        Airway management
        Anaesthesia
        Cardiovascular medicine
        Ethics
        Fluids and electrolytes
        Gastroenterology

Haematology/transfusion
Monitoring devices
Neurology
Obstetrics and Gynaecology
Pain medicine
Perioperative medicine
Quality
Renal medicine
Respiratory medicine
Resuscitation and cardiac arrest
Sedation
Sepsis
Steroids
Toxicology
Trauma
Paediatric Critical Care Literature

Recall cases
Lab data
ECG data
Imaging data
Monitoring data
Clinical photo cases
Paediatric cases
Index of cases

Useful resources

Flow-man diagrams
Blank template
Abdominal catastrophe
Abdominal catastrophe with VAC dressing
Cardiogenic shock
High frequency oscillatory ventilation (HFOV)
Multiorgan failure (MOF)
Polytrauma
Traumatic brain injury (TBI)
Obstetric
Post CABG or valve surgery

Pharmacology quiz

References

Copyright & Legal

About the DVD

This edition of *Examination Intensive Care Medicine* is accompanied by a complementary DVD. It contains a wide range of extra information, and reflects the growth of intensive care as a specialty area since the publication of *Examination Intensive Care and Anaesthesia* in 2006. By presenting this information on DVD we have avoided creating a large, unwieldly book or multiple volumes. Also, the format allows us to present the information in a more interactive, portable and user-friendly manner.

The content of the DVD is easily navigable by clicking on the section or topic of interest.

Foreword

Medical specialist examinations, in the milieu of a busy clinical workload and a young family, can be all-consuming and soul destroying. With motivation, careful planning and regular revision, climbing this Everest can become more manageable, exacting a lesser cost in relationships and physical and mental health. How best to do this?

Educators have devised techniques in 'active learning' such as SQ3R (Survey, Question, Read, Recite, Review), PQRST (Preview, Question, Read, Summary, Test) and the KWL Table (what we know, want to know, learned), with tips on passing examinations. While these have undoubtedly helped high school and university students, the more mature medical specialists-to-be require approaches more substantive than sublime, basic 'how to' methods to pass a more demanding clinical examination. While textbooks on the specialty of intensive care are plentiful, those that address preparing and 'fronting' intensive care examinations are as rare as the proverbial hen's teeth. *Examination Intensive Care Medicine* fills this gap.

The book first addresses training programs and their examination formats in Australia and New Zealand (College of Intensive Care Medicine), the United Kingdom (Intercollegiate Board for Training in Intensive Care Medicine), and Europe (European Society of Intensive Care Medicine). The other chapters (ten in all) discuss strategies and tips on studying (e.g. health, study notes, study groups), presentation (e.g. travel, dress), and performance at vivas and clinical cases. The pragmatic pearls are not limited to the above examinations, but are universally useful for other intensive care examinations, or indeed (in many parts), for other specialty examinations.

Apart from strategies and tips on studying for, and presenting at, intensive care examinations, this book also provides a mountain of relevant factual information to help pass these examinations (i.e. SQ3R and PQRST material), including basic sciences, equipment, procedures, clinical cases and investigations. Chapter 3, 'Basic Sciences for Intensive Care Medicine', offers a superbly comprehensive and useful revision for candidates of all acute medical specialty examinations. The icing on the cake is an accompanying interactive DVD, replete with a wealth of material, including ECGs, images, laboratory profiles, monitoring data and supplementary facts.

Any resource that can guide a candidate to pass an intensive care examination is good, but it *must* be good to succeed. *Examination Intensive Care Medicine* is impressively good. The first tip in this journey to be a specialist intensivist should be: *Read this book before paying your examination fee.*

Professor Teik E. Oh
AM, MBBS, MD(Qld), FCICM, FRACP, FRCP, FANZCA, FRCA,
Hon FCA(SA), Hon FCA RCSI,
Emeritus Professor, University of Western Australia

Preface

In the last two decades intensive care medicine (ICM) has rapidly evolved into a medical speciality in its own right. The Australian and New Zealand College of Anaesthetists and Royal Australasian College of Physicians Joint Faculty of Intensive Care Medicine (ANZCA/RACP JFICM) developed a Fellowship training and examination process that is widely recognised as a premier training program for intensivists worldwide. In 2008 they moved to establish the first independent training college for ICM in the world and on 1 January 2010 the College of Intensive Care Medicine of Australia and New Zealand (CICM) became formally operational.

In 2006 Elsevier published *Examination Intensive Care and Anaesthesia* (Nikki Blackwell, Carole Foot and Christopher Thomas) for both Australasian ICM and anaesthesia trainees, reflecting a historic close relationship between the two specialities. This highly successful book was the first examination guide to help meet the needs of these two groups of clinicians.

There are increasing numbers of individuals training in ICM in Europe and Australasia. They now come from a diversity of backgrounds, including anaesthesia, emergency medicine, medicine and surgery. Recently, a pathway has evolved in Australasia for training in ICM alone and the first primary examination was held in 2007. There are strong relationships between the intensivists working in these regions, many of whom have trained and/or worked in several countries. To standardise training in ICM the CICM in Australasia, the European Society of Intensive Care Medicine (ESICM) and the Intercollegiate Board for Training in Intensive Care Medicine (IBTICM) in the United Kingdom have all introduced competency-based training programs and formative assessment. The first EDIC exam was held in 1989, the first UK diploma in 1998, and the modern, revised JFICM in 2002. Not unexpectedly, there are many similarities in the topics covered and methods of assessment prescribed in the training and examination syllabuses for the three training programs.

There is a need for high-quality, exam-focused resources to facilitate the passage of candidates through these various ICU Fellowship examinations, which are universally demanding and stressful career progression requirements. This book covers the key components of the syllabuses of EDIC, UK ICM diploma and the CICM Primary and Fellowship exams. It also provides material to assist trainees approaching the CICM Paediatric ICM Fellowship exam. Comprehensive strategies for dealing with each of the specific components of the exams are covered in detail using a structured approach that is evident from the table of contents. The purpose of this book is not to replace didactic intensive care textbooks but to provide exam candidates with all the necessary tailored information they require to successfully and more easily pass their examinations. This book will also be extremely useful as an update and/or reference guide for supervisors of training, established intensivists and all non-training doctors practising critical care medicine.

The first two chapters deal with training requirements in intensive care medicine as well as providing some hints for surviving the pre-exam period. These are followed by a summary of the essential basic sciences facts underpinning ICM practice, which is relevant to a greater or lesser degree to all of the examinations. Chapters 4 to 6 cover equipment, practical and procedural skills, and data interpretation, addressing the breadth of material related to the practical side of practice. This area is fundamental for intensivists and is frequently examined.

The vivas and clinical cases are then addressed in Chapter 7 and 8, with an emphasis on preparing candidates for interactive sessions with examiners and patients. The aim of these sections is not to produce 'intensivist clones'; instead we hope that readers will be able to use these suggestions as a framework to develop their own individual clinical/exam style.

Familiarity with key journal articles is essential for the practising intensivist. Understanding the state of the literature surrounding ICM not only facilitates exam performance, but also enables candidates to move beyond the process with a foundation on which to contextualise new developments during their future career as a specialist. Chapter 9 summarises the important tools needed to evaluate such material.

Finally, Chapter 10 addresses the needs of CICM Paediatric Fellowship exam candidates. This material is also relevant for candidates approaching the CICM Adult and European examinations as adult intensivists may be called upon to resuscitate and manage young patients until transfer can be made to paediatric centres. Key paediatric knowledge is therefore expected. This is a common source of stress for candidates with limited paediatric critical care experience.

The accompanying DVD complements the book by providing a wealth of additional resources and material. In particular, there is an extensive equipment and procedure library, a summary of important papers intensivists need to be aware of, a range of recall cases and a pharmacology quiz to facilitate self-assessment and guide further study.

We are all practising intensivists with a passion for education and training. We have written the book for our future colleagues. We sincerely hope that this book makes the reader's journey to a long and rewarding career in ICM somewhat less daunting and helps them present their hard-won knowledge and clinical competence to the best possible advantage.

Carole Foot
Liz Steel
Kim Vidhani
Bruce Lister
Matthew Mac Partlin
Nikki Blackwell

April 2011

About the authors

Carole Foot MBBS (Hons), FACEM, FCICM, MSc International Health Management (Distinction)
Clinical Associate Professor, University of Sydney, NSW, Australia; Staff Intensive Care Specialist, Royal North Shore Hospital; Visiting Medical Officer and Co-Supervisor of Training, North Shore Private Hospital, Sydney, NSW, Australia; Winner of the Joint Faculty of Intensive Care Medicine GA (Don) Harrison Medal for the highest Fellowship Examination mark for 2004.

Liz Steel BMedSci, MBChB (Hons), MRCP, FCICM
Staff Intensive Care Specialist, Royal North Shore Hospital; Visiting Medical Officer and Co-Supervisor of Training, North Shore Private Hospital, Sydney, NSW, Australia. New Fellows Representative on the Board of the College of Intensive Care Medicine (CICM) of Australia and New Zealand.

Kim Vidhani MBChB, FRCA, FCICM, FANZCA
Staff Specialist (Anaesthesia), Princess Alexandra Hospital, Brisbane; Staff Specialist (Intensive Care), Ipswich Hospital, Qld, Australia.

Bruce Lister MBBS, FANZCA, FCICM, MBA
Associate Professor, Griffith University Medical School, Qld. Staff Paediatric Intensive Care Specialist and Supervisor of Training, Mater Children's Hospital, Brisbane, Qld, Australia; Board Member, College of Intensive Care Medicine of Australia and New Zealand.

Matthew Mac Partlin LRCP&SI, MB, BCh, BAO, MRCPI, FACEM, FCICM
Intensive Care Staff Specialist, Wollongong Hospital, NSW; Visiting Medical Officer, Intensive Care Unit, Figtree Private Hospital, NSW; Casual Academic Lecturer, Graduate School of Medicine, University of Wollongong; Joint Deputy Chief Medical Officer, Rally Australia.

Nikki Blackwell MBBS, BSc, FRCP, FRACP, FAChPM, FJFICM, DTMH, PSM
Senior Staff Specialist, The Prince Charles Hospital, Brisbane, Qld, Australia; Clinical Associate Professor Critical Care, The University of Queensland, Brisbane; Qld, Medical Director, ALIMA (Alliance for International Medical Action) Paris, France.

Acknowledgements

Special thanks to Dr Pascale Gruber, Head of Intensive Care, The Royal Marsden Hospital, NHS Foundation Trust, UK—We thank you, particularly for your detailed insights and explanations of the examination processes in Europe and the UK.

The authors also wish to thank the following:

Daniel Steel

Thomas Czarniecki

Dr Jan Kelly, Paediatric Intensive Care Registrar, Starship Children's Hospital, New Zealand

Dr Joseph Ting, Staff Emergency Medicine Specialist, Mater Children's Hospital, Queensland, Australia

Dr Richard Piper, Senior Staff Intensive Care Specialist, Royal North Shore Hospital, New South Wales, Australia

Associate Professor Richard Lee, Senior Staff Intensive Care Specialist, Royal North Shore Hospital, New South Wales, Australia

Dr Hawn Trinh, Intensive Care Registrar, Royal North Shore Hospital, New South Wales, Australia

Dr Gordon Flynn, Intensive Care Specialist, Prince of Wales Hospital, New South Wales, Australia

Dr Mark De Neef, Intensive Care Senior Registrar, Royal North Shore Hospital, New South Wales, Australia

Dr Andrew Hooper, Intensive Care Senior Registrar, Royal North Shore Hospital, New South Wales, Australia

Dr Clare Richards, Emergency Medicine Registrar, Royal North Shore Hospital, New South Wales, Australia

Dr Caroline Orr, Neurologist, Royal North Shore Hospital, Sydney, Australia

Matt Tinker, Clinical Nurse Consultant, Royal North Shore Hospital, New South Wales, Australia

Francis Bass, Intensive Care Research Co-ordinator, Prince of Wales Hospital, New South Wales, Australia

Dr Hergan Buscher, Staff Intensive Care Specialist, St Vincent's Hospital, New South Wales, Australia

Dr Jonathan Egan, Paediatric Intensivist, The Children's Hospital at Westmead, Sydney, Australia

Clare Davies, CNC Paediatrics, Northern Sydney Health, Sydney, Australia

Dr Christina Liang, Neurophysiology Fellow, Royal North Shore Hospital, New South Wales, Australia

Mandy Smith, Critical Care Consultant, MAQUET – Datascope, Australia

Debbie Broderick, Business Manager, Edwards Lifesciences, Australia

Kerrie Eurell, Marketing Manager, Edwards Lifesciences, Australia

Dr Ian Seppelt, Senior Intensive Care Staff Specialist, Nepean Hospital, New South Wales, Australia

Dr Marek Nalos, Intensive Care Staff Specialist, Nepean Hospital, New South Wales, Australia

Dr Arvind Rajumani, Intensive Care Staff Specialist, Nepean Hospital, New South Wales, Australia

Ms Janet Scott, Intensive Care Clinical Nurse Consultant, Nepean Hospital, New South Wales, Australia

Dr Stephen Huang, Intensive Care Research Scientist, Nepean Hospital, New South Wales, Australia

Mr Richard Huang, Cardiovascular Ultrasound Technician, Nepean Hospital, New South Wales, Australia

Nikki Blackwell and Carole Foot also wish to thank **Dr Christopher Thomas**, Anaesthetist, Ipswich Public and Private Hospitals, Queensland, Australia – for his major contribution to *Examination Intensive Care and Anaesthesia.*

The following individuals not only reviewed sections of this book, but also made significant contributions to our early professional development in ICM:

Dr Greg Comadira, Senior Staff Intensive Care Specialist, The Gold Coast Hospital, Queensland, Australia

Dr Dan Mullany, Senior Staff Intensive Care Specialist, The Prince Charles Hospital, Queensland, Australia

Associate Professor Bala Venkatesh, Senior Staff Intensive Care Specialist, The Princess Alexandra Hospital, Queensland, Australia

Dr Chris Joyce, Director of Intensive Care Medicine, The Princess Alexandra Hospital, Queensland, Australia

We also wish to thank the following people for their select inputs to the manuscript:

Dr Meng Tan, Neurology Fellow, The Mayo Clinic, Rochester, Minnesota (Neurologist, Royal Melbourne Hospital, Victoria, Australia)

Dr Marc Ziegenfuss, Director of Intensive Care Medicine, The Prince Charles Hospital, Queensland, Australia

Associate Professor John Fraser, Senior Staff Intensive Care Specialist, The Prince Charles Hospital, Queensland, Australia

Jennifer Fahy, Instructor and Perinatal Outreach Co-ordinator, University of Maryland School of Medicine, Baltimore, Maryland, USA

Thanks and acknowledgement for the support and input of the Intensivists who travelled the path to success in the 2004 FJFICM exam with us and made valuable contributions to this project:

Dr Hayden White, Director of Intensive Care Medicine, Logan Hospital, Queensland, Australia

Dr Shawn Sturland, Director of Intensive Care Medicine, Wellington Hospital, New Zealand

Dr Enda O'Connor, Staff Intensivist, St James' Hospital, Dublin, Ireland

Dr Chris Graves, Staff Specialist Anaesthesia and Intensive Care, Nambour Base Hospital, Queensland, Australia

Reviewers

Dr Annette Forrest, ICU Middlemore Hospital, Auckland, New Zealand

Dr Dale Gardiner, Adult Intensive Care Unit, Queen's Medical Centre Campus, Nottingham University Hospitals, Nottingham, UK

Dr Nhi Nguyen, Department of Intensive Care Medicine, Nepean Hospital, New South Wales, Australia

Dr Timothy Wigmore, Clinical Lead Critical Care, Royal Marsden Hospital, London, UK

Disclaimer

The authors have taken considerable care in ensuring the accuracy of the information contained in this book and DVD. However, the reader is advised to check all information carefully before using it in clinical practice. The authors take no responsibility for any errors which may be contained herein, nor for any misfortune befalling any individual as the result of action taken using information in this book.

DVD Acknowledgements

Special thanks to Dr Pascale Gruber, Head of Intensive Care, The Royal Marsden Hospital, NHS Foundation Trust, UK—We thank you, particularly for your detailed insights and explanations of the examination processes in Europe and the UK.

The authors wish to thank the contributions of:

Daniel Steel

Thomas Czarniecki

Dr Jan Kelly, Paediatric Intensive Care Registrar, Starship Children's Hospital, New Zealand

Dr Joseph Ting, Staff Emergency Medicine Specialist, Mater Children's Hospital, Queensland, Australia

Dr Richard Piper, Senior Staff Intensive Care Specialist, Royal North Shore Hospital, New South Wales, Australia

Associate Professor Richard Lee, Senior Staff Intensive Care Specialist, Royal North Shore Hospital, New South Wales, Australia

Dr Hawn Trinh, Intensive Care Registrar, Royal North Shore Hospital, New South Wales, Australia

Dr Gordon Flynn, Intensive Care Specialist, Prince of Wales Hospital, New South Wales, Australia

Dr Mark De Neef, Intensive Care Senior Registrar, Royal North Shore Hospital, New South Wales, Australia

Dr Andrew Hooper, Intensive Care Senior Registrar, Royal North Shore Hospital, New South Wales, Australia

Dr Clare Richards, Emergency Medicine Registrar, Royal North Shore Hospital, New South Wales, Australia

Dr Caroline Orr, Neurologist, Royal North Shore Hospital, Sydney, Australia

Mr Matt Tinker, Clinical Nurse Consultant, Royal North Shore Hospital, New South Wales, Australia

Francis Bass, Intensive Care Research Co-ordinator, Prince of Wales Hospital, New South Wales, Australia

Dr Hergan Buscher, Staff Intensive Care Specialist, St Vincent's Hospital, New South Wales, Australia

Dr Jonathan Egan, Paediatric Intensivist, The Children's Hospital at Westmead, Sydney, Australia

Clare Davies, CNC Paediatrics, Northern Sydney Health, Sydney, Australia

Dr Christina Liang, Neurophysiology Fellow, Royal North Shore Hospital, New South Wales, Australia

Ms Mandy Smith, Critical Care Consultant, MAQUET – Datascope, Australia

Ms Debbie Broderick, Business Manager, Edwards Lifesciences, Australia

Ms Kerrie Eurell, Marketing Manager, Edwards Lifesciences, Australia

Dr Ian Seppelt, Senior Intensive Care Staff Specialist, Nepean Hospital, New South Wales

Dr Marek Nalos, Intensive Care Staff Specialist, Nepean Hospital, New South Wales

Dr Arvind Rajumani, Intensive Care Staff Specialist, Nepean Hospital, New South Wales

Ms Janet Scott, Intensive Care Clinical Nurse Consultant, Nepean Hospital, New South Wales

Dr Stephen Huang, Intensive Care Research Scientist, Nepean Hospital, New South Wales

Mr Richard Huang, Cardiovascular Ultrasound Technician, Nepean Hospital, New South Wales

Chapter 1

Training in intensive care medicine in Europe and Australasia

You are rewarding a teacher poorly if you remain always a pupil.
FRIEDRICH NIETZSCHE

European Diploma of Intensive Care Medicine (EDIC)

The European Diploma of Intensive Care Medicine (EDIC) is a two-part exam organised and conducted by the European Society of Intensive Care Medicine (ESICM). The EDIC is awarded to candidates who have successfully passed both parts of the exam and completed training in their primary specialty. The EDIC exam is intended to complement specialist postgraduate intensive care medicine training.

Part 1 of the EDIC exam is a multiple choice question (MCQ) paper in English. The objective of the MCQ paper is to test candidates' knowledge across a broad range of topics in intensive care medicine (ICM). Candidates who have successfully passed the Part 1 exam may then choose to sit Part 2 of the exam after 24 months of intensive care medicine training (including complementary specialty training). Part 2 of the EDIC is a clinical and oral exam. The standard expected for Part 2 is of a senior intensive care medicine trainee nearing the completion of their training. The syllabus for the EDIC exam is drawn from the international Competency-Based Training in Intensive Care Medicine in Europe (CoBaTrICE), which covers a broad spectrum of intensive care medicine, including resuscitation, diagnosis, disease management, perioperative care, transport, paediatrics, professionalism and end-of-life care. The CoBaTrICE website (www.cobatrice.org) offers useful links to educational resources.

The website of ESICM has information on registering for the EDIC and the EDIC exam guidelines (www.esicm.org). The ESICM website also offers the Patient-centered Acute Care Training (PACT), which is a modular-based long-distance learning program. The PACT contains 44 modules covering the intensive care curriculum, which is divided into four categories: clinical problems, skills and techniques, organ-specific problems and professionalism. Each module consists of scientific content, patient challenges or task-based learning, where users are given a clinical scenario and asked to interpret the nature of the problems and make management decisions, followed by MCQs for self-assessment. Access to PACT is available to all ESICM members free of charge; for non-ESICM members access is also permitted for a fee.

The ESICM also offers candidates access to sample MCQs used in previous EDIC exams and run a number of educational courses throughout the year that are useful for candidates preparing for the exam.

EDIC Part 1: Multiple choice question (MCQ) paper

The EDIC Part 1 exam is a 100-question MCQ paper over 3 hours. To achieve minimum entry criteria to the Part 1 exam, applicants must have evidence that they are:

- a fully registered Medical Doctor
- participating in a national training program in a primary specialty (anaesthesia, general medicine, emergency medicine, general surgery, paediatrics or intensive care medicine)
- participating in a national training program in intensive care medicine or completion of at least 12 months intensive care medicine training, of which a maximum of 6 months may be in a complementary specialty (acute or emergency medicine other than the candidate's primary specialty).

The MCQs are equally divided into two types: type A and type K questions. Type A questions consist of a stem with five possible answers, from which the candidate may only select one correct answer. A correct answer in a type A question scores one point; a wrong or blank answer scores no points. An example of a type A question is shown in Table 1.1.

TABLE 1.1 Type A question		
Which ONE of the following statements about dopamine is FALSE?		
A	The cardiovascular effects of dopamine are dependent on its rate of infusion	
B	Dopamine attenuates the response of the carotid body to hypoxia	
C	Dopamine can be used to prevent nausea and vomiting	X
D	Dopamine has been shown to vasodilate mesenteric vessels	
E	Dopamine is a precursor to noradrenaline and adrenaline	

Type K questions require candidates to choose either a T (true) or F (false) response to four statements labelled A to D. For type K questions all four responses must be correct to score a full mark, with a half mark scored if three out of four responses are correct. An example of a type K question is shown in Table 1.2.

TABLE 1.2 Type K question		
In tumour lysis syndrome the following biochemical abnormalities can be found:		
A	Hyperkalaemia	T
B	Hyperphosphataemia	T
C	Hypercalcaemia	F
D	Hyperuricaemia	T

The MCQs cover a broad range of topics in intensive care medicine. The exam questions broadly follow the EDIC 'content blueprint' as shown in Table 1.3, although the content blueprint may be changed annually.

Blueprint number	Blueprint topic	Number of type A and K questions
TABLE 1.3 Distribution of questions according to blueprint topic		
1	Cardiovascular	12
2	Respiratory	16
3	Neuro-critical care	10
4	Gastrointestinal/nutritional	8
5.1	Renal	4
5.2	Urology, obstetrics and gynaecology	4
6.1	Endocrine and metabolic	4
6.2	Bleeding and coagulation disorders	4
6.3	Oncology	4
7	Environmental hazards, poisoning and acute pharmacology	8
8	Severe infection and sepsis	10
9	Surgery and trauma	6
10.1	Ethics, law and quality assurance	4
10.3	Intensive care management	4
10.4	Transplantation	2
Total		100

Source: *EDIC Guidelines 2008*

Candidates may also choose to sit the 'dummy exam', which replicates the real exam conditions without it counting. Candidates sitting the 'dummy exam' are not eligible to sit the real exam for at least 1 year.

The pass mark is variable each year and based on a calculation using the mean value and standard deviation for each group of candidates. The pass mark is approximately 56%, with about 70% of candidates passing the exam in any one sitting. Results take 1–2 months, to arrive by post. Candidates who fail Part 1 of the EDIC exam are not allowed to re-sit it for 12 months. A total of three attempts is allowed.

EDIC Part 2: Clinical and oral examination

The Part 2 exam consists of a clinical and an oral component. Candidates who have successfully passed Part 1 may sit the Part 2 exam. It is anticipated that most candidates will take Part 2 within 24 months of passing Part 1, and no later than 4 years after passing Part 1. Candidates may choose the country/centre in which they wish to sit the exam and, depending on availability, the EDIC committee will allocate the candidate a centre and date 1 month prior to the exam.

The minimum entry criteria for the Part 2 examination are evidence of:
• successful completion of the Part 1 exam
• 24 months' intensive care medicine training, of which a maximum of 6 months may be in complementary specialties.

The Part 2 exam takes approximately 2 hours and consists of clinical and oral components. The candidate may be assessed by a number of examiners, some of whom may be external and invited from another European country. The clinical examination takes place at the bedside, lasts 60–90 minutes and consists of one long case and two or three short cases. The oral component takes approximately 30–40 minutes.

Clinical component

During the long case the candidate has 30–40 minutes to familiarise themselves with the patient. Candidates have access to the patient's notes, charts and bedside monitoring, blood results, radiology and other relevant investigations, and will also have the opportunity to examine the patient. The objective is to enable examiners to assess candidates in a real-life environment where candidates must assimilate information in the allocated time period and decide on the appropriate therapeutic options. Candidates will be expected to initially summarise the clinical course of the patient and will then be questioned on specific areas of management. For the clinical exam, candidates are assessed in each of the following areas: approach to the patient, eliciting clinical information, clinical capacity in the intensive care environment and presentation of clinical findings. The long case is preceded or followed by two or three bedside short cases. These commonly focus on clinical signs (e.g. bronchial breathing), equipment (e.g. pulmonary artery catheter) or clinical examination (e.g. neurological examination).

Oral component

This takes place away from the bedside and commonly includes data interpretation (arterial blood gases, haematology and biochemical results, ECGs, echocardiograms, radiographs, CT and MRI scans), abbreviated case histories, hot topics and ethical dilemmas. Certain themes are common and include ventilation strategies in ARDS, care bundles, the surviving sepsis campaign, therapeutic hypothermia, blood glucose control, steroids and sepsis, nutrition, trauma management, brain stem testing, renal replacement therapy, management of head injury, and issues around consent and ethics. A sound knowledge of the evidence base in these areas is expected in the discussion.

The candidate receives a mark for both the clinical and oral parts of the examination (severe failure, failure, bare fail, pass, good pass or excellent) by each pair of examiners. A fail in any component ensures failure overall and a bare fail in one component may be compensated for by a good pass or excellent grade in another component at the discretion of the examiners. Candidates are notified of their results by the ESICM administrative office by post. Two attempts are allowed initially and if a candidate has not succeeded after the second attempt, a further two attempts are allowed 12 months later.

UK Intercollegiate Diploma in Intensive Care Medicine (DICM)

The training program in ICM in the United Kingdom is supervised by the new Faculty of Intensive Care Medicine (FICM) and is currently undergoing a number of changes. Training in ICM in the UK has traditionally been undertaken within a main specialty training program (anaesthesia, medicine, surgery, emergency medicine). ICM training consists of Basic ICM training (3 months of ICM at senior house officer/core trainee 1–2 level), Complementary Specialty training (6 months of general medicine for anaesthetists or 6 months of anaesthesia for physicians, surgeons or emergency medicine physicians at senior house officer/core trainee 1–2 level), Intermediate ICM training (6 months of general adult ICM at registrar/specialty trainee 3+ level) and Advanced ICM training (12 months of general and/or specialised ICM undertaken during the final 2 years of specialty training). Candidates completing the program receive recognition for ICM and their primary specialty training (anaesthesia, medicine, surgery, emergency medicine). In the future there will be the option for candidates to undergo training in ICM as a primary specialty. Up-to-date and detailed information can found on the FICM website (www.ficm.ac.uk). The exam structure is also changing. The current United Kingdom Intercollegiate Diploma in Intensive Care Medicine (DICM) will have its last sitting in June 2012 and will be replaced by a new high level final exam.

Currently the DICM is an optional exam, available to doctors who have completed Intermediate training in ICM. The DICM consists of two modules:

- Module 1 is a 4000–6000 word dissertation relevant to the field of ICM and an oral exam of the dissertation. Candidates who have taken a relevant higher degree are allowed to submit their thesis and, with confirmation of award of the degree, may be excused from the dissertation viva.
- Module 2 involves a series of oral exams based on case scenarios, structured questions and expanded case summaries. The 10 expanded case summaries are a required component of Intermediate training in ICM.

The diploma is awarded on successful completion of both modules. Currently there are no limitations on the number of attempts allowed to pass the exam, but candidates must be aware that they will be unable to re-sit any part of the exam after June 2012.

The entry criteria for the DICM are:

- possession of a postgraduate qualification in a primary specialty (i.e. MRCP, FRCA, FRCS, FCEM or equivalent)
- registration with the FICM (or previous Intercollegiate Board for Training in Intensive Care Medicine) for either Intermediate/Advanced ICM training or the ICM Certificate of Completion of Training (CCT) program
- satisfactory completion of the Intermediate ICM training or other training acceptable to the FICM (this usually equates to a minimum of 3 months ICM training at senior house officer/core trainee 1–2 level, 6 months at registrar/specialty trainee 3+ level and 6 months of a complementary specialty at senior house officer/core trainee 1–2 level)

Of note, the FICM does not accept applications from overseas trainees for the DICM. The exam is conducted twice a year (June/November) and dates of the exam are published on the FICM website. The FICM website also provides guidance on the exam regulations, dissertation, expanded case summaries and exam syllabus. The syllabus is extensive and has a heavy emphasis on basic sciences, which is arguably misleading and not representative of the exam.

Dissertation

Candidates are initially required to submit a summary of their planned dissertation to the FICM for approval (ficm@rcoa.ac.uk). The intention of the summary is to provide the examiners with an opportunity to ensure that the dissertation is in an appropriate subject area and of adequate depth and breath for the exam. Once approval has been granted the candidate is allowed to submit a formal 4000–6000 word dissertation. This is done electronically via the DICM Manuscript Central site. The dissertation may be a review, research paper, audit or based upon a higher degree in a subject relevant to ICM. The philosophy behind the dissertation is that candidates have the opportunity to become 'an expert' in an area of ICM that is of particular interest to them. The range of potential topics is wide and candidates should choose a topic of interest that is broad enough to justify exploration. The candidate should have discussed the topic with their regional advisor in ICM and nominate a dissertation supervisor.

The dissertation is marked against six domains: defining a question for a structured review, accessing relevant and up-to-date resources in the area of study, appraising the current status of the field of study, drawing pertinent conclusions from the results of the review or study, appraising limitations and future directions in the field of study, and demonstrating effective written communication skills. If examiners find that the dissertation is of marginal standard it may be returned to the candidate for revision. If the candidate fails to reach an adequate standard their supervisor is notified of the areas that need revision.

Expanded case summaries

All candidates are required to complete 10 expanded case summaries as part of Intermediate ICM training. The expanded case summaries should be approximately 750–1500 words in length and examine one aspect of the patient's clinical problem in depth. Each case summary should address a different clinical problem. The subheadings for each case summary are standardised and are as follows: clinical problem, relevant management, further information, changes to future management and references. Examples of expanded case summaries can be found at the FICM website.

Exam format

- Dissertation viva (45 minutes): candidates should have in-depth knowledge of their topic and are required to discuss their dissertation with the examiners.
- Clinical scenario and data interpretation viva (30 minutes): this typically consists of one long case (15 minutes) and up to three short cases (5 minutes each). For the long case candidates are asked to review a written clinical case history and discuss various management options. The short cases comprise data interpretation involving biochemistry results, arterial blood gases, ECGs and radiology.
- Case summaries viva (30 minutes): candidates will be required to discuss their expanded case summaries. As candidates are able to select the cases they submit it is expected that they will have a reasonable depth of knowledge.
- Structured oral vivas (2 × 30 minutes): topics are diverse and can cover several aspects of ICM. The examiners use structured questions based on a predetermined list of domains to maximise consistency and objectivity. Previous topics have included: blood transfusion in the critically ill, management of ARDS, transfusion-related lung injury, scoring systems in intensive care, medical emergency teams, acute coronary syndromes, cardiac output monitoring, management of status epilepticus, diagnosis of community-acquired pneumonia, definitions of SIRS/sepsis/MOF, Stewart's hypothesis of acid base, renal replacement therapy, management of subarachnoid haemorrhage, antibiotic-associated diarrhoea, endocarditis, ethics and difficult management decisions. A good knowledge of the recent literature is essential.

Examiners assign an independent mark based on their assessment of the candidate's performance in each of the different vivas above. To pass the exam, candidates must submit a satisfactory dissertation, obtain a pass in the dissertation viva and obtain a pass in at least two of the three remaining vivas.

Fellowship of the College of Intensive Care Medicine (FCICM) training requirements

Core knowledge and resources

To be admitted to Fellowship of the College of Intensive Care Medicine of Australia and New Zealand it is necessary to have:

- completed advanced training with five out of six satisfactory training assessments, including the final one
- spent 12 months in approved posts in both medicine and anaesthesia

- submitted a formal project and had it accepted
- spent at least 6 months of advanced training working at senior registrar level
- completed an ADAPT course (for trainees who registered on or after 1 November 2004)
- been successful at the Fellowship examination.

Regulation 4 of the College of Intensive Care Medicine: Admission to Fellowship of the College of Intensive Care Medicine by Training and Examination (available on the college website: www.cicm.org.au) describes in detail the process necessary to be admitted to Fellowship.

All trainees registered after 1 January 2010, when the College of Intensive Care Medicine (CICM) of Australia and New Zealand was formally established, are governed by Regulation 5: Program for Training and Certification in Intensive Care Medicine. Those trainees who commenced their training before this date are governed by the Joint Faculty of Intensive Care Medicine (JFICM) regulations that applied at the time of their registration.

The Administrative Officer (Training and Examinations) at CICM can provide guidance through the various aspects of the paperwork and requirements needed during the different phases of training.

The CICM website contains a description of some of the desirable abilities required to practise as a competent, caring specialist in intensive care under Training/Training resources, in the document titled 'Trainee selection policy' (www.cicm.org.au). The abilities include excellent clinical skills, good management skills, an aptitude to cope with stress, a motivation to behave professionally in a manner that earns respect, an understanding of medical ethics and a commitment to undertake continuing education and quality assurance activities. Given that the FCICM Fellowship Examination is an exit exam for intensivists it is obvious that it will aim to give candidates the chance to demonstrate their possession of these desired qualities.

Successfully completing the CICM Primary examination is one way to advance towards becoming an intensive care specialist. The journal, *Critical Care and Resuscitation* (the college house journal), is available online, with editorials on key topics in intensive care. You will also find an education module on the website. It contains practical advice on how to approach studying, as well as tips on how to avoid common pitfalls.

CICM Primary examination

The requirements of basic training must be completed before progress to advanced training can occur. Basic training consists of 12 months of general hospital experience plus 36 months of approved basic training positions. This is explained in detail on the college website.

The rate-limiting step for most trainees to complete their basic training is the requirement to pass either the CICM Primary examination or an acceptable alternative primary examination.

The regulations currently state that success at the ANZCA, ACEM and RACS Primary examination or basic physician training and success at the RACP written and clinical (adult or paediatric) examinations are acceptable alternatives to the college's Primary examination.

Applications for exemption from the Primary exam are individually assessed by the college censor. However, the process is time-consuming and should be started early to avoid the loss of training time.

Trainees must have completed 12 months' general hospital experience and be registered as a trainee of the college in order to apply for the CICM Primary examination. They do not, however, have to have started approved training in order to present for the exam. The Primary examination may be taken at any time during basic training.

The syllabus for the CICM Primary is available on the college website. The subject areas are described in-depth but it should be noted that the content is examined in an integrated fashion. This is different from some of the other primary examinations, where different subjects can be sat at different sittings.

Format of the CICM Primary examination

The CICM Primary examination consists of two parts: a written section followed by an oral examination. The written section is held in the major cities of Australia and New Zealand or other countries at the discretion of the Board. The oral exam is usually held in Melbourne. The College must receive applications before the closing date, 2 months before the date of the exam. The exam is held twice a year. The written section usually occurs in March and September, with the orals held 2 months later.

In the written paper a score of at least 45% must be obtained in order to be invited to sit the oral section. Candidates who are subsequently unsuccessful in the overall exam can proceed directly to the oral examination at the next two sittings, provided they have achieved a score of 50% or over in the written section. If a fail is obtained at the third attempt, the written section will need to be taken again on the next attempt.

The written section

This consists of two 150-minute papers. Both papers consist of 12 short-answer questions (SAQs) and 20 short-fact questions (SFQs). The college advises that 120 minutes are allocated to the SAQs (10 minutes per question) and 30 minutes to the 20 SFQs. Eighty per cent of the overall marks for the written are allocated to the SAQs and 20% to the SFQs. The written section makes up 50% of the total marks for the entire exam (see Table 1.4 for a breakdown of the marks).

The usual advice about written exams applies for these papers. Marks are divided equally between the SAQs, so allocate the time accordingly. Answers should be planned, writing legible and diagrams, lists and notes utilised to save time. Pre-planned generic skeleton answers (e.g. for a 'critically evaluate' question, a 'pharmacology question', a 'compare and contrast' question) will help organisation of answers under pressure. A mock exam is available on the CICM website, which gives an indication of the format, level of difficulty and scope of the questions.

The oral section

This comprises eight stations, each of 10 minutes. There are also one or two rest stations. The stations are a mixture of cross-table vivas and objective structured clinical examinations (OSCEs). All of the stations carry equal marks. Normal laboratory values will be given with investigation results. The examiner(s) assess performance using a predetermined marking grid.

Thirty minutes before the start time of the exam the chairman gives an overview of the process and logistics of the oral stations. Two minutes are allowed for movement between stations and for reading the introductory scenario outside the station. Ten minutes are allocated for the actual station.

Each station is marked individually, and the examiners are different for each station with no knowledge of your previous performance. The questions are graded in terms of difficulty, to allow a good assessment of knowledge. It is therefore possible that a point will be reached when candidates are unable to answer all the questions posed. In reality this means that, although they may not have answered all the questions correctly, they may still have passed the station.

Marking components

TABLE 1.4 Breakdown of the marks in the CICM Primary examination

Topic	Maximum mark	Pass mark
Written section		
2 × 150-minute papers		
SAQs	40	20
SFQs	10	5
Total	50	25
Oral section		
8 × 10-minute stations	50	25
Total	100	50

Results
After the examination has concluded, an examiners meeting takes place. Immediately after this, results are handed to each candidate in a sealed envelope at a designated time and place.

CICM Fellowship examination
The breadth and depth of knowledge, skills and attitudes required to pass the CICM Fellowship examination are well described in the college documents, 'Objectives of Training in Intensive Care', which can be downloaded from the college website (www.cicm.org.au).

A thorough knowledge of the basic sciences and a broad-based understanding of general medicine, surgery and other disciplines as they relate to ICM form part of the core knowledge required by the examination.

Many trainees in adult intensive care worry about paediatric questions in the Fellowship exam. The level of knowledge expected is well described in the document 'Objectives of Training and Competencies for Advanced Training in Paediatric Intensive Care' and further explored in Chapter 10 of this book. The CICM Paediatric Intensive Care Medicine Fellowship examination is also specifically addressed in Chapter 10.

The exam takes place twice a year, with the written section usually occurring in April and August, and the oral section 6 weeks later. Completed application forms for the exam should be received by the faculty office 56 days before the written section. Exam dates and closing dates are available on the college website. The written section takes place in the capital cities of each state, with the location of the oral section rotating between the major metropolitan centres.

Basic training and at least 12 months core intensive care training must be completed before presenting for the Fellowship examination.

A new prerequisite to presenting for the Fellowship examination was introduced in August 2010 to assist candidates to prepare for the clinical examination. In the 6 months leading up to the date of the written examination every candidate must be formally assessed by their supervisor of training (or an appropriate delegate who is a Fellow of the CICM) as having achieved a satisfactory standard during an observed clinical assessment of a critically ill patient, on four separate occasions. This replaces the previous requirement for candidates to have performed four separate observed clinical assessments without a stipulation of the standard required. The cases should be performed under the same conditions as the exam. Extra time should be used after the case to discuss the clinical problem(s) and for the candidate to receive feedback on their performance. In order to complete the four satisfactory assessments, generally more than four cases will need to be covered. This means the cases should be started 6 months prior to the written exam.

Satisfactory completion of these four assessments does not guarantee success in the clinical component of the examination. However, the college believes the process will ensure that candidates receive feedback during these assessments, allowing them to adequately prepare and present for the exam at the best time to ensure success.

Candidates who are unsuccessful in the clinical part of the Fellowship examination will need to repeat the four observed satisfactory clinical assessments prior to each subsequent attempt at the clinical component of the exam.

The management of a large number of intensive care patients is one of the best ways to prepare for the examination. This ensures the development of a considered approach to clinical and non-clinical issues that occur in the intensive care unit. Before attempting the examination, a frank assessment by the supervisor of training can be useful in determining the appropriate time to sit, not forgetting that this is an exit examination for consultant intensivists.

Format of the Fellowship examination

Candidates are required to pass the written section of the examination with a mark of 50% or more before being invited to the clinical section. A pass at the written exam with failure in the clinical allows direct entry to the oral section of the examination at the next two sittings. A breakdown of the marks for the different components of the Fellowship examination is shown in Table 1.5.

Written examination

The written exam consists of two 150-minute papers held on the same day. Each paper consists of 15 questions. The marks are allocated equally between the 30 questions. Consequently, time must be divided equally between each question, with 10 minutes to answer each question.

All the usual commonsense examination advice applies. Read the question carefully and only answer the question posed. Write legibly and be concise. Plan your answers and use lists, tables and diagrams to save time. One approach is to spend 2 minutes planning your answer, and 8 minutes writing it. Practising by completing past papers will help candidates develop useful strategies.

The content of the written papers has changed in recent years. Data interpretation, radiology and equipment questions are now all possible in the written papers, alongside questions on every aspect of intensive care practice, including the literature, management and basic sciences.

Clinical examination – Cross-table vivas

The viva section consists of eight cross-table vivas, each lasting 10 minutes. There are 2 minutes between each viva for candidates to move to the next station and read the introduction to the next viva, apart from the radiology station where candidates enter directly into the viva station and spend the 2 minutes looking at the radiology images before the questioning starts. Each viva is allocated equal marks. Do not despair if a viva does not seem to have gone well. The examiners at each station have no knowledge of your performance at other stations. Questions range in difficulty in order to test candidates' depth of knowledge. When you are tested to the limits of your knowledge you will probably encounter questions that you cannot answer, nevertheless you may have already gained sufficient marks to pass the station.

Clinical examination – Clinical cases
The exam features two clinical cases. These are patients currently in the intensive care unit of the hospital(s) hosting the exam. Each case lasts 20 minutes and is examined by a different pair of examiners. The examiners direct candidates to assess a specific problem or system. The first 10 minutes of each case should be spent performing a purposeful examination to allow evaluation and assessment of clinical signs present and allow the development of a management strategy. The second 10 minutes is spent discussing an appropriate diagnosis and management plan, as well as interpreting relevant investigations.

Marking components

TABLE 1.5 Breakdown of the marks in the CICM Fellowship examination		
Topic	Maximum mark	Pass mark
Written section		
2 × 150-minute papers	30	15
Clinical section		
Clinical cases	30	15
Cross-table vivas		
8 × 10-minute vivas	40	20

To pass the examination a total score of at least 50% must be achieved. Only one section may be failed. Due to the importance placed on clinical examination and assessment a pass in the Fellowship examination cannot be achieved with a 'poor fail' (12/30) in the clinical cases section, however well an individual has scored overall.

Results
After the examination has concluded an examiners meeting takes place, which usually lasts at least 2 hours. Immediately after this, results are handed to each candidate in a sealed envelope at a designated time and place.

Chapter 2

Strategies for success

Luck is what happens when preparation meets opportunity.
    SENECA

Timing

Candidates should begin studying for the exam sooner rather than later and ideally with a year's run up to the event. In reality, preparation starts with your first training position. This is not as onerous as it sounds, as it will help you to learn how to do your job well. It is much easier to attempt the exam while you are working in an intensive care medicine post rather than trying to do it from another rotation such as anaesthetics or medicine. Do not be pressured into sitting the exam too early. The only way to learn the tricks of the trade is to learn the trade properly. If you have not learnt enough or seen enough patients then you will not pass. It is recommended that candidates study for all parts of the exam at the same time, rather than leaving the clinical and oral sections until after the written exam. That time is for finessing and polishing your personal style, not deciding what it is.

It is easy to feel quite overwhelmed by the amount of studying required when you first begin contemplating the exam. Preparing an exam study timetable will break the process down into manageable portions so that you can avoid feeling swamped. This way you can systematically cover the material required without panicking at the extent of the task. Systematic learning in this way will raise your confidence and morale as you look back over the areas you have successfully covered in the past, knowing that you can apply the same process to the topics that lie ahead.

There is an absolute goldmine of information to be found on various websites and you would be most unwise not to be familiar with the resources available, especially those associated with the examining bodies (see Chapter 1).

Preparation courses

There are several courses available for trainees in ICM who want to progress towards becoming a specialist intensivist. There are many benefits in attending some of these as they not only contain a high level of educational content, but more importantly provide an opportunity to meet and mix with other trainees. They also provide the chance to meet and be taught by senior specialists in the field, many of whom are also examiners.

EDIC/DICM
Scientific meetings
Attending the ESICM Annual Scientific Congress is a high-yield activity. A number of education workshops are held prior to and during the Congress. The Pre-Congress Critical Care Refresher course is popular. Aside from the educational merits of

attending the Congress, it is usually held in a European city where hard work may be rewarded with a break. Other useful meetings are the annual International Symposium of Intensive Care and Emergency Medicine (Belgium) and Intensive Care Society Meetings (United Kingdom). These conferences provide up-to-date information and give a guide to the current hot topics in ICM.

National Intensive Care exam revision course (Bristol/Bath, UK)
This one-day course is predominantly aimed at candidates sitting the EDIC or DICM. It provides candidates viva practice and up-to-date literature in critical care. The course consists of lectures, vivas, data interpretation and small group tutorials. Detailed information is available online at www.cardiff.ac.uk/pgmde/wimat or you can email wimat@cardiff.ac.uk.

Diploma of the Irish Board of Intensive Care Medicine preparatory course (Dublin, Ireland)
This three-day course covers topics relevant to the DICM and EDIC. Detailed information is available at www.icmed.com.

FCICM
The CICM website has a list of current courses and conferences that is regularly updated.

Scientific meetings
If you are fortunate enough to have the opportunity to attend a CICM Annual Scientific Meeting or the Australian and New Zealand Intensive Care Society (ANZICS) conference, you will be provided with up-to-date information as well as a guide to the current controversies in the specialty.

CICM Primary exam courses
Courses are evolving that are designed to assist primary exam candidates (e.g. Royal Adelaide Hospital Primary short course).

ANZICS Intensive Care Registrars course
This course is conducted in Melbourne in July every year. It does not aim to prepare participants for the FCICM exam; rather, it provides a sound theoretical basis to current practice in intensive care. Eminent leaders in the field regularly give excellent interactive lectures on core intensive care topics. The best time to attend this course is early in your advanced training (i.e. first core year). Further details are available on the ANZICS website: www.anzics.com.au/education_courses.htm.

ADAPT workshop (Australian Donor Awareness Program Training)
The aim of the Australian Donor Awareness Program is to increase awareness of organ and tissue donation and grief counselling among health professionals who care for patients and their families. It is hoped that it will provide health professionals with the knowledge and skills to support potential donor families, so that they are able to make a decision about organ donation that is right for them. The course runs for one day in centres around Australia and New Zealand. Attendance is now compulsory for all trainees in intensive care prior to being awarded Fellowship. Further details are available on the website: www.adapt.asn.au/activities.

Advanced Paediatric Life Support (APLS) course
This three-day course is run frequently all around Australia and New Zealand. The coursebook essentially covers the syllabus of paediatric knowledge required by adult intensivists, and the scenarios cover most of the practical skills. At the very least you

should be familiar with the coursebook, and track down local APLS instructors to take you through some scenarios. Course information can be found at www.apls.org.au and www.resus.org.uk.

Emergency Management of Severe Trauma (EMST) course
The EMST (Advanced Trauma Life Support) course teaches a systematic practical approach to the trauma patient. Unfortunately the waiting list for courses is long and it may not be possible for candidates to complete one before their examination. However, familiarity with the course manual will provide an excellent framework on which to base the initial assessment of the severely injured patient. The course webpages can be found via the Royal College of Surgeons websites in your respective regions.

Exam courses
There are a number of excellent courses available to help prepare candidates for all of the components of the second part of the FCICM exam. Each of the courses below offers an opportunity to practise all the parts of the Fellowship exam. The experience gained by attending these courses is invaluable and you should aim to attend at least one of them before sitting the exam. A limited number of places are available so you should plan well ahead, both in terms of applying for a place on the course and in booking leave from work, especially if you are sitting the exam with several other colleagues from the same ICU. The format of the courses changes in response to feedback from participants, but currently all are offering interactive lectures and insight into exam techniques followed by real-time exam practice of clinical cases and vivas.

Australian Short Course in Intensive Care Medicine
This course is held in Adelaide, just before the FCICM exam in April/May.

The Australian Intensive Care Medicine clinical refresher course
This course is held in Brisbane, between the written and clinical parts of the examination in August/September. It is also run under the umbrella of the Australasian Academy of Critical Care Medicine, with further details available on the College website.

The Sydney Short Course in Intensive Care Medicine
This course is held in Sydney in November. Although this course is newer than the Adelaide and Brisbane courses, it has been highly recommended by past participants. A long course is also held with regular structured evenings, including moving between different units for clinical cases and practice vivas.

The Canberra ICU course
This most recent addition targets trainees commencing their approach to the Fellowship exam and includes lectures as well as mock exam practice.

Sydney Intensive Care Equipment course
This new course aims to provide trainees with an up-to-date practical refresher on ICU equipment.

Textbooks, journals and online resources

Investing in a comprehensive textbook to establish a broad basic knowledge of intensive care cannot be overemphasised. Suggestions include Oh's Intensive Care Manual; Irwin and Rippe's Intensive Care Medicine; Critical Care Secrets; Key Topics in Critical Care (less detailed); Intensive Care: A Concise Textbook (less detailed);

and Core Cases in Critical Care (less detailed). For Part 1 of the EDIC exam a useful book is Multiple Choice Questions in Intensive Care. Data interpretation is well covered in Data Interpretation in Critical Care Medicine, and radiology in Radiology for Anaesthesia and Intensive Care and Diagnostic Imaging in Critical Care.

Candidates are expected to be up-to-date and journals such as The Lancet, The New England Journal of Medicine, Current Opinion in Critical Care, Intensive Care Monitor, Intensive Care Medicine, Critical Care and Critical Care Medicine are important resources.

Useful online resources include the European Society of Intensive Care Medicine (www.esicm.org), CoBaTrICE (www.cobatrice.org), Medscape (critical care section) (www.medscape.com), the Intensive Care Society (UK) (www.ics.ac.uk), Anaesthesia (UK) (www.frca.co.uk), the Evidence-based medicine group of the Scottish Intensive Care Society (www.sicsebm.org.uk), Crit-IQ (www.crit-iq.com.au) and the Society of Critical Care Medicine's Resident Intensive Care Unit program (www.sccm.org).

For those training in Australasia, detailed exam reports for previous Primary examinations and the Fellowship examination, including the written paper questions, are available on the website. These provide a wealth of information that can help you prepare for the examination. Not only do you have access to the questions that have been asked over the years, allowing you to identify key recurring themes, but you can also gain an insight into the approach and level of knowledge the examiners are seeking. **You would be well advised to use these past papers as the keystone for your exam preparation**. Plan perfect answers to the questions as an open-book exercise early in your study to provide a task-based focus as opposed to directionless reading of textbooks. Later on, attempt the questions without access to your textbooks under time pressure. This will allow you to highlight the gaps in your knowledge, as well as to develop the crucial skill of disciplined time management.

Study notes

Compiling study notes is a very individual practice and most candidates will have established a style they are happy with; abbreviated cards, longhand notes or electronic files prepared on computer are all useful ways of covering the syllabus. It is now recognised that preparing notes is an important exercise in itself and often more constructive than just reading and underlining textbooks.

As you start to synthesise the information you accumulate from numerous sources, it is often wise to summarise it all in one document. An example for toxicology is given overleaf. Further study notes in the toxicology series would include management and antidotes.

Developing your own logical headings, as shown in the study notes for Principles of toxicology, which you can also use when answering short answer questions and viva answers, is a useful way of encouraging thinking in a structured manner. These notes can also be used as a resource for considering the answers to multiple choice and short answer question answers from previous exam papers and to help predict future questions.

Those who find diagrams more helpful than written notes may find that preparing diagrams or mind maps is helpful. For example, preparing a diagram specific to each of the possible major clinical scenarios may be helpful when approaching the clinical cases. Figure 2.1 provides an example of a generic approach to performing clinical case assessments (also provided on the DVD). Candidates can print out this template and annotate key items that are important for each type of case they encounter. Figure 2.2 shows an example of this approach applied to the patient with cardiogenic shock and multiple organ failure.

Study notes for Principles of toxicology

History	Examination	Investigations
What was taken? How much? – Dose (work out mg/kg and/or exposure duration) When did it occur? Allows estimation of expected symptom profile, decay times, timing of investigations (e.g. paracetamol level at 4 hours post acute ingestion) Symptoms to date – Allows estimation of progression, likely severity, disposition planning Treatment to date and effect (e.g. administration of O_2 following carbon monoxide exposure) Co-morbidities Intent of exposure – accidental, intentional, non-accidental injury in children	Vital signs – HR, BP, SpO_2, RR, GCS, Temp Appearance/odours (e.g. cyanosis in methaemoglobinaemia, garlic odour in organophosphate toxicity) Toxicology-specific examination (e.g. catecholaminergic, cholinergic toxidrome; envenomation signs) There may not be much to find	Few toxicology-specific investigation results are returned quickly enough to be clinically relevant to the acute management of the toxicology patient. Majority of investigations are performed to assess for complications of the exposure or to exclude differentials for: • bedside (BSL, ABG, ECG) • lab (FBC, electrolytes, LFT, coagulation profile, CK, urinalysis) • imaging (CXR, CT brain)

Toxicology-specific investigations		
Toxic agent	**Investigation**	**Rapid result**
Anticonvulsants	Serum total and free levels	Relatively rapid turn-around time. Take care with slow-release preparations (e.g. carbamazepine)
Carbon monoxide	Carbon monoxide level on blood gas co-oximeter	Yes, but level rapidly lowered by administration of O_2 making initial exposure level difficult to ascertain
Cyanide	i) Blood cyanide level ii) Gastric content + $FeSO_4$ + NaOH + boiled + cooled = Green precipitate	i) No. Confirmatory test only ii) Usually not available and only relevant if ingested
Digoxin	Serum digoxin level	Yes, but correlates with severity in acute toxicity only
Ethylene glycol	Serum ethylene glycol level	No, but used for monitoring progress during therapy
Iron	Serum iron	Yes. If level >90 mmol/L then desferrioxamine indicated

Continued

Toxicology-specific investigations—cont'd		
Toxic agent	**Investigation**	**Rapid result**
Lithium	Serum lithium level	Yes. Correlates with severity in chronic toxicity, but not acute toxicity
Methaemoglobinaemia	MetHb level on blood gas co-oximeter	Yes
Methanol	i) Serum methanol ii) Serum formic acid	No, but used to assess likelihood of toxicity, prognosis and progress of therapy
Organophosphates	i) Plasma pseudocholinesterase ii) RBC acetylcholinesterase	i) Yes. Sensitive screening test, but poor correlation with severity ii) Result takes >24 hours. Limited availability. Better predictor of severity
Paracetamol (acetaminophen)	Serum paracetamol level at 4 hours post ingestion, plotted to nomogram	Yes. Plotted to Rumack-Matthews nomogram
Paraquat	A clinical diagnosis, but can do: i) Serum paraquat level ii) Urinary paraquat level iii) Urine + 1 mL 1% Na Dithionate blue colour	i) and ii) No iii) Rapid, if available
Salicylate	Serum salicylate level at 6 hours	Yes. Plotted to Done nomogram
Snake venom	Venom detection kit (VDK) using bite site swab and urine	Takes about 20–30 minutes to process
Tricyclic antidepressants	Serum TCAD level	No and poor correlation with severity

Looking after yourself

As the date for the exam approaches it is imperative that you have a strategy to contain stress, particularly as you will need to balance ongoing work and personal commitments with studying for the exam. Some people find that a written study program reassures them that they will cover everything in time. Taking blocks of leave for consolidated study can also be helpful. Scheduled *guilt-free* time away from work and study, for yourself and significant others in your life, is crucial. The exam process tests even the most stable of partnerships to the absolute limit.

The usual advice about a healthy diet, adequate exercise and sleep applies. Some candidates have found hypnosis and sessions with a sports psychologist to be useful for controlling overwhelming feelings of anxiety or nervousness that can hamper the presentation of knowledge.

In order to improve performance you will have to develop a mechanism to cope with constructive criticism. Sometimes this can cause feelings of inadequacy and deflation. One of the ways to deal with this is to develop a robust attitude as quickly as possible

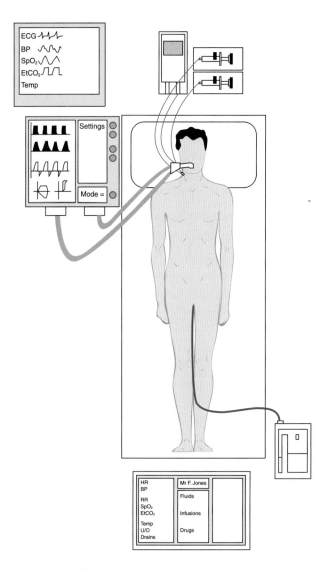

FIGURE 2.1 The generic clinical case assessment

(however, see comments about excess anxiety above). If there are specialists whom you find particularly intimidating, time your practice orals or clinical cases carefully. Wait until you have gained enough experience to be able to make a reasonable effort, but do not wait so long that if the experience is very negative you do not have time to recover before the exam itself.

Study groups

There is a lot of ground you have to cover by yourself. However, having contact with other candidates is not only reassuring when you are riding the 'emotional rollercoaster' associated with preparation, but is helpful in practical ways. You should arrange to visit as many other units as possible and be examined by as many

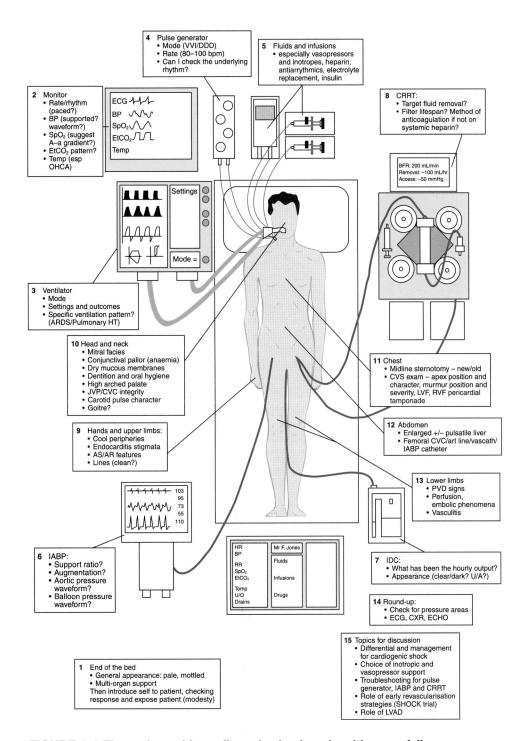

FIGURE 2.2 The patient with cardiogenic shock and multi-organ failure

people as possible. This is time-consuming to arrange and it can be useful to share the organisation. Desensitisation to unfamiliar physical environments, equipment, examiners and case mixes makes it less likely that the actual exam will throw you off-track. Furthermore, there is much to be gained from watching your colleagues perform and learning from them. Taking the opportunity to act as an examiner for each other provides an invaluable insight into ways you can improve your own performance as a candidate. For those candidates taking the EDIC and FCICM, do not forget to schedule in a session with a paediatric intensivist on topics relevant to the exam (see Chapter 10).

Clinical cases

The best way to become good at clinical cases is to have examined and managed a large number of intensive care patients with a broad spectrum of problems. Initially this should happen in a tightly supervised fashion, which becomes increasingly relaxed as you grow in expertise and clinical wisdom towards becoming an independent practitioner. This forms the basis which you can then modify and perfect for the clinical cases. The examiners may give you a clinical problem: 'This patient is day 5 post cardiac surgery and has been slow to wean from mechanical ventilation. Please could you examine him with a view to planning his ongoing management', or simply they can ask for the examination of a particular organ system. It is almost impossible to look comfortable and experienced when examining patients and addressing weaning problems and other common issues after cardiac surgery if you have limited clinical experience and have not prepared adequately. It is necessary to have a systematic approach to examining each organ system. Make good use of your normal working day, for example, turning the daily ward round into a succession of clinical cases. Familiarity with the types of patients that have featured in previous examinations (see the examiners' reports on past papers) should help the way you approach patients and organise your thoughts and management plans in day-to-day practice. On night duty, the bedside nurses will often offer to listen patiently as you rehearse your presentations.

Like all theatrical performances an essential part of getting it right on the day is to have rehearsed adequately. Make use of your study group colleagues, practise being the examiner and examinee for each other. Arrange clinical case teaching sessions with your consultants and senior colleagues who have recently sat the exam. It is far better to make embarrassing mistakes before the exam than in the middle of it.

Vivas

Any topic related to intensive care medicine may appear in a viva, but it is essential you have knowledge of core intensive care topics. Questions may range from the evidence base of current practice to complex ethical issues, to the management of a critically ill obstetric patient. The key in answering clinically based viva questions is to start with big picture, all-encompassing statements, e.g. 'I would commence with a rapid simultaneous history/evaluation of the patient while ensuring a safe airway, adequate ventilation and perfusion', becoming progressively more specific as the case history unfolds. It is excellent, for example, to discuss recent molecular research into the mechanism of eclampsia, but not before resuscitation and treatment modalities, and the marks will be weighted accordingly. This is discussed in more detail in Chapter 7.

Creating the right impression

Dress standards need to be smart but suitable for making a thorough physical examination of the patient, just like on the ward round. When selecting what to wear you need to consider looking professional while also taking heed of comfort and sleeve length. If you wear a suit most ICUs will require you to remove the jacket before entering. It is a good idea to have several dress rehearsals in your chosen outfit to make sure you appear and feel completely comfortable. Revealing or unusual clothing are inappropriate. For candidates with long hair, make sure it is off your face and tied back. All jewellery, including wristwatches, should be avoided, with the exception of a plain wedding band.

Most ICUs will have stethoscopes by the patient's bedside. Some candidates may prefer to use their own stethoscope and bring all their own equipment. This is perfectly acceptable but may not be permitted at all examination venues, so an element of flexibility is required. All items of equipment required for examination should be available on request at the venue. If you choose to take your own assortment of tools, ensure that you have practised accessing and using them.

The measures utilised for infection control (e.g. aprons, handwashing versus alcohol hand rub, gloves) will vary between locations. Be guided by the examiners. Some things remain universal, however: if you put your apron on with your stethoscope already around your neck it will end up in a tangled mess.

Candidates are often intimidated by the clinical components of the exam. Although clinical cases can be daunting this is the opportunity to showcase the skills that you have been working so hard to acquire. Do not be surprised if you leave the exam having enjoyed yourself!

Travel considerations

Make sure you book travel and accommodation requirements well in advance of the exam to minimise any further stress. Try to arrive during daylight the day before the exam so you can determine the best method and the correct amount of time you will need to arrive at the venue with plenty of time to spare before the exam. Invest in the best hotel you can afford as you will be staying for a few long and gruelling days there.

The decision of whether to attend the exam on your own or with your supportive family is an individual one. These important people may be welcome to attend the congratulatory drinks and this goes some way towards acknowledging their role in your success.

On the day

It is likely that you will be quarantined between sections of the exam. This involves staying in an area with other candidates, invigilated by official personnel. The purpose is to prevent candidates from sharing their experiences at different stages of the proceedings. Take advantage of the refreshments on offer, but avoid post mortems of questions with other candidates in the room.

There may be rest stops interspersed with active testing stations. They provide an excellent opportunity for you to re-focus on the examination, especially after a station that has not appeared to go well. Inevitably you will encounter some parts of the examination where your knowledge and performance seem to be weaker. Actively try to move on after any experiences that have appeared to be negative so that you don't sabotage further opportunities to perform well through negative self-talk.

Coping with failure

The best way to avoid failing is to be adequately prepared before you sit the exam. Candidates will be notified of failure in the written or MCQ paper within 2 to 8 weeks by post, depending on the exam. It is also at this time that successful candidates will receive their invitation to present for the clinical exam and/or vivas. Generally the reason for failure in the written or MCQ section is insufficient work with the core books and past exam papers, or under-preparation for the discipline of spending only the allocated time on each question. Remember that the law of diminishing returns applies here: spending a lot of time on one question is unlikely to outweigh the loss of marks incurred when a question is missed out completely. It is therefore essential to practise writing answers to questions and completing MCQs under strict exam conditions.

Candidates who fail the EDIC Part 1 will be notified by post within 8 weeks. Candidates who have failed can receive feedback from the ESICM administrative office in Brussels. Some centres inform candidates of the outcome after the 'court of examiners' meeting and allow feedback at this time. The exam co-coordinator or an agreed designated examiner will normally counsel candidates who have failed more than once and this will often include specific information on where the candidate performed poorly and advice on how they can improve.

Candidates who are unsuccessful in the DICM dissertation component receive feedback from the Regional Advisor in ICM on the areas that need attention. If the candidate is unsuccessful during the exam but has submitted a satisfactory dissertation they are permitted to resubmit the same dissertation for a further four sittings of the exam. Candidates who have failed are strongly recommended to get advice from their Regional Advisors in ICM, who will have details of the examiner's assessments.

Candidates who fail the FCICM Fellowship exam receive a telephone call from the Chair of the Examiners shortly after the exam. This gives guidance on areas for improvement and areas of particularly poor performance. This is kept sufficiently anonymous to prevent individual examiners from being identified. Other helpful information may include such things as the examiners felt that the candidate possessed the required knowledge but was missing structure, or that the relevant clinical signs were demonstrated but coherent synthesis and division of a management plan was not achieved. If the issue is that the candidate is unprepared, they may suggest he or she gain more clinical experience before re-sitting. After this an appointment with the supervisor of training can be useful so that the candidate can discuss feedback received about the examination and help devise strategies to address the specific areas of concern, e.g. vivas. Attending an exam-focused course prior to the next attempt can also be very useful.

Failing the exam can be a devastating (and expensive) experience. For many this will be the first time they have not succeeded at a professional exam. Each exam is challenging in different ways, but all are very searching and demanding, which seems entirely appropriate for such a searching and demanding specialty. Furthermore, it should not be forgotten that several of the world's foremost intensivists did not pass their exam the first time around.

References

Bersten A, Soni N (eds). Oh's Intensive Care Manual. Elsevier; 6th edn: 2009.

Cameron P, Jelinek G, Kelly A, et al. Textbook of Adult Emergency Medicine. Elsevier; 3rd edn: 2009.

Craft T, Nolan J, Parr M. Key Topics in Critical Care. Taylor and Francis; 2nd edn: 2004.

Dunn R, Dilley S, Brookes J. The Emergency Medicine Manual. Venom Publishing; 3rd edn: 2003.

Hinds C, Watson D. Intensive Care: A Concise Textbook. Saunders Elsevier; 3rd edn: 2008.

Irwin R, Rippe J. Intensive Care Medicine. Lippincott Williams and Wilkins; 6th edn: 2008.

Parsons P, Weiner-Kronish J. Critical Care Secrets. Mosby Elsevier; 4th edn: 2007.

Ridley S, Smith G, Batchelor A. Core Cases in Critical Care. Cambridge University Press; 1st edn: 2002.

Tintinalli J. Tintinalli's Emergency Medicine: A Comprehensive Study Guide. McGraw-Hill Professional Publishing; 7th edn: 2010.

Chapter 3

Basic sciences for intensive care medicine

If I have seen further than others, it is by standing upon the shoulders of giants.
ISAAC NEWTON

Introduction

Central to the understanding of intensive care medicine (ICM) and the interventions that form the specialty is a requirement for trainees to be familiar with the basic sciences. Physiology, pharmacology, research methods/statistics and physics/clinical measurement are core subjects that may be covered in any of the exams described in this book. The CICM Primary examination is the most likely to require detailed factual recall of concepts, although questions are generally designed with a clinical focus. The other exams are more likely to explore concepts with a stronger relevance to ICM practice.

For example, in a search on how pharmacology is tested, analysis of past CICM Primary examination papers reveals that approximately one-third of the questions directly tested generic pharmacology topics. These frequently required examples of drugs to be supplied that explained the concepts. The remaining questions were concerned with specific drugs or classes, with a comparison of agents used to explore diverse elements of pharmacodynamics and pharmacokinetics. By contrast, the exit examinations, such as the EDIC and the CICM Fellowship examination, tend to be much more targeted towards eliciting clinically relevant information, including an understanding of the evidence basis for prescribing certain medications.

This chapter does not claim to cover all of the material necessary to satisfy each exam syllabus. The emphasis is on empowering exam candidates to prepare themselves for specific exams with the breadth and depth of knowledge needed to meet the standards reflected in past exam papers. It aims to demonstrate approaches that will maximise efficient study time.

Approaching the study of these topics is somewhat daunting due to the diversity of the type and quantity of information that needs to be absorbed. We suggest different strategies be considered when tackling each component.

- **Physiology**
Recall rests with firstly understanding the concepts, followed by being able to explain them to others, typically using diagrams. In this chapter we therefore focus on explaining, in simple terms, some of the most important topics in each body system. Diagrams that have been drawn specifically at the level expected from a trainee under examination conditions supplement these summaries. It is essential to be able to rapidly produce simple diagrams when under pressure, but candidates are not expected to be able to reproduce complex, detailed figures.

- **Pharmacology**
  Recall is linked to being able to digest and memorise facts and link the concepts to medications or fluids that are prescribed to patients. In this chapter we therefore present a range of ways of codifying this knowledge.
- **Research methods/statistics**
  Recall is linked to analysing papers in order to grasp the relevance of the approaches used, which may be examined. In Chapter 9 we therefore summarise the most important basic statistical approaches to data analysis that should be understood. We encourage the reader to supplement this material with an appraisal of journal articles of various kinds to consolidate understanding. By seeing and interpreting items such as Forest plots in actual systematic reviews, the concepts can be more easily remembered.
- **Physics/clinical measurement**
  This material is important and will be examined, as it encompasses the fundamental principles, laws and concepts governing the behaviour of matter that underpin how equipment works. In Chapter 4, an approach to learning about equipment and preparing for related basic science exam questions is covered in detail.

Physiology

The core areas of emphasis in physiology are the respiratory and cardiovascular systems. However, breadth of knowledge is required in the areas of renal, neurological and gastrointestinal physiology. Less common areas, such as the musculoskeletal system and obstetrics, are also assessed. These may provide high-yield areas for study, as there are limited topics to be examined, but a requirement for them to be assessed.

SAMPLE QUESTION

Describe the physiological changes in prone ventilation in a patient with normal lungs. How might this differ in a patient with ARDS?

Answer
This is focused on the physiological changes in relation to ventilation and perfusion in the lung unit.
    The following changes occur with the prone position:

In the normal lung
Cardiovascular
- Decreased CI
- Decreased SV
- Maintained heart rate
- Increased SVR
- Increased PVR
- Decreased arterial filling following increased intrathoracic pressure
- IVC obstruction.

Respiratory
- Increased FRC
- FEV_1/FVC unchanged
- Tidal volume, inspiratory flow rates unchanged
- Static compliance unchanged
- Airway resistance unchanged
- Perfusion directed to dorsal lung areas

- More uniform distribution of flow
- Possible lower PVR in dorsal areas
- Pleural pressure gradient reduced
- More even distribution of ventilation.

In the ARDS lung
- Lung weight – ventral lung dependent, hence collapse under hydrostatic pressures
- Cardiac mass effect – less alveolar compression
- Cephalad diaphragmatic displacement – changed due to less compression by abdominal contents
- Alveolar inflation more homogeneous
- Decreased thoraco-abdominal compliance
- Respiratory compliance unchanged, but improved when supine position assumed
- Primary ARDS – no change in lung volume and alveolar recruitment, but secondary ARDS improvement seen
- V/Q improved by increased lung volume, redistribution of perfusion, recruitment of dorsal lung regions, more homogeneous ventilation
- More triangular shape of thorax in supine position; more improvement in oxygen in prone position
- Secretion mobilisation
- Dorsal areas maintain perfusion.

The following descriptions are aimed at covering often examined but poorly understood areas. Diagrams are crucial to help efficiently answer questions in physiology. We suggest that it is easiest to reproduce these rapidly by drawing the curve first and labelling the axes second.

Respiratory system
Examination favourites, such as the oxygen-haemoglobin dissociation curve, oxygen cascade and spirometry (Figs 3.1–3.3), are basic concepts in respiratory physiology. Following this there is a discussion of various other material, essential for a core understanding of this subject. Emphasis on applied physiology and interaction with other organ systems is now expected.

Venous admixture
The venous admixture is a theoretical value. It provides a simplified approach to explaining the difference between the alveolar and arterial oxygen values. An admixture refers to the reduction of value of something when another component is added. Also known as a shunt, and calculated by the shunt equation (shown in Fig 3.4), it is the amount of mixed venous blood combined with pulmonary end-capillary blood. It produces an observed difference between arterial and alveolar pO_2 (taken to be end-pulmonary capillary blood).

Airway resistance
Airway resistance is related to pressure difference divided by flow rate. It is affected by flow characteristics (laminar or turbulent) of the large and small airways (see Chapter 4). The normal value is about 2 $cmH_2O/L/sec$. Lung volume versus resistance is a hyperbolic relationship, as shown in Figure 3.5.

Pulmonary vascular resistance (PVR)
Pulmonary vascular resistance has a normal value of 144 dyn s cm^{-5} (these are the traditional units used in describing PVR and SVR from the centimetre–gram–second measuring system used, predating the SI units. 1 dyn = 10^{-5} Newtons). The resistance

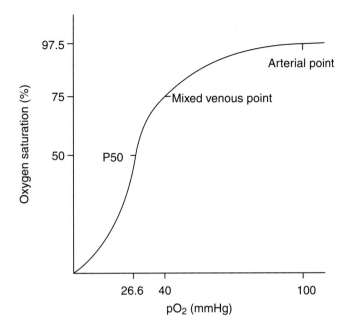

FIGURE 3.1 Oxygen-haemoglobin dissociation curve
Source: Guyton A, Hall J. Textbook of Medical Physiology. Saunders; 11th edn: 2005,
Fig 40-8, p. 506.

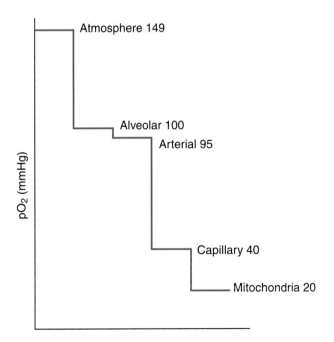

FIGURE 3.2 Oxygen cascade
Source: West J. Respiratory Physiology: The Essentials. Lippincott Williams & Wilkins;
8th edn: 2000, Fig 5-1, p. 56.

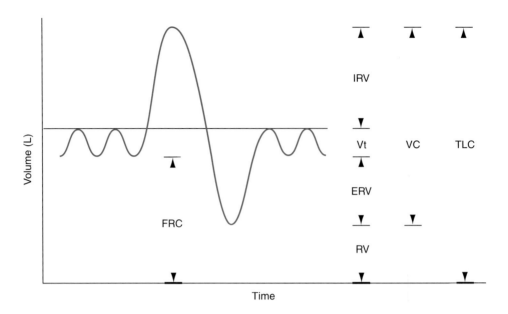

FIGURE 3.3 Spirometry
Source: West J. Respiratory Physiology: The Essentials. Lippincott Williams & Wilkins;
8th edn: 2000, Fig 2-2, p. 14.

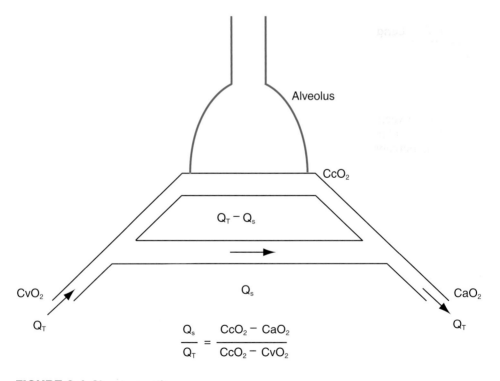

$$\frac{Q_s}{Q_T} = \frac{CcO_2 - CaO_2}{CcO_2 - CvO_2}$$

FIGURE 3.4 Shunt equation
Source: West J. Respiratory Physiology: The Essentials. Lippincott Williams & Wilkins;
8th edn: 2000, Fig 5-3, p. 60.

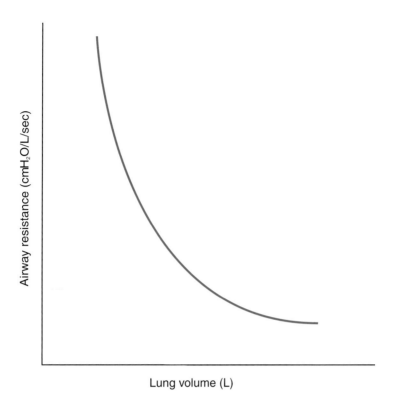

FIGURE 3.5 Lung volume versus airway resistance
Source: West J. Respiratory Physiology: The Essentials. Lippincott Williams & Wilkins; 8th edn: 2000, Fig 7-15, p. 113.

is shared between arteries, arterioles, venules and capillaries, which in turn are affected by alveolar pressures. Factors affecting the PVR include recruitment, posture, hypoxia, hypercapnia, autonomic and local mediators. In a graph of lung volume versus PVR (Fig 3.6), it is clear that there are low volumes near RV (residual volume) leading to increasing PVR from HPV (hypoxic pulmonary vasoconstriction) or compression of capillaries with increasing PVR near TLC (total lung capacity) due to alveolar capillary compression.

Compliance
Compliance is the change in volume per unit pressure change. Normal value is 200 mL/cmH$_2$O for the lung and thoracic cage, hence 100 mL/cmH$_2$O for total system (1/total compliance = 1/thoracic cage compliance + 1/lung compliance). It is described as *dynamic* when flow is occurring and *static* if there is no flow. Factors that affect compliance include surfactant, lung volume, pulmonary blood volume, lung size (lung compliance per functional residual capacity i.e. specific compliance), lung elastic recoil or lack thereof (in disease) and frequency dependence.

Surfactant reduces the surface tension in the alveoli and hence by the Law of Laplace applied to the alveolus: alveolar pressure = 2 × surface tension/alveolar radius the tendency for alveolar collapse is reduced. Thus, less pressure is required to inflate the alveolar unit and so compliance is improved.

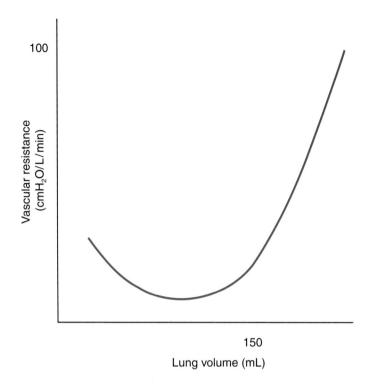

FIGURE 3.6 Lung volume vs pulmonary vascular resistance
Source: West J. Respiratory Physiology: The Essentials. Lippincott Williams & Wilkins; 8th edn: 2000, Fig 4-6, p. 41.

Dead space

The normal value of the anatomic dead space is 150 mL and equates with the volume of the conducting airways that does not take part in respiration. Anatomical dead space is measured using Fowler's method (with a rapid nitrogen analyser, as demonstrated in Fig 3.7). The physiological (functional) dead space is the volume that does not eliminate CO_2 and is similar to anatomical, but is affected by disease states and is usually larger. It is measured using the Bohr equation:

$$V_D / V_T = P_{ACO2} - P_{ECO2} / P_{ACO2}$$

V_D is dead space volume; V_T is tidal volume; P_{ACO2} is alveolar CO_2 and P_{ECO2} is mixed expired CO_2.

Alveolar dead space is that volume beyond the anatomical dead space, which still does not take part in ventilation.

Physiological dead space = alveolar dead space + anatomical dead space

Carbon dioxide dissociation curve

Compared with the O_2 dissociation curve (Fig 3.8) the curve for CO_2 is more linear, reflecting a higher CO_2 concentration for pCO_2 and also the Haldane effect, which describes the higher CO_2 binding at lower pO_2.

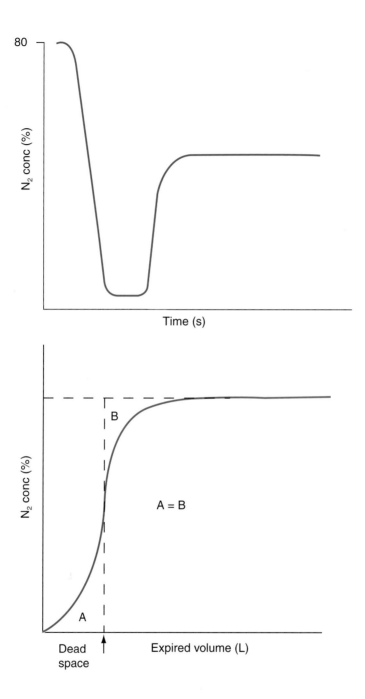

FIGURE 3.7 Fowler's method of estimating anatomical dead space
Source: West J. Respiratory Physiology: The Essentials. Lippincott Williams & Wilkins;
8th edn: 2000, Fig 2-6, p. 19.

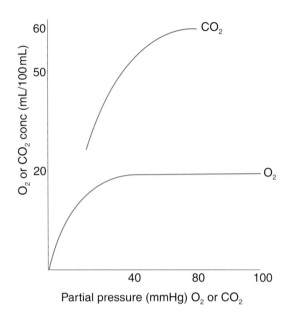

FIGURE 3.8 Oxygen and carbon dioxide dissociation curve
Source: West J. Respiratory Physiology: The Essentials. Lippincott Williams & Wilkins;
2000: 8th edn, Fig 6-7 p. 83.

Causes of the difference in arterial and end-tidal pCO_2

The normal gradient is between 5 and 10 mmHg (1–2 kPa). Alveolar pCO_2 is related to alveolar ventilation and blood CO_2 output. The difference occurs due to underperfused alveoli, i.e. shunting of blood and variable ventilation: perfusion ratios of different lung units. The larger the shunt, the greater the difference between $PaCO_2$ and $EtCO_2$. Non-physiological (in this case, equipment) causes of a difference include circuit leaks and sampling line problems. Pathological causes may be due to poor lung perfusion from pulmonary emboli and cardiac arrest.

Effects of changes of posture on ventilatory function

The functional residual capacity (FRC) is reduced when supine. When upright the upper alveoli are more open due to more negative intrapleural pressures, but they undergo less ventilation than basal alveoli.

Physiological effects of positive end expiratory pressure (PEEP)

These can be divided into:
- respiratory – increased FRC, increased compliance, decreased work of breathing, decreased airway resistance, increased ventilation in dependent lung areas, increased physiological dead space
- cardiovascular – decreased systemic venous return due to increased right ventricular afterload (hence, increased pulmonary vascular resistance); decreased left ventricular afterload
- renal – decreased renal blood flow, decreased glomerular filtration rate, increased antidiuretic hormone (ADH).
- gastrointestinal – decreased hepatic blood flow.

Physiological effects of invasive positive pressure ventilation (IPPV)
- Respiratory – alteration in distribution of ventilation but minimal functional change; dead space increased with circuits in both invasive ventilation and non-invasive ventilation (larger increase); no effect on physiological dead space in the short term; no effect on FRC; improves pO_2 in pathological states but not in healthy lungs.
- Cardiovascular – decreases effect of thoracic pump similar to PEEP, leading to reduced cardiac output (as negative intrathoracic gradient is removed).

Changes of the respiratory system in obesity
In obesity various effects are seen in the respiratory system, including upper airway obstruction from pharyngeal fat deposition, decreased compliance and increased resistance, and the associated syndromes of obstructive sleep apnoea and hypoventilation, both of which cause decreased FRC.

Key features of the pulmonary blood flow
The pulmonary circulation has limited ability to control regional flow, meaning that gravity has significant effects (Starling resistors in areas I, II and III). On moving from the supine to erect posture, the pulmonary blood volume decreases by one-third. Increased systemic vascular resistance will increase pulmonary blood volume. This is reliant on the fact that pulmonary arterial pressure is one-sixth of systemic pressure.

Factors affecting respiratory control
- Central medullary chemoreceptors are CO_2 sensitive and increase the rate and depth of respiration in response to a CO_2 increase.
- Peripheral chemoreceptors in carotid bodies are O_2 sensitive and respond to the partial pressure and not total content. Minute ventilation is proportional to arterial pCO_2 but varies in gradient according to pO_2 (steeper gradient with lower pO_2).

Factors determining oxygen flux
DO_2 = cardiac output × {oxygen saturation × haemoglobin concentration × 1.31 [volume of oxygen in mL which combines with 1 g haemoglobin]} + 0.3 mL/dL (oxygen in solution)

Cardiovascular system
Common exam favourites are the Valsalva manoeuvre, cardiac cycle and central venous pressure waveform (Figs 3.9–3.10). These are all well explained with accurate diagrams (with the emphasis on timing) and it is well worth spending time practising drawing these to aid both understanding and answering questions when you sit the exam.

Electrochemical basis of the ECG
The cardiac action potential has five phases (0–4), of which the fast phases – 1 and 2 – are absent in the SA and AV nodes (Fig 3.11). Automaticity of the SA node is due to slow inward calcium movement and a fall in potassium permeability. The resting membrane potential of the SA node is less negative than ventricular muscle. A steady leak of calcium into the node causing threshold voltage needs to be achieved, causing an action potential that spreads throughout the atria. The AV node has slower depolarisation than the SA node.

The summation of all the action potentials is recorded on the surface ECG. Convention dictates that the depolarisation waves cause positive deflections approaching the electrodes and repolarisation waves cause negative deflections. This accounts for the predominantly positive deflected ECG.

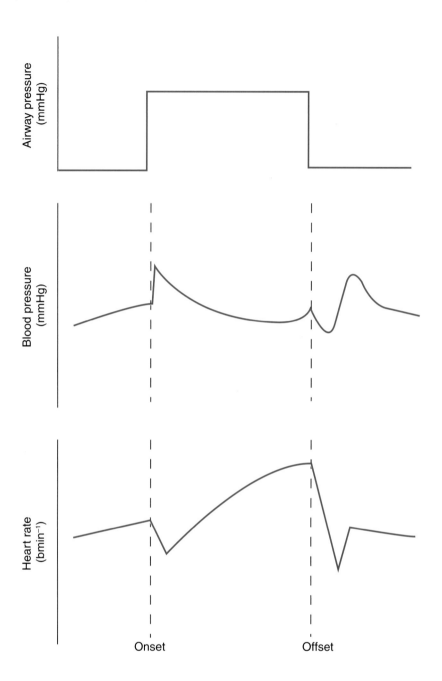

FIGURE 3.9 Valsalva manoeuvre
Source: Power I, Kam P. Principles of Physiology for the Anaesthetist. Hodder Arnold, 2001, Fig 4-47, p. 157.

Special features of the coronary circulation

The high resting oxygen extraction (75%) means that increasing blood flow is the only method of increasing overall oxygen delivery. Resting flow is 80 mL/min/100 g tissue, which can increase up to 400 mL/min/100 g. Aortic diastolic pressure is the main

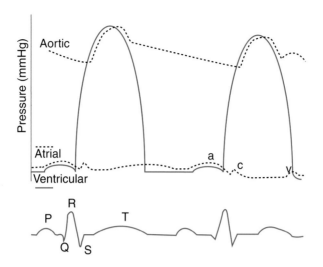

FIGURE 3.10 Events of the cardiac cycle
Source: Guyton A, Hall J. Textbook of Medical Physiology. Saunders; 11th edn: 2005, Fig 9-5, p. 107.

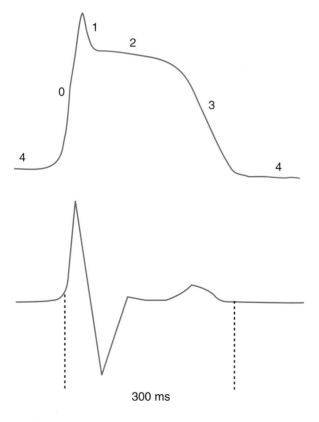

FIGURE 3.11 The ECG and cardiac action potential
Source: Guyton A, Hall J. Textbook of Medical Physiology. Saunders; 11th edn: 2005, Figure 11-3, p. 125.

driving pressure. Left ventricular flow occurs mainly in diastole and is intermittent, whereas right ventricular flow is higher in systole and is pulsatile. High resting tone of coronary vessels (from systolic compression) results in local mediators affecting autoregulation, such, as nitric oxide, adenosine, lactic acid and hydrogen ions. Autonomic innervation of coronary vessels exists, but sympathetic vasoconstrictor effects and parasympathetic vasodilator effects are secondary phenomena to local mediator effects. There is a very low oxygen saturation of coronary sinus blood, which drains the left ventricle mainly of about 30–35%.

Aspects of ventricular pressure–volume relationships

This relationship describes the changes that occur during the cardiac cycle (Fig 3.12). Work (area under curve), contractility (end-systolic p–v relationship) and stiffness (end-diastolic p–v relationship) can be determined from this.

Four phases exist:
- filling
- isovolaemic contraction
- ejection
- isovolaemic relaxation.
  To understand these relations an appreciation of the following concepts is essential:
- Pre-load: left ventricular end-diastolic volume prior to initial contraction.
- After-load: left ventricular wall tension developed after the onset of myocardial fibre shortening or the tension needed to overcome the impedance to ejection of blood and opposition of wall shortening.
- Contractility: independent from both pre- and afterload, and related to the amount of shortening intrinsic to the myocardial fibres and the velocity of that shortening.

The end-systolic pressure–volume line gradient reflects the contractility with an increase in gradient (positive inotrope) and depressed slope (with negative inotropy).

Physiological response to haemorrhage

The response is dependent on the rate and amount of blood loss. The main objective is to preserve flow in vital areas, which include the myocardial and cerebral territories. The response can be divided into:
- immediate: baroreceptor and thoracic stretch receptor activation causes sympathetic activation, which results in arterio- and veno-constriction. This mainly occurs in tissues with high sympathetic innervation, e.g. splanchnic and cutaneous beds. This is associated with tachycardia and increased contractility. Autoregulation occurs in cerebral, coronary and renal vascular beds down to mean pressures of approximately 75 mmHg.
  Large blood loss may stimulate a CNS sympathetic mediated response.
  Endocrine responses include increased ADH and renin pathway activation. This occurs over a period of minutes.
- prolonged: fluid absorption from the interstitial compartment occurs over a period of hours.
  Erythropoietin increases to stimulate red cell production and adrenal glucocorticoid stimulation occurs.

Frank-Starling mechanism of the heart

The Frank-Starling concept, in relation to the heart, describes the force of contraction as proportional to initial applied (diastolic) resting length and can be expressed as a cardiac function curve (Fig 3.13), where stroke volume is related to left ventricular end-diastolic volume. Note that this differs from contractility, which refers to the *intrinsic* shortening of the fibre not *applied* shortening.

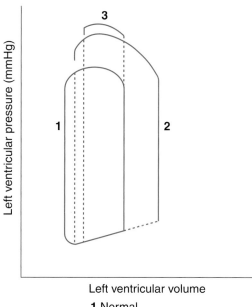

1 Normal
2 Increase preload
3 Increase afterload

FIGURE 3.12 Left ventricular pressure–volume loop with changes in preload, afterload and contractility
Source: Power I, Kam P. Principles of Physiology for the Anaesthetist. Hodder Arnold; 2001, Figs 4-22, 4-23, p. 118.

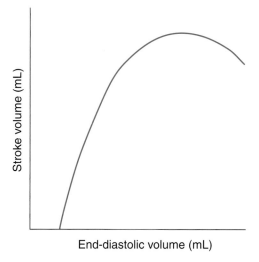

FIGURE 3.13 Starling curve applied to the left ventricle of the heart
Source: Power I, Kam P. Principles of Physiology for the Anaesthetist. Hodder Arnold; 2001, Fig 4-15, p. 115.

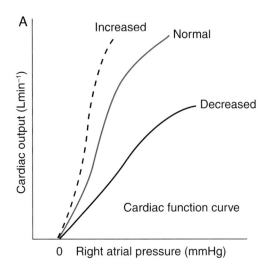

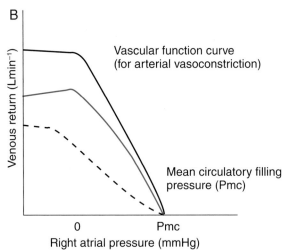

FIGURE 3.14 A) Cardiac output and venous return versus right atrial pressure and then: B) The same relationship as a vascular function curve
Source: Guyton A, Hall J. Textbook of Medical Physiology. Saunders; 11th edn: 2005, Fig 20-4, p. 234; Fig 20-9, p. 239.

Cardiac output and the relationship with central venous pressure

A graph of cardiac output versus central venous pressure (Fig 3.14a and b) expresses the inverse relationship of the two and can be described as a vascular function curve.

Physiological response to change in posture

From supine to standing, the arterial baroreceptor-mediated sympathetic response results in reduction of venous compliance (venoconstriction) and increased tone of resistance vessels (peripheral vasoconstriction), along with direct myocardial stimulation (increased heart rate and contractility). Skeletal muscle also contributes to maintenance of mean blood pressure by rhythmic contraction of the veins. Arterial to venous cerebral perfusion gradient is maintained due to similar drops in venous and CSF pressures.

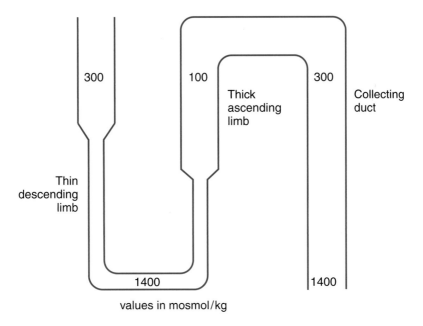

FIGURE 3.15 **Osmolality through the nephron**
Source: Power I, Kam P. Principles of Physiology for the Anaesthetist. Hodder Arnold; 2001, Fig 7-16, p. 209.

Renal system

Regional circulations are a favourite exam topic, with the kidney being no exception. Knowledge of functional anatomy from glomerulus to collecting duct and applied aspects, such as handling of electrolytes, is expected.

Features of renal blood flow

The main feature is the high flow relative to oxygen consumption. Flow is predominantly to the cortex rather than the medulla. A diagram of the main functional unit of the kidney, the nephron, and the osmolality gradients throughout is shown in Figure 3.15. Normal renal function requires that the flow through the kidney be kept within a narrow range and relies on afferent arteriole smooth muscle changes (not efferent). A rise in glomerular perfusion pressure leads to increased flow of Na and Cl in the ascending loop of Henle, detected by the macula densa, which releases adenosine and causes afferent arteriole vasoconstriction. This process is called tubuloglomerular feedback and is an important mechanism whereby the kidney is able to regulate glomerular filtration rate. Large sympathetic stimulation can cause both afferent and efferent arteriolar constriction. Angiotensin II is an afferent and efferent constrictor. Prostacyclin and some prostaglandins provide vasodilation in balance to circulating vasoconstrictors.

What are the counter-current mechanisms?

- Multiplier: increases the osmolar gradient in the loop of Henle, achieving a maximum concentration of 1400 mosmol/kg H_2O at the tip by counter-current flows in the descending and ascending loops of Henle.
- Exchanger: maintains the gradient via slow flowing vasa recta, which are vessels that have their own counter-current exchange of solutes and water, preventing washout of the gradient.

Sodium handling by the kidney

Sodium handling by the kidney is complex. The proximal tubule reabsorption of sodium predominates (65%) by co- and counter-transport means and is energised by passive sodium flow down its concentration gradient. Glomerulotubular balance matches GFR with sodium reabsorption as a constant fraction. The ascending limb of loop of Henle provides 25% active reabsorption of sodium with a chloride pump.

Endocrine factors involved are:
- aldosterone: increases reabsorption of sodium in distal convoluted tubule and collecting duct
- angiotensin II: directly stimulates sodium reabsorption in proximal convoluted tubule
- ADH: increases reabsorption of sodium and water in collecting ducts
- atrial natriuretic factor: increases excretion of sodium.

Neural factors involve the renal sympathetic nerves, which act by increasing the reabsorption of sodium.

Potassium handling by the kidney

Potassium is tightly controlled in the ECF. Potassium is mainly an intracellular ion, but small changes in extracellular concentrations cause cardiac arrhythmias, hence the requirement for tight control. Intake, distribution and output affect potassium levels.

Key control features include:
- rapid redistribution into cells, e.g. insulin, aldosterone, adrenaline
- filtration: usually constant with stable GFR
- reabsorption: proximal tubule (55%), ascending loop of Henle (30%), intercalated cells of collecting duct
- secretion: performed by principal cells of the late distal convoluted tubule and collecting duct. Aldosterone increases secretion of potassium via Na/K pump production and potassium channels in basolateral membrane. The plasma potassium levels directly stimulate the Na/K pump and influence this process, along with luminal membrane permeability and potassium's electrochemical gradient from cell to tubule
- tubular flow rate is directly proportional to potassium secretion
- indirect effects of ECF volume and sodium content via aldosterone and tubular flow rate balance the secretion processes, similarly with ADH and tubular flow rate
- alkalosis stimulates the Na/K pump due to low hydrogen ion concentration.

Glomerular filtrate factors

$$GFR = Kf \times NEP$$

where Kf is the filtration coefficient = the product of glomerular surface area and permeability of the glomerular capillary.

Compared to other locations, blood flow is very high in these capillary beds, allowing rapid filtration.

$$NFP = \text{net filtration pressure} = pGC + \pi BC - pBC = \pi GC$$

where p is hydrostatic pressure, π is oncotic pressure, GC is glomerular capillary and BC is the Bowmans capsule.

Solving the equation gives:

$$NEP = 1 * [60 + 0 - 15 - 21] = 24 \text{ mmHg at afferent end and}$$

$$NFP = 1 * [58 + 0 - 15 - 33] = 10 \text{ mmHg at efferent end.}$$

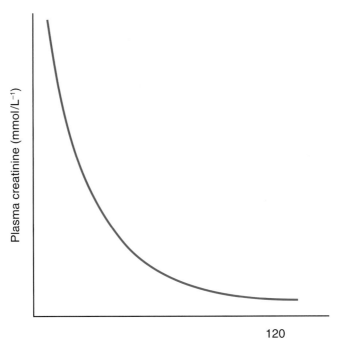

FIGURE 3.16 Plasma creatinine vs glomerular filtration rate
Source: Guyton A, Hall J. Textbook of Medical Physiology. Saunders; 11th edn: 2005, Fig 27-19 p. 346.

The NFP can be determined for the proximal and distal ends of the glomerulus, giving an average NFP sufficient to produce the 180 L/day required to remove the 600 mosmol of waste products/day.

Glomerular filtrate is an ultrafiltrate (proteins removed due to size, hence πBC is zero).

Filtration fraction = GFR/renal plasma flow = 125/600 = 20% of renal plasma flow that is filtered into the tubule.

Creatinine as a marker of renal function

$$GFR \approx C_{cr} = U_{cr} \times V / P_{cr}$$

where C_{cr} is creatinine clearance, U_{cr} is urinary creatinine concentration, V is urine volume and P_{cr} is plasma creatinine concentration.

Creatinine is a naturally occurring metabolite that is filtered and secreted (almost, but not quite the ideal marker, as the amount excreted exceeds the amount filtered, as seen in Figure 3.16). However, plasma measurement of creatinine usually overestimates the level, therefore elevation of U_{cr} and P_{cr} cancel each other out. Also the creatinine level changes with production and excretion, creating a lag time for measurement. In the steady state, production = excretion. A non-linear relationship exists between the serum level and clearance.

Total body water (TBW) and its composition

TBW = 60% of body weight
60% of 70 kg = 42 L

The 42 L is distributed into 28 L of intracellular fluid (ICF) and 14 L of extracellular fluid (ECF). ECF is further subdivided into plasma (3 L) and interstitial fluid (11 L). Transcellular fluid (minimal) is not kinetically very active, e.g. synovium and CSF.

Sodium is ≈ 6 mmol/L higher in the plasma compared with the interstitial fluid (ISF) due to the effect of negatively charged plasma proteins confined to the plasma (Donnan effect). This is countered by a measurement effect that measures sodium in the plasma water as though it is in the whole plasma (i.e. that which contains proteins). The combination of these processes leads to the ECF and ISF sodium concentrations being roughly equal. Potassium, calcium, magnesium and chloride are in equal concentrations between ECF and ISF. The ICF concentration of ions is quite different: low sodium (14 mmol/L) because of the Na pump and poor solubility of the membrane. Potassium (140 mmol/L), calcium (zero), magnesium (20 mmol/L) and chloride (4 mmol/L). The osmolarity of plasma is slightly higher than the ISF and ICF due to plasma proteins.

Tonicity refers to water movement changing the cell volume.

Effect of fluid infusion on fluid spaces

The four types of infusion are shown in Figure 3.17.
- Saline infusion is isotonic, so no osmosis occurs as the membranes are impermeable to solutes, so the fluid remains in the ECF.
- Dextrose 5% infusion is hypotonic, so osmosis leads to intracellular fluid movement with ICF volume increasing to a greater extent than ECF volume.
- Saline 3% infusion is hypertonic, so osmosis of water out of cells occurs into the ECF causing increased ECF volume, decreased ICF volume and an increase of osmolarity in both compartments.
- Albumin solutions are isotonic, so no osmotic changes occur but protein is confined to ECF so expansion of this compartment occurs initially, with subsequent long-term redistribution of fluid into other compartments.

Note the traditional view of a colloid to crystalloid ratio of plasma expansion = 1:3 was dispelled by the SAFE study (for details, see Chapter 9), which reflected a ratio of 1:1.4 as more accurate.

Renal control of acid–base balance

The maximum urinary pH achievable is 4.4. Mechanisms to excrete acid load occur in the proximal tubule, which is a low-gradient, high-capacity system. These include hydrogen ion secretion allowing bicarbonate reabsorption of about 90% of the filtered load. Also, formation of titratable acidity with non-volatile or fixed acid buffering of hydrogen phosphate happens here. Re-absorption occurs in the distal tubule hydrogen ion secretion for bicarbonate. Ammonium ion secretion occurs in both proximal and distal tubules.

The distal tubule, which is a high-gradient, low-capacity system, achieves net acid excretion as secreted proximal tubular hydrogen ions are converted to water, so no *net* excretion occurs from here.

Titratable acidity is defined as the amount of alkali required to titrate the acid bound to filtered buffers to a pH of 7.4. Other filtered buffers include β hydroxybutyrate and creatinine, which play a role mainly at low tubular pH.

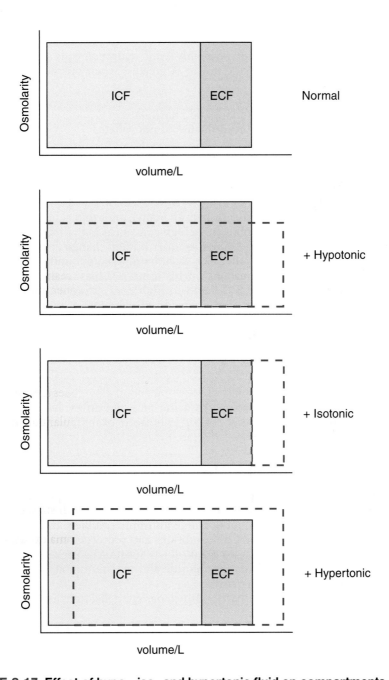

FIGURE 3.17 Effect of hypo-, iso- and hypertonic fluid on compartments Intracellular fluid (ICF) and extracellular fluid (ECF)
Source: Guyton A, Hall J. Textbook of Medical Physiology. Saunders; 11th edn: 2005, Fig 25-6, p. 30.

Buffer systems in the body

A buffer is a substance that can reversibly bind hydrogen ions (usually a weak acid and conjugate base). Buffering power is greatest when operating within ± of 1 pH unit.

In the blood:
- plasma: bicarbonate (70%), proteins and phosphates
- red cell: haemoglobin (90%), bicarbonate and phosphates
- interstitial fluid: bicarbonate
- intracellular fluid: proteins and phosphates.

The main buffers are:
- bicarbonate: carbonic acid system: pK_a 6.1 (low); low concentration but open system
- haemoglobin: pK_a 6.8; powerful system as many imidazole side chains exist on the histidine sites of haemoglobin and a high concentration of red cells is present. Isohydric buffering (no change in pH as other buffers change in balance) occurs with deoxygenated Hb. Also buffer CO_2 as carbamino compounds.
- proteins: pK_a 6.8, imidazole groups on histidine residues; mainly intracellular buffer so effective as pH is 6.8–7.1 and in high concentrations, but takes time to buffer ECF changes due to slow diffusion of elements of bicarbonate buffer system
- phosphate: pK_a 6.8 of biphosphate; low concentration in ECF, closed system in ECF – mainly intracellular buffer (higher concentrations) and urinary buffer.

Neurological system

Factors affecting, and measurement of, cerebral blood flow are popular topics in neurophysiology. Substances involved in acute pain are an evolving subject. The differences between plasma and CSF constituents are an exam favourite.

The blood brain barrier (BBB)

The main characteristics of the BBB can be divided into:
- physical: tight junctions between capillary endothelium and ependymal cells. Astrocyte foot processes exist beyond the basement membrane, which has clefts. Allows small Mwt substances, but not large non-lipid soluble substances
- functional: provides controlled CSF conditions and protects from substances such as bilirubin. Enzymatic processes break down substances preventing entry, e.g. L-dopa. Active transport occurs for chloride and magnesium at the BBB (higher concentrations in CSF than in plasma).

Note there is also a blood–CSF barrier, which has epithelial tight junctions between cells of the choroid plexus

Circumventricular organs, such as the posterior pituitary, pineal gland, area postrema near the third and fourth ventricles, are exposed to the systemic circulation.

Factors influencing cerebral blood flow

Numerous factors affect the cerebral blood flow as shown in Figure 3.18. These include oxygen, carbon dioxide, mean arterial pressure, metabolic rate, intracranial pressure, central venous pressure, flow characteristics of the blood, altitude (increased due to lower pO_2) and regional variations in the brain (grey matter flows four times faster than white matter due to metabolic requirements of cell bodies). Measured by Kety-Schmidt method using N_2O derived from Fick principle. Normal value 50 mL/min/100 g tissue.

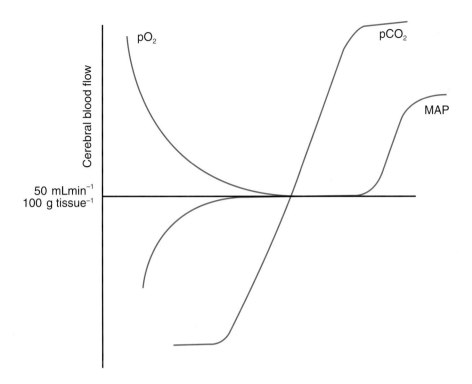

FIGURE 3.18 Effect of PaO$_2$, PaCO$_2$ and mean arterial blood pressure (MAP) on normal cerebral blood flow

Nerve axon conduction

Resting membrane potential (RMP: -70 mV) is established by the electrochemical balance of potassium inside and outside the membrane. Gradients are created by selective membrane permeability and ionic concentration differences. A sodium pump counters the passage of sodium down its electrochemical gradient into the cell, preventing loss of the RMP. The Nernst equation for individual ions calculates the potential difference across the membrane created by that ion. The Goldman equation accounts for the potential difference of all ions across the membrane.

Threshold potential (-55 mV) is reached on initial depolarisation allowing a positive feedback process of sodium influx into the cell. Subsequent increases in potassium return the cell to the RMP.

Propagation occurs in a unidirectional manner (by local currents advancing the membrane to threshold potential). Refractory periods (absolute and relative) exist behind the advancing conduction, and prevent subsequent depolarisations. Factors decreasing the rate of propagation include smaller diameter fibres, lack of myelin and electrolyte disturbances.

Pain pathways and mediators

Acute pain is an unpleasant sensory and emotional experience associated with actual or potential tissue damage.

Mediators of noxious stimuli act via metabotropic receptors (prostanoids, histamine, serotonin), ionotropic receptors (NMDA, purine, acid sensing) or directly on ligand-gated ion channels.

Nociceptors are the peripheral sensory organs. Nociceptor afferents conduct action potentials to the CNS and consist of Aδ fibres, which are myelinated, and C fibres which are unmyelinated. Cell bodies of peripheral (limb, trunk) afferents (Aδ and C fibres) are located in the superficial Rexed laminae I and II of the dorsal root ganglion of the spinal cord. Head and neck cell bodies are located in the trigeminal ganglion. Excitatory amino acids (glutamate) and peptides (substance P) act as neurotransmitters in the primary afferent terminals.

Wind-up phenomenon describes the progressive increase in output of the dorsal horn action potentials. Descending inhibitory influences are mediated by endorphins and enkephalins.

The spinothalamic tracts project pain to the thalamus and somatosensory cortex (site and pain type) from laminar V of the dorsal horn; the spinoreticular and spinomesencephalic tracts project to the medulla (integrate autonomic, homeostatic and arousal functions) and central areas (emotional component).

The rostroventromedial medulla integrates descending input to the dorsal horn from areas such as the peri-aqueductal grey matter and nucleus tractus solitarius. A classification of nerve fibres is outlined in Table 3.1.

Gastrointestinal system

The main areas candidates should review are bilirubin metabolism and enzymatic and endocrine aspects of the gut.

Blood flow to the liver

The blood flow to the liver accounts for 25% of cardiac output, including both hepatic arterial and portal venous supply.

- Hepatic artery: contributes 30% flow (degree of autoregulation present), high-resistance vessels. Has α and β adrenergic receptors, along with dopaminergic receptors.
- Portal vein: contributes 70% flow (linearly related to pressure), is valveless and drains the gastrointestinal tract; a low-resistance system; has α and dopaminergic receptors.

TABLE 3.1 The classification of nerve fibres			
Type	Myelination	Function	Conduction velocity (m/s)
Motor			
Aα	Yes	Motor	60–120
Aβ	Yes	Deep pressure/touch	40–70
Aγ	Yes	Proprioception	15–30
Aδ	Yes	Sharp pain, temperature	10–30
B	Yes	Autonomic	3–15
C	No	Aching pain, temperature	0.5–2
Sensory			
I	Yes	Vibration, touch, pressure	70–120
II	Yes		20–70
III	Yes	Cold, touch, pressure	5–25
IV	No	Warm, touch, pressure	0.5–2

A decrease in portal flow leads to an increase in arterial flow and vice versa. The hepatic veins drain into the IVC via left and right branches. The portal triad is made up of the hepatic artery and portal vein with bile canaliculi. The sinusoids are the terminal anastomosis of inflow supply, which eventually drains into the hepatic vein via central veins.

Features of hepatic blood flow:
- Increased with feeding, expiration, hypercapnia and glucagon.
- Reduced with inspiration, hypocapnia, positive-pressure ventilation and intravenous induction agents (dose-dependent).

Urea cycle

Urea excretion occurs in the kidneys after being formed in the liver from amino acid degradation. Ammonia is a toxic intermediary that combines with CO_2 to form citrulline. Arginine is then formed when ammonia and citrulline combine; then following hydrolysis, it forms urea and water along with ornithine, and is recycled back to combine with ammonia and CO_2. Excess ammonia may also build up due to shunting of blood from the portal vein to the IVC, preventing it from taking part in the above process.

Bile, bilirubin and bile salts

Bile contains water, bile salts (glycol- and tauro-conjugated bile acids), bilirubin, electrolytes, cholesterol, fatty acids and lecithin.

Bile salts are formed from cholesterol, emulsification of fats and acid absorption of lipids from the intestine via micelles. Enterohepatic circulation exists for these. An inner lipid area is hydrophobic, the outer area is hydrophilic (hence water soluble), and hence bile salts are amphipathic.

Bilirubin is formed by the reduction of biliverdin (a breakdown product of the haem ring). It is transported conjugated mainly with albumin and eventually absorbed by hepatocytes. Conjugation then occurs to become water soluble, mainly with glucuronic acid, after being released from albumin. This is then excreted in bile, with 50% being converted into urobilinogen. Urobilinogen is re-absorbed through the intestine back to the liver and re-excreted. A small amount passes in the urine. Oxidation in the urine forms urobilin and in the faeces stercobilin.

Consequently, with obstructive jaundice, conjugated bilirubin is present in the plasma and haemolytic jaundice leads to 'free' bilirubin in plasma and increased urobilinogen in the urine.

Gastric secretion – electrolyte composition and their functions

- Oxyntic glands secrete mucus, pepsinogen, hydrochloric acid and intrinsic factor.
- Pyloric glands secrete mucus and gastrin.

Gastric juice is produced in quantities of about 2.5 L/day and contains hydrogen ions, potassium and chloride ions, and small amounts of sodium ions relative to plasma. It has a low pH (1–1.5) and is hyperosmolar. Production is stimulated by three phases called cephalic, gastric and intestinal, but also inhibited by the negative feedback of the intestinal phase.

Gastric juice has various functions and achieves this by the production of various substances:
- hormones
  ○ gastrin: produced in G cells of the antrum; stimulates histamine secretion, pepsinogen secretion and force of peristaltic contractions. Inhibited by hydrogen ions and glucagon
  ○ somatostatin: inhibits gastrin release and is inhibited itself by vagal activation
- enzymes

◦ pepsinogen: released by vagal stimulation throughout all three phases and is converted to pepsin in the presence of acid to act as a proteolytic enzyme
◦ α amylase: hydrolyses carbohydrates until inactivated by low stomach pH
◦ gastric lipase: acts on triglycerides
• glycoprotein
◦ intrinsic factor: produced in parietal cells of the fundus to aid vitamin B12 absorption in the ileum.

Gastric emptying factors

Control of gastric emptying is necessary to coordinate chyme entering the small intestine. Gastric-promoting factors are balanced with duodenal inhibitory factors.
• Antral distension causes local reflexes enhancing the pyloric pump.
• Gastrin promotes stomach emptying.
• Food entering the duodenum stimulates reflexes via the enteric nervous system, using inhibitory sympathetic nerves and inhibition of vagal system.
• CCK released in the jejunum in response to fats inhibits gastrin-induced, enhanced motility.
• Secretin inhibits emptying when acid is detected in the duodenum and gastric inhibitory peptide may have a weak effect.

Thermoregulation

A commonly asked, yet small section of the syllabus. Popular questions focus on definitions and mechanisms of heat loss, along with measurement.
The system consists of:
• sensors, which are located in the skin and hypothalamus
• a central integrator located in the hypothalamus with the *a*nterior (*w*arm) stimulating heat loss and *p*osterior (*c*old) stimulating heat gain mechanisms
• effectors, mainly behavioural, but also sympathetically driven, such as shivering and endocrine mechanisms, e.g. thyroid.
Other important concepts are:
• thermoneutral zone: temperature range in which temperature regulation may be maintained by changes in skin blood flow alone
• interthreshold range: core temperatures not triggering autonomic thermoregulatory responses (normally 0.2°C)
• mechanisms of heat transfer:
◦ radiation: transfer of heat from one surface to another
◦ convection: heat transfer through bulk motion of air
◦ conduction: heat loss between two adjacent surfaces
◦ evaporation: heat loss through the slow vaporisation of a liquid.
• Other definitions:
◦ hypothermia: core temperature below 36°C
◦ threshold: temperature at which the effector is activated
◦ gain: rate of response to a given decrease in core temperature
◦ maximum response: response intensity no longer increasing with further deviation in core temperature.

Musculoskeletal system

This represents a small area of the syllabus, but comparisons of cardiac and smooth muscle are important.
The main functional components of the skeletal system:
• The motor unit consists of one motor neuron and multiple muscle fibres.
• Muscle fibres contain myofibrils, which consist of thick myosin and thin actin filaments surrounded by cytoplasm.

- The sarcomere is the unit of contraction and consists of two half I bands and an A band enclosed by Z lines (where actin is fixed):
  - I band is actin filament containing only
  - H band has myosin only
  - A band formed by myosin and actin
  - M line is where myosin is attached together.

The sliding filament theory refers to the myosin head crossbridges bringing actin filaments towards the centre of the sarcomere. Muscle shortening is brought about by repetitive cycling of this process. Initial muscle length determines tension developed by optimum crossbridging.

The muscle action potential stimulates calcium release from the sarcoplasmic reticulum via T tubules at the A–I junction of the sarcomere. Dihydropyridine and ryanodine receptors are thought to be involved in this process to cause muscle contraction via troponin C interacting with troponin I. This results in tropomyosin moving and allowing crossbridge formation. Inhibition by actomyosin ATPase is removed and contraction proceeds.

Troponin (Tn), along with actin and tropomyosin make up the actin filament. Troponin has three subunits: T, C and I. Troponin T has affinity for tropomyosin; C has affinity for calcium; and I has affinity for actin and also inhibits interaction between calcium and TnC. The three subunit troponin complexes attach along the tropomyosin molecule.

Immunology and host defence
The hypersensitivity reactions
In-depth knowledge of the hypersensitivity reactions is an essential element of the syllabus as it enables an understanding of anaphylaxis and other problems seen clinically.

Hypersensitivity describes an exaggerated reaction to an allergen.

There are four types:
- Type 1: immediate; IgE reacts with antigen causing mast cell sensitisation, degranulation releases mediators such as SRS (slow-releasing substance), histamine and bradykinin resulting in bronchoconstriction and vasodilatation. Atopic reactions and anaphylaxis (especially with parental administration of antigen) is the consequence.
- Type 2: IgG- or IgM-mediated cytotoxic reaction with antigen. Classical complement pathway activation and cell lysis. Transfusion reactions and autoimmune haemolytic anaemia are clinical examples.
- Type 3: IgG-, IgM- or IgA-mediated immune complex reaction. Antigen–antibody complex deposition in tissues or locally. Serum sickness and SLE are examples.
- Type 4: T-cell antigen-mediated reaction releasing interleukins. Macrophages appear after 24 hours (hence delayed). This results in granuloma formation, such as with sarcoid and tuberculosis.

Haematological system
There is an increased focus on the cell-based view of coagulation and therefore the constituents of blood and their properties.

Cross-matching of blood
This is the process used to prevent the reaction of donor red cell antigens agglutinating with recipient plasma antibodies. Many antigens exist, but only two types dominate reactions (ABO and rhesus).

Looking at Type A and Type B antigens (agglutinogens), most of the population have one, both or neither on the surface of their red cells. The blood group is denoted by surface antigen/s present. Those who are Type A antigen positive will have anti-B agglutinins in the plasma. By comparison, people who are Type AB antigen positive will have no agglutinins in their plasma. In terms of the antigens present, the following is seen, with the most common first: O (47%), A (41%), B (9%), AB (3%).

IgG and IgM make up the agglutinins that have more than one binding site, so clumps of red cells form on agglutination. Haemolysis may also occur if IgM (haemolysins) predominate.

The saline agglutination test involves taking red cells separated from plasma, diluted with saline and then mixed separately with known anti-A agglutinin and known anti-B agglutinin. Other antibodies are also tested this way, such as anti-P and anti-M.

The albumin agglutination test looks for IgG antibodies.

The LISS test enhances antibody activity to increase the sensitivity of antibody detection.

The antiglobulin test is also known as a direct or indirect Coombs test, which detects Kidd and Duffy antibodies. It is also used for diagnosis of autoimmune haemolytic anaemia.

Haemostasis

A delicate balance exists between bleeding and coagulation. The normal haemostatic response is linked through vasoconstriction of the vessel wall, platelet activation and a coagulation cascade, of which there are two main theories: the traditional cascade (intrinsic/extrinsic) system and cell-based (initiation: amplification: propagation).

- Cell-based theory (Fig 3.19)
  - Initiation: vascular injury causes membrane-bound tissue factor reaction with factor VIIa (normally circulating in small quantities); TF-VIIa (also known as extrinsic factor Xase) complexes (formed on cell surfaces) activate factors X and IX; Xa forms thrombin from prothrombin. Thrombin activates platelets, factor V and factor VIII.
  - Amplification: extrinsic Xase is rapidly inactivated by TFPI (tissue factor pathway inhibitor). Intrinsic Xase formed by factors IXa and VIIIa causes more Xa to be produced.
  - Propagation: factor Xa and factor Va form a prothrombinase which causes massive thrombin production from prothrombin and ultimately fibrin from fibrinogen.

In normal physiological states, fibrinolysis (activated by plasmin), flow of blood and inhibitors of coagulation (TFPI, antithrombin III, protein C and cofactor protein S) prevent uncontrolled coagulation.

The role of platelets in blood clotting

The main function of platelets is to form a plug via interactions with other platelets and the vessel wall.

They react with glycoproteins, including:
- GPIa: adherence to collagen
- GPIb–GPIIb/IIIa: attachment to von Willebrand factor (VWF), which aids binding to vessel wall and other platelets
- GPIIb/IIIa also binds fibrinogen.

Platelet activation occurs, leading to a change to spherical shape, secretion of granules and GPIIb/IIIa activation.

Platelet aggregation occurs via crosslinking with fibrinogen bridges. The process is stabilised by α granules. ADP and thromboxane A2 provide positive feedback for the amplification process.

Obstetrics

This is a high-yield area in which the following topics are focused on: applied aspects of physiology affected by pregnancy, along with changes of fetal physiology (particularly circulatory, respiratory and haematological) at birth.

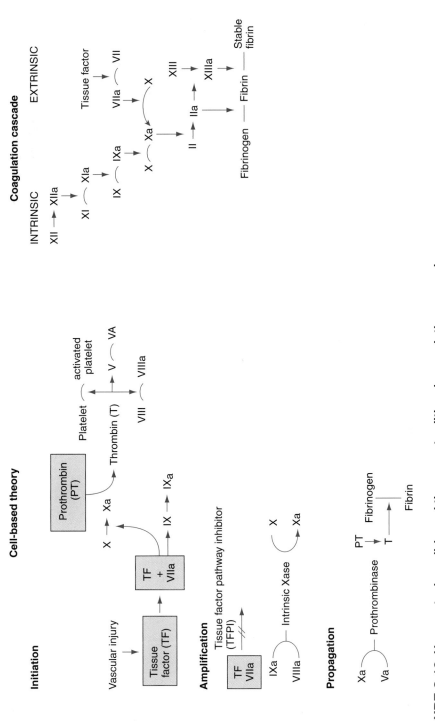

FIGURE 3.19 Haemostasis: cell-based theory vs traditional coagulation cascade
Source: Power I, Kam P. Principles of Physiology for the Anaesthetist. Hodder Arnold; 2001, Fig 9-15, p. 250.

Gas exchange across the placenta

Many factors are involved. Both oxygen and carbon dioxide must be considered.

Oxygen flows down a concentration gradient according to Fick's law of diffusion:

Flow ≈ area of placental gas exchange/thickness x diffusion constant of gas
x partial pressure gradient across the placenta

$$\{ \text{Flow} \approx A/T \times D \ (P_1 - P_2) \}$$

where Dgas ∞ solubility/$\sqrt{}$ molecular weight.

The placental surface area is increased by chorionic villi and the blood flow is high (600 mL/min). The gradient between the maternal intervillous space (PaO_2 50 mmHg (or 6.7 kPa)) and the fetal uterine artery (PaO_2 20 mmHg (or 2.7 kPa)) is the diffusion driving force.

Fetal Hb: high Hb content (17 g/dL) and left shifted O_2–Hb dissociation curve allows (i.e. lower p50) increased O_2 affinity and higher SaO_2 for PaO_2.

Double Bohr effect: higher $PaCO_2$ in maternal intervillous sinus blood aids oxygen offloading. Lower $PaCO_2$ in fetal blood increases oxygen affinity.

Double Haldane effect: maternal blood offloads oxygen-enhancing carbon dioxide transfer from fetus, which has less ability to bind carbon dioxide because of enhanced oxygen binding.

Maternal pCO_2 lowers secondary to hyperventilation, which favours carbon dioxide transfer.

Endocrine and nutrition

These areas of physiology are less frequently asked about; however, a focus on glucose in terms of metabolism and body requirements is essential.

Pharmacology

This is a massive topic with a large amount of pure facts to recall, particularly when learning about specific drugs and classes. Candidates are also required to be able to demonstrate understanding of generic pharmacology concepts, which may be best achieved by using examples of drugs that possess specific characteristics.

In this section we provide a range of approaches to assist exam preparation and mastery of pharmacology. These techniques are also relevant to approaching other subjects, but are demonstrated well here, where there is such diversity of information types to learn.

Diagrams and graphs

The topic of 'interaction between drugs and receptors' is a favourite in written and viva parts of primary exams and is based on the classical 'occupation theory' of drug and receptor interaction: in a constant population of receptors, as drug concentration increases, fractional occupation of receptors increases, with a directly proportional response until there is 100% receptor occupancy (related to the Law of Mass Action, which states that the concentration of reacting components proportionately determines the rate of reaction).

Diagrams and graphs are a useful way to approach this topic. The diagrams and graphs in Figure 3.20 and Table 3.2 summarise these concepts and aid revision.

Explaining anomalies to the 'occupation theory'

To remember important concepts such as these, we suggest making specific short study notes to accompany diagrams, or making annotations on the back of the diagrams or graphs that can easily be reviewed later:

DRUG–RECEPTOR RESPONSES

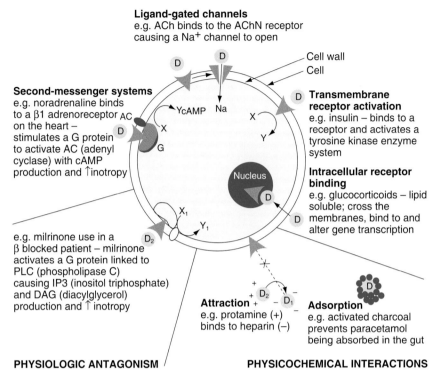

Ligand-gated channels
e.g. ACh binds to the AChN receptor
causing a Na$^+$ channel to open

Cell wall
Cell

Second-messenger systems
e.g. noradrenaline binds
to a β1 adrenoreceptor
on the heart –
stimulates a G protein
to activate AC (adenyl
cyclase) with cAMP
production and ↑inotropy

**Transmembrane
receptor activation**
e.g. insulin – binds to a
receptor and activates a
tyrosine kinase enzyme
system

**Intracellular receptor
binding**
e.g. glucocorticoids – lipid
soluble; cross the
membranes, bind to and
alter gene transcription

e.g. milrinone use in a
β blocked patient – milrinone
activates a G protein linked to
PLC (phospholipase C)
causing IP3 (inositol triphosphate)
and DAG (diacylglycerol)
production and ↑ inotropy

Attraction
e.g. protamine (+)
binds to heparin (–)

Adsorption
e.g. activated charcoal
prevents paracetamol
being absorbed in the gut

PHYSIOLOGIC ANTAGONISM   **PHYSICOCHEMICAL INTERACTIONS**

FIGURE 3.20 Mechanisms of drug responses

Receptor reserve ('spare receptors')
This occurs for different reasons. In some settings not all receptors need to be activated for a maximal response to occur (e.g. *numeric* spareness – when phenoxybenzamine, an irreversible alpha-adrenoreceptor antagonist, binds to its receptor there is a maximal effect, even when there is low receptor occupancy). The effect of receptor binding can also be shorter than the duration of the triggered response (e.g. *temporal* spareness – when noradrenaline binds to a receptor and activates a G protein, adenyl cyclase activation continues after the noradrenaline–receptor interaction ceases).

Transducer molecules
This may explain why partial agonists cannot produce a maximal response. Partial agonist–receptor complexes bind with a low affinity to a 'transducer molecule' and hence only elicit a partial response. A full agonist binds with high affinity and hence elicits a full response. This affinity of binding with a transducer molecule is called *intrinsic efficacy*.

Non-linear receptor binding
The modern view that describes receptor occupation by drugs in a non-linear way related to cooperativity in molecule binding (e.g. sigmoidal binding of ACh to the nicotinic receptor), where, as in haemoglobin binding with oxygen, allosteric changes occur that affect sequential binding of molecules.

TABLE 3.2 Drug receptor responses

Graph	Notes
Concentration vs effect Effect (y-axis) vs Conc. (x-axis); curve rising to E_{max}; dashed lines at C_{50}	*Agonist* = a substance (drug) that binds to a receptor and causes an effect C_{50} = the concentration of a drug at which 50% of the maximal possible effect occurs E_{max} = the maximal effect that may be caused by a drug
Potency and efficacy Effect (y-axis) vs Conc. (x-axis); curves A, B, C Efficacy A = B > C Potency C > A > B	*Potency* = relates to the C_{50}; lower C_{50} the more potent the drug *Efficacy* = relates to the E_{max}; the higher the E_{max} the more efficacious the drug *Specificity* = the ability of a drug to bind to a specific receptor *Affinity* = the degree to which a drug binds to a specific receptor; related to potency
Agonist and partial agonist Effect (y-axis) vs Conc. (x-axis); Agonist curve and Partial agonist curve	*Partial agonist* = a drug that binds to a receptor but only has partial efficacy compared to a full agonist (e.g. buprenorphine vs morphine)
Receptor antagonism Effect (y-axis) vs Conc. (x-axis); curves for Agonist, Reversible competitive antagonist, Irreversible antagonist	*Competitive antagonists:* *Reversible* = binds with a receptor at the same site as the agonist, but an agonist is able to overcome its effects in sufficient concentrations (e.g. vecuronium on the nicotinic ACh receptor competing with ACh) *Irreversible* = binds with a receptor at the same site as the agonist and reduces the number of receptors available for agonist binding due to slow dissociation from the receptors; behave like reversible antagonists at low doses and non-competitive at high doses (e.g. phenoxybenzamine on alpha-receptors competing with endogenous catecholamines) *Non-competitive antagonists* = bind to a site near the receptor and reduce the effectiveness of the agonist; can be reversible (e.g. ketamine and glutamate at the NMDA receptor) or irreversible (e.g. benzodiazepines and GABA at the $GABA_A$ receptor)

Tables

These are extremely efficient ways of summarising information about individual drugs, classes and comparison of specific aspects of interest. Tables 3.3 and 3.4 have been prepared to demonstrate this. These tables are the synthesis of information taken from a variety of origins and the equivalent information might otherwise have taken many pages of written notes, the result being less suitable for rapid review and contrast. Study notes are seldom satisfactory if only one source of information is used. Part of the process of preparing for exams involves tapping into a range of sources, including those of your supervising consultants, and practical approaches, such as looking at the printed information on the side of fluid bags and reading product information.

TABLE 3.3 Comparison of intravenous fluids used in the ICU								
	pH	Na mmol/L	K mmol/L	Cl mmol/L	Other mmol/L	Osmolality mosm/L	Cost	Potential problems
Crystalloids								
Normal saline (0.9%)	5.0	154	0	154	0	308	⇓	Hyperchloraemic acidosis
5% Dextrose	4.0	0	0	0	Glucose 278 (50 g/L)	252	⇓	Fluid overload Caution in renal and cardiac failure
Hartmann's	6.5	131	5	111	Lactate 29	279	⇓	Hyperkalaemia
Plasmalyte 148	5.0	140	5	98	Bicarbinate 29 Acetate 27 Gluconate 23	294	⇓	Hyperkalaemia
Sodium bicarbonate 8.4%	7.8	1000	0	0	Bicarbinate 1000	200	⇑	Fluid overload
Colloids								
Albumin 4%	7.4	130–160	<1	130–160	Albumin 40 g/L	309	⇑⇑	Hypersensitivity reactions
Albumin 20%	7.4	130–160	<1	130–160	Albumin 200 g/L	312	⇑⇑	May be harmful in brain injury
Gelofusine™	7.4	154	<0.4	125	Succinylated gelatin 40 g/L	308	⇑	Hypersensitivity reactions
Voluven™	4–5.5	154	0	154	6% HES 130/0.4	308	⇑	Hypersensitivity reactions Starches are associated with pruritis, coagulopathy and renal failure

TABLE 3.4 Drugs with specific antidotes

Antidotes

Toxin	Antidote (dose)	Mechanism
Benzodiazepine	Flumazenil 0.1–0.2 mg IV repeated as required to a total of 2 mg	Competitive inhibition at receptor. Generally not used in polypharmacy overdose, or when exact nature of toxicity is uncertain, as acute reversal of benzodiazepine effect may precipitate refractory seizures
Beta-blocker	i) Glucagon 50–150 mcg/kg IV bolus (max. 10 mg), then 50 mcg/kg/hr IV infusion (max. 5 mg/hr) ii) Atenolol, nadolol and sotalol are dialysable. The others are not	i) Bypasses beta receptor and stimulates production of cAMP through nonadrenergic pathways
Calcium channel blocker	i) 10–30 mL 10% $CaCl_2$ IV, then 20–50 mg/kg/hr IVI ii) Glucagon 50–150 mcg/kg IV bolus (max. 10 mg), then 50 mcg/kg/hr IVI (max. 5 mg/hr) iii) Anecdotal reports of benefit from insulin/dextrose infusions	i) Overwhelms calcium channel blocker activity ii) Bypasses calcium channel and stimulates production of cAMP iii) Possibly through adrenergic effect of insulin
Carbamazepine	1–2 mEq/kg $NaHCO_3$ 8.4% IV if widened QRS complex	Mechanism unclear; possibly via sodium channel action
Carbon monoxide	100% oxygen. Role of hyperbaric oxygen is controversial and becoming smaller. Significant symptoms and/or pregnancy warrant discussion with hyperbaric centre	Reduces CO–Hb half-life from 250 min to 50 min for 100% O_2 and to 22 min for 100% O_2 at 2.4 atm Also, bypasses haemoglobin-based oxygen delivery via plasma dissolved O_2
Cyanide	i) Australia = dicobalt edetate 300 mg in 50 mL 5% dextrose over 1–5 min + sodium thiosulfate 12.5 mg IV ii) Europe = Hydroxocobalamin iii) USA = induced Met-Hb using 10 mL of 3% sodium nitrite + sodium thiosulfate 12.5 mg	i) Thiosulfate provides substrate for metabolism of cyanide by liver rhodenase ii) Calcium edetate binds free plasma (but not tissue-bound) cyanide, enhancing renal elimination iii) Hydroxocobalamin + cyanide combine to form cyanocobalamin, which is renally cleared iv) Induced Met-Hb results in release of bound cyanide to be metabolised. Relies on patient's ability to tolerate Met-Hb up to 25%

Continued

TABLE 3.4 Drugs with specific antidotes—cont'd

Antidotes

Toxin	Antidote (dose)	Mechanism
Digoxin	Digoxin antibody fragments 1 vial binds 0.6 mg and 1 nmol/L of digoxin Dose in vials = (mg × 0.8)/0.6, or (serum level × weight kg)/100, or 5 vials in acute toxicity and 2 vials for chronic toxicity Given as infusion over 40 min unless arrest	Binds free digoxin and facilitates renal elimination Can be dialysed
Ethylene glycol & Methanol	i) Ethanol infusion, 10 mL/kg IV of 10% ethanol (V/V) in dextrose 5% over 30 min, then continue infusion at 1–1.5 mL/kg/hr to maintain serum levels of 100–150 mg/dL (20–30 mmol/L). Monitor q2 h BSL ii) Fomepizole 15 mg/kg in 100mL 0.9% saline over 30 min, then 10–15 mg/kg over 12 hrs for 4 doses iii) Dialysis – aim for serum ethylene glycol < 10 mg/dL (1.5 mmol/L) iv) Also give thiamine, pyridoxine and folic acid to divert metabolism from toxic metabolites	i) Competes for metabolism by alcohol dehydrogenase, preventing excess production of glycolic and oxalic acids, while dialysis is used to clear the ethylene glycol ii) Inhibits alcohol dehydrogenase iii) Reduces ethylene glycol's half-life from 10 to 2.5 hrs
Iron	Desferrioxamine – 1000 mg IM then 500 mg IM q4h × 2, max. 6 g/24 hrs – 1000 mg IV at 5–15 mg/kg/hr, then 500 mg q4h × 2, max. 6 g/24 hrs	Chelates free iron for renal elimination (vin-rosé urine) or dialysis
Local anaesthetic agent (lignocaine, bupivacaine, ropivacaine etc)	100 mL Intralipid 20% IV	Mechanism unclear, but thought to act as a sink for lipophilic agents. Ongoing investigation into its use for treating non-dialysable toxins
Methaemoglobin	10% Methylene blue 0.1–0.2 mL/kg IV over 5 min. Repeat after 1 hour if required. (Contraindicated if G-6-PD deficient; consider HBO_2)	Accelerates reduction of Met-Hb

Continued

TABLE 3.4 Drugs with specific antidotes—cont'd

Antidotes

Toxin	Antidote (dose)	Mechanism
Opiates	Naloxone 0.4–2 mg IM/IV	Competitive inhibition at receptors. Beware that naloxone half-life is shorter than most opiates and repeated doses or infusion may be required
Organophosphate	i) Atropine 1–2 mg IV q 5 min, for the excess muscarinic effects. Repeated boluses generally preferred over infusion ii) Pralidoxime 30 mg/kg IV bolus, then 10–20 mg/kg/hr IVI for the neuromuscular effects. Duration and adequacy assessed by the serial cholinesterase test and cholinesterase mixing test respectively iii) Benzodiazepine therapy has been shown to reduce the incidence of the long-term neuropsychological syndrome	i) Antimuscarinic effect by inhibiting competitive inhibition at muscarinic receptors ii) Regenerates acetyl cholinesterase iii) Unknown
Paracetamol	N-acetylcysteine. 150 mg/kg in 100 mL 5% dextrose over 30–60 min (slower rate reduces incidence of hypotension), then 50 mg/kg in 250 mL 5% dextrose over 4 hrs, then 100 mg/kg in 1000 mL 5% dextrose over 16 hrs	Provides glutathione substrate, diverting metabolic pathway away from NAPQI generation
Salicylate	Urinary alkalinisation: 100 mmol $NaHCO_3$ in 1000 mL 5% dextrose over 4 hrs. Aim for urine pH approx 7.5–8.0	Increases urinary elimination
TCAD	50 mL $NaHCO_3$ 8.4% IV	Indicated for unstable arrhythmias and cardiac arrest. Mechanism uncertain, but may be related to sodium channel activity

Lists

Lists may be helpful when there are a series of causes of a problem (e.g. mechanisms of drug interactions), or to bring together equations and/or definitions (e.g. pharmacokinetic terms). Where possible, incorporating acronyms as aide memoirs is a helpful strategy for many candidates.

Mechanisms of drug interactions – the Ps and PASS

- *Pharmaceutical* – chemical (e.g. calcium precipitates with bicarbonate if infused in the same line; intravenous phenytoin preparations are stabilised in a vehicle containing propylene glycol and this is implicated in causing hypotension if administration is too rapid) or physical (e.g. GTN absorbed into PVC therefore prepared in a glass bottle).
- *Pharmacodynamic* – various mechanisms:
  - **Potentiation** = drugs with different actions enhance each other's effects on an end-point (e.g. diuretics and ACE inhibitors in heart failure)
  - **Antagonism** = one drug reduces or prevents the action of another (e.g. naloxone prevents the effects of fentanyl)
  - **Summation** = drugs with similar actions have additive effects (e.g. amlodipine and nifedipine may have additive effects on lowering BP by blocking calcium channels of vascular smooth muscle)
  - **Synergism** = the combined effects are greater when two drugs are used together than would be expected from simple addition of their effects (e.g. the effect of vasodilators, such as amlodipine, when combined with a beta-blocker, such as metoprolol, produces a greater drop in BP than would be expected; related to the beta–blocker blunting the reflex tachycardia seen with vasodilators, which can attenuate the resulting BP lowering response).
- *Pharmacokinetic* (e.g. amiodarone reduces warfarin and digoxin clearance through inhibition of liver cytochrome P450 enzyme pathways).

Pharmacokinetic terms

To demonstrate how, after understanding is achieved through reading, large amounts of information may be distilled into lists of facts, the following material has been prepared on pharmacokinetics. The following information is a summary of concepts and equations described in Katzung et al. Basic and Clinical Pharmacology.

Volume of distribution (V_D) = the volume of bodily fluid in which a drug appears to be dissolved. Larger volume for lipid-soluble drugs and lower for water-soluble drugs.

$$V_D = \frac{\text{Amount of drug in the body}}{\text{Concentration of drug C}}$$

where C is described in terms of blood, plasma or plasma water.

Clearance (CL) = elimination of a drug from the body

$$CL = \frac{\text{Rate of elimination}}{C}$$

where rate of elimination is described in terms of the total or the amount by a specific mechanism (e.g. renal or hepatic).

Half-life ($t_{\frac{1}{2}}$) = time for the amount of drug in the body to change by half

$$t_{\frac{1}{2}} = \frac{0.7 \times V_D}{CL}$$

Extraction ratio (ER) = the amount of drug, after oral absorption, that is removed by the liver on 'first pass' to the systemic blood

$$ER = \frac{CL_{hepatic}}{\text{Hepatic blood flow}}$$

Bioavailability (F) = amount of drug to reach the blood after administration by a given route

$$F = f \times (1 - ER)$$

where f is the extent of absorption.

Loading dose (LD) = the amount of drug needed to be administered to achieve a desired drug concentration in the blood

$$LD = V_D \times TC$$

where TC is the target concentration.

Dosing rate (DR) = the dose and frequency needed to maintain a desired drug concentration in the blood

$$DR = CL \times TC$$

First-order kinetics = elimination of a drug from the body is constant and proportional to concentration; rate of elimination is equal to the area under the curve of the concentration versus time curve after a dose of drug is administered

$$\text{Rate of elimination} = CL \times C$$

Zero-order kinetics = elimination of a drug from the body is saturable, non-constant, concentration dependant (Michaelis-Menton)

$$\text{Rate of elimination} = \frac{V_{max} \times C}{K_m + C}$$

where V_{max} is the maximum elimination capacity and K_m is the drug concentration at which the rate of elimination is half of the maximal rate.

Applying concepts to consolidate learning

Applying difficult-to-remember dry facts, such as mathematical equations, to a clinically relevant issue can also assist recall. For example, applying some of the pharmacokinetic equations to considering vancomycin prescribing (see Box 3.1).

Mind maps

After reading and researching large amounts of information on a subject, it can be helpful to organise these thoughts into a visual diagram that can be used to stimulate recall when revising. An example of a mind map (a term attributed to Tony Buzan), is included in Figure 3.21.

BOX 3.1 Vancomycin pharmacokinetics

Looking up information about the pharmacokinetic properties of vancomycin (e.g. L. Bauer, Applied Clinical Pharmacokinetics, pp. 187–8) reveals that for a 70-kg male with a creatinine clearance of 100 mL/min, there is an expected CL 73 mL/min and V_D 49 L.

For a hypothetical patient with an MRSA infection the desired TC is 20 mg/L. Calculate LD, DR and $t_{1/2}$.

$$LD = V_D \times TC = 49\ L \times 20\ mg/L = 980\ mg\ (\text{approx. 1 g})$$

$$DR = CL \times TC = 0.073\ L/min \times 20\ mg/L = 1.46\ mg/min = 87.6\ mg/hr$$
$$= \text{approx. 2 g/day as an infusion or 1 g bd as boluses}$$

$$t_{\frac{1}{2}} = \frac{0.7 \times V_D}{CL} = (0.7 \times 49\ L)/0.073\ L/min = 469\ min - \text{approx. 8hrs}$$

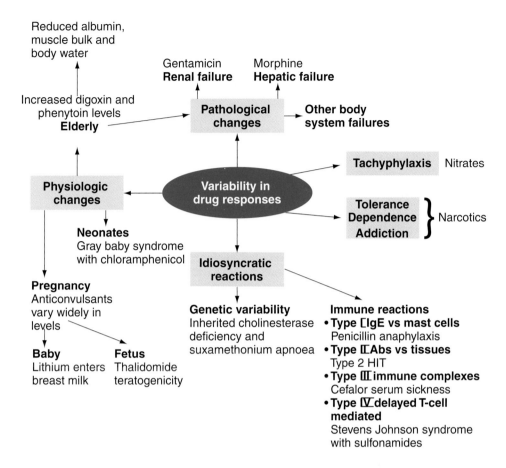

FIGURE 3.21 Mind map: sources of variability in drug responses

Facts cards

A card system lends itself well to preparing study material for subsequent revision. Some people use cardboard index cards and, increasingly, electronic devices have equivalent filing systems that enable convenient access to the information anywhere at any time (e.g. tablet computers such as the Apple iPad2).

For example, an individual card could contain the summarised information shown in Box 3.2 (overleaf).

Past papers

Analysing and attempting past paper questions will assist in obtaining an appreciation for where the 'yard stick' is set in terms of the breadth and depth of knowledge expected of exam candidates. As the exam approaches, completing questions under exam conditions can help the development of discipline and practice in writing rapidly, legibly and managing time pressure. Examples are provided of possible approaches to two different types of questions that have featured in the CICM Primary exam. These have been selected because they illustrate the importance of pausing to consider a plan for answering questions rather than aimlessly starting to expel a stream of unorganised material.

BOX 3.2 Isomerism

ISOMERISM

Refers to drugs with the same number of atoms, molecular weight, molecular formula, but different arrangements.

Structural = different order of atomic bonds; *tautomerism* is used to describe a drug's ability to change to a different structural isomer as its environment, such as pH, changes (e.g. glibenclamide)

Stereo = different 3-D configuration; may be:

• geometric – different orientation of functional groups within a molecule with a non-rotating double bond; conformation around this double bond called *cis* (if the groups are on the same side of the double bond) or *trans* (if on opposite sides) (e.g. cisatracurium is one of 10 isomers of atracurium)

• optical – paired molecules that are the same, except they are non-superimposable mirror images of each other as they have chiral centres (e.g. a carbon atom surrounded by four groups). Historically termed *optical isomers,* as they rotated polarised light differently. Now described by the arrangement of groups around the chiral centre (R and S pairs, named depending on whether the largest to smallest atomic number groups occur in a clockwise or anticlockwise direction; the pair are called *enantiomers*). Drugs are available as a single enantiomer (e.g. Chirocaine™ - levobupivacaine the S enantiomer of bupivacaine) or as racemic mixtures with both in equal amounts (e.g. Marcain™ – standard bupivacaine).

SAMPLE QUESTION

Compare and contrast the pharmacology of noradrenaline and vasopressin.

Answer
Pharmacokinetics
Noradrenaline
• Catecholamine
• IV route. Not active orally.
• Plasma protein bound, but therapeutic doses exceed binding capacity.
• Metabolised by COMT (liver, kidneys) and MAO (synapses) to VMA and MHPG.
• Renal excretion of metabolites.
• $t_{1/2}$ 2 min.
Vasopressin
• Nanopeptide hormone.
• IV route.
• Plasma protein bound, but therapeutic doses exceed binding capacity.
• Metabolised by plasma, liver and kidney endopeptidases.
• Renal excretion of metabolites.
• $t_{1/2}$ 8–15 min.

Pharmacodynamics
Majority of data derived from animal models and healthy volunteers.
Noradrenaline
• $\alpha > \beta$ adrenergic receptor activity. Little $\beta2$ effect.
• Promotes cGMP-mediated vasoconstriction and inotropic effect.
• ↑ diastolic BP, systolic BP and MAP.

- ↑ mean pulmonary artery pressure.
- ↑ SVR.
- Unchanged, raised or lowered CO; depending on balance of SV and afterload.
- Can result in splanchnic ischaemia due to vasoconstriction.
- ↑ myocardial O_2 demand.
- Pro-arrhythmogenic.

Vasopressin
- Acts at $V1_A$ receptors, via G-protein coupling to phospholipase C, to increase intracellular Ca^{2+}, resulting in vasoconstriction.
- $V1_B$ receptors stimulate ACTH release from the anterior pituitary and V2 receptors mediate antidiuretic and platelet aggregation effects.
- ↑ diastolic BP, systolic BP and MAP
- ↑ SVR
- Can result in splanchnic and coronary ischaemia
- Often used as catecholaminergic-sparing agent, especially in severe septic shock.

This is a common type of question where two drugs with some similarities but important differences need to be compared. The approach taken in this sample answer is simply structured and well set out. It deliberately avoids using a table, as some candidates struggle with using tables for answers, a more commonly used approach. This answer demonstrates that there are effective alternatives.

Others would have answered this question by drawing a table with columns for the two drugs and individual characteristics on a series of rows. If tables are to be used it is important to maintain a structured ordering of facts and some people might use a series of smaller tables spread out over a few pages so they can add to sections as they think of additional facts. Candidates will need to practise using tables if this is to be done effectively under exam conditions.

SAMPLE QUESTION

Describe the factors that are important when interpreting plasma drug concentrations.

Answer
Need to be able to measure levels using reliable methods:
- Not all drugs have readily available assays available.
- Commonly measured drug levels include:
  ○ antimicrobials (e.g. gentamicin, vancomycin)
  ○ anticonvulsants (e.g. phenytoin, carbamazepine)
  ○ antiarrhythmics (e.g. digoxin)
  ○ antipsychotics (e.g. lithium)
  ○ anti-rejection drugs (e.g. cyclosporin).

There needs to be clinically relevant, known reference ranges to compare a result against or a given result may be meaningless.

The result needs to be available rapidly or delayed results may lack relevance and no longer reflect a patient's situation.

Need to have an appropriate clinical indication for ordering levels to ensure the correct tests are ordered:
- Monitor drugs where:
  ○ the level is important for effectiveness (e.g. antibiotics)
  ○ there is a drug being administered with a narrow therapeutic index with associated risk of toxicity (e.g. lithium, phenytoin)
  ○ there are pathological conditions that are likely to make dosing of drugs difficult (e.g. renal failure, hyperexcretion in critical illness).

- Monitor levels when:
  - drug interactions are likely to complicate dosing
  - toxicity may be difficult to detect (e.g. risk of gentamicin causing ototoxicity in sedated patients).

Need to take samples at an appropriate time consistent with the required information sought:

- Peak levels: dependent on mode of delivery such that after oral dosing at least 2 hours is required before taking a level (to assume adequate absorption), but after intravenous administration about 1 hour is adequate. Levels reflect the efficacy of the dose prescribed (e.g. aminoglycoside levels).
- Steady state levels: three half-lives are usually required before obtaining an accurate level, which is defined by when the rate of elimination = rate of administration (e.g. patients on a vancomycin infusion).
- Trough levels: taken immediately prior to the next dose. Reflect the safety of the dose prescribed (e.g. aminoglycoside, cyclosporin levels).

Need to be aware of the limitations of the level:

- The level, even when within reference range, may not correspond with therapeutic efficacy (e.g. phenytoin levels do not always correlate with seizure control).
- Reference ranges generally reflect population norms and may not be appropriate for individual patients (e.g. some patients can tolerate higher levels of drugs without side effects or have adequate efficacy at subtherapeutic levels).

Other practical considerations:

- The level should be rechecked if it seems inappropriate for the clinical situation (e.g. a very low level in the setting of a very high dose).
- An unexpected level should prompt review of factors why this might be real (e.g. unappreciated drug interactions).

This is a reaching question that cannot be answered simply with recall of a list of facts. It requires the candidate to consider a range of factors from first principles using commonsense mixed with knowledge and aided by some clinical experience. It is an excellent question as it is highly relevant to everyday intensive care practice. It is tough as it crosses over different areas of the pharmacology syllabus (pharmacokinetics, pharmacodynamics and individual drug properties) and an obvious structure is not easy to develop. Using examples to support statements is important for this type of question. Questions of this type may be used to discriminate between candidates and warrant practice.

Making your own questions

Composing questions of your own generally requires thinking like an examiner. After reading a topic, try to think of how this material might be examined. Formulate possible questions. Answer your questions to see if they seem reasonable and comparable in difficulty and style to past paper questions. Also answer them to check your recall, both straight after you complete topics to confirm that you have understood it, and also later as a revision exercise.

SAMPLE QUESTION

Describe the difference between fentanyl and remifentanil. What are the advantages and disadvantages of using remifentanil in critical care?

Answer

The main difference is the context-sensitive half-time: The time taken for the plasma concentration of the drug to fall by 50% after termination of an infusion (context is reference to infusion duration).

Factors involved in the above are peripheral compartmental distribution, infusion duration and clearance.

As the ratio of distribution clearance to elimination clearance increases, the range of the context-sensitive half-time increases (ratio is 4 for fentanyl, compared with remifentanil which is <1). This explains how the context-sensitive half-time of fentanyl increases with infusion duration.

For remifentanil the half-life is consistently short (3 minutes, contrasted with elimination half-time, which is clearance dependent, and the time for plasma concentration to decrease by half in the elimination phase).

Both illustrate a three-compartment model of decay.

Remifentanil is considered to be more expensive.

	Fentanyl	Remifentanil
Presentation	Clear, colourless 50 mcg/mL solution and transdermal patches	1, 2 or 5 mg powder with glycine
Dose	1–2 mcg/kg bolus	0.05–2 mcg/kg/min infusion
Chemical group	Phenylpiperidine derivative	Anilidopiperidine
pKa	8.4 Exists >90% in the ionised form	7.1 Un-ionised form at physiological pH
Protein binding	80%	80%
Relative lipid solubility (cf morphine)	600	20
First-pass effect	Lung-significant	Nil
Volume of distribution (L/kg)	4	0.3
Clearance (mL/min/kg)	10–20	40
Elimination half-time (min)	190	10
Metabolism	Hepatic (N-dealkylation and hydroxylation) to nor-fentanyl	Extra-hepatic esterases–plasma, red cell, interstitial tissue to a carboxylic acid metabolite (explains why its high clearance is greater than hepatic blood flow)
Excretion	Renal	Renal
Effects	Respiratory depression. In high-dose bradycardia, chest rigidity. Analgesia	Bradycardia, chest rigidity. Analgesia

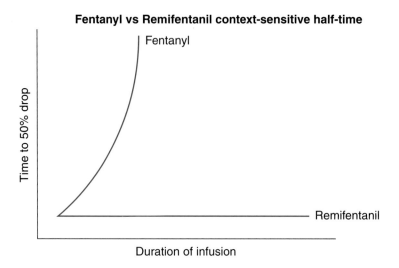

Fentanyl vs Remifentanil context-sensitive half-time

Exam templates
Some questions lend themselves well to a template approach that can be used to answer questions that share the same style.

Some examples include:

Describing specific drugs
Used when describing, comparing and contrasting drugs to generate a table or flow of points. It comprises headings that include:
• Presentation
• Use(s)
• Mechanism of action
• Pharmacodynamics
• Pharmacokinetics (absorption, distribution, metabolism, elimination)
• Side effects (organ system approach)

Approach to managing specific drug overdoses
Key headings to consider include:
• Supportive care
• Specific care
  ○ Decrease absorption
  ○ Enhance elimination
  ○ Antidotes

Quizzes
Some candidates find it useful to make and/or perform quizzes as a break from reading. This is often a more engaging way of approaching material, particularly useful during the phase of revision, when fatigued or during group study sessions. A common, simple example of this is making and/or answering multiple-choice questions, but activities are only limited by motivation and creativity.

On the DVD there is a pharmacology quiz section. This has been designed to allow self-testing of knowledge about individual drugs. It has been designed to include memorable facts about medications, as it is unusual or 'quirky' facts that are often best recalled, and these can be linked with learning and memory of less interesting but important information.

References

Bauer L. Applied Clinical Pharmacokinetics. McGraw-Hill Professional; 2001.

Bersten AD, Soni N (eds). Oh's Intensive Care Manual. Elsevier; 6th edn: 2009.

Brandis K. The Physiology Viva: Questions And Answers. Alderbury House; rev. edn: 2003.

Calvey T, Williams N. Principles and Practice of Pharmacology for Anaesthetists. Blackwell Science; 4th edn: 2001.

Cameron P, Jelinek G, Kelly A, et al. Textbook of Adult Emergency Medicine. Elsevier; 3rd edn: 2009.

Craft T, Nolan J, Parr M. Key Topics in Critical Care. Taylor and Francis; 2nd edn: 2004.

Dhillon S, Kostrzewski A. Clinical Pharmacokinetics. Pharmaceutical Press; 2006.

Dunn R, Dilley S, Brookes J. The Emergency Medicine Manual. Venom Publishing; 3rd edn: 2003.

Farrand P, Hussain F, Hennessy E. The efficacy of the 'mind map' study technique. Medical Education 2002; 36(5): 426–31.

Faunce T. The Australian Intensive Care and Anaesthesia Primary Exam. Panther; 3rd edn: 2001.

Guyton A, Hall J. Textbook of Medical Physiology. Elsevier Saunders; 11th edn: 2006.

Hardman J, Limbird L, Gilman A. Goodman and Gilman's The Pharmacological Basis of Therapeutics. McGraw-Hill, New York; 11th edn: 2006.

Hinds C, Watson D. Intensive Care: A Concise Textbook. Saunders Elsevier; 3rd edn: 2008.

Katzung B, Masters S, Trevor A. Basic and Clinical Pharmacology. McGraw-Hill, New York; 11th edn: 2009.

Lumb A. Nunns. Applied Respiratory Physiology. Elsevier Butterworth Heinemann; 6th edn: 2005.

Neal M. J. Medical Pharmacology at a Glance. Wiley-Blackwell; 6th edn: 2009.

Paw H, Shulman R. Handbook of Drugs in Intensive Care. Cambridge University Press; 4th edn: 2010.

Peck T, Hill S, Williams M. Pharmacology for Anaesthesia and Intensive Care. Greenwich Medical Media; 3rd edn: 2008.

Power I, Kam P. Principles of Physiology for the Anaesthetist. Hodder Arnold; 2nd edn: 2008.

Power I, Kam P. Principles of Physiology for the Anaesthetist. Hodder Arnold; 1st edn: 2001.

Sidebotham D, Mckee A, Gillham M, et al. Cardiothoracic Critical Care. Butterworth Heinemann Elsevier; 2007.

Tintinalli J. Tintinalli's Emergency Medicine: A Comprehensive Study Guide. McGraw-Hill Professional Publishing; 7th edn: 2010.

Tomlin M. Pharmacology and Phamacokinetics: A Basic Reader. Springer; 2010.

West J. Respiratory Physiology: The Essentials. Walters Kluwer/Lippincott Williams and Wilkins; 8th edn: 2008.

Chapter 4

Equipment

It matters little how much equipment we use; it matters much that we be masters of all we do use.
   SAM ABELL

Equipment overview

It is daunting to consider the vast range of items that an intensivist needs to be familiar with. There is a multitude of potential pieces of equipment that could feature in the examinations in numerous ways. An understanding of some of the key physics principles underpinning these is essential and may be the focus of the question (e.g. CICM Primary examination). In contrast, there may be a more clinically relevant focus to the task (e.g. CICM Fellowship examination). This chapter outlines how questions about equipment may feature and introduces the equipment library, which appears on the DVD.

SAMPLE QUESTION 1

Describe the principles of invasive blood pressure monitoring on the ICU.

Answer
- Invasive blood pressure monitoring most commonly utilises a transducer. This consists of an intravascular catheter connected to low-compliance tubing, which moves a diaphragm connected to a Wheatstone bridge. This converts mechanical to electrical energy, which is amplified and displayed.
- Once the system oscillates from the pulse pressure waveform further oscillations occur due to the resonant frequency of the system (F_0), causing distortion of the recorded waveform.
- The pressure waveform is a graphical representation of a complex wave, consisting of the summation of mechanical pressure signals at different frequencies.
- The summation of between 6 and 10 harmonics are required to create an accurate arterial pressure waveform.
- The longer the fluid-filled tubing, the lower the natural frequency of the monitoring system and the greater the chance of signal distortion.
- 30 Hz is thought to be the minimum desirable natural frequency of an optimally damped monitoring system (1 Hz = 1 cycle/second).
- Fundamental frequency = square of the pulse rate.
- Fourier analysis is the process used to sum the series of waves, which are harmonics of the fundamental frequency.
- Most arterial pressure monitoring systems are underdamped.
- System frequency response and system damping coefficient help define the monitoring system's characteristics.

Wheatstone Bridge

Used to measure resistance
R1 + R2 are known

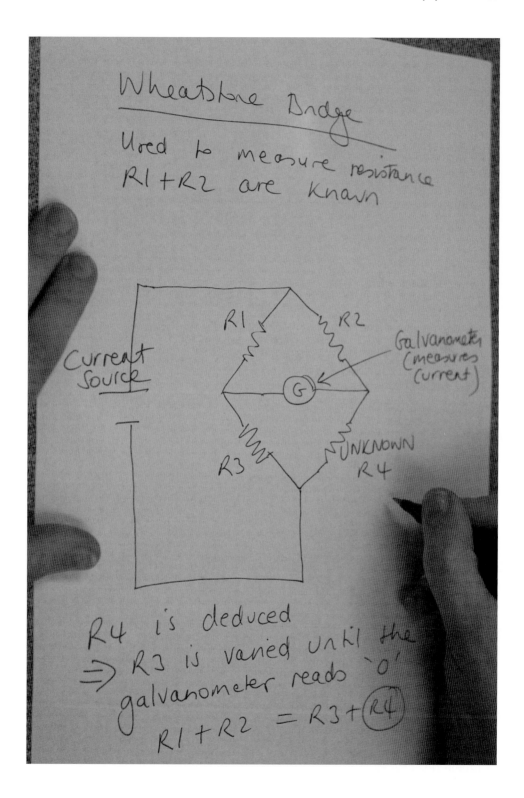

R4 is deduced
⇒ R3 is varied until the
galvanometer reads `0`
R1 + R2 = R3 + (R4)

- Damping is the absorption of oscillatory energy by frictional forces and hence reduces artefacts that can distort the pressure waveform.
- Air bubbles in the system aid damping but also lower the natural frequency of the system.
- If the damping coefficient = 1, only the MAP is recorded, as there is no resonance at all.
- Optimal damping (DC = 0.6 – 0.7) is when all oscillatory forces (of the monitoring system) are diminished such that only the pulse pressure waveform is recorded.

SAMPLE QUESTION 2

A patient is being ventilated on a high frequency oscillatory ventilator. List four possible mechanisms of gas transport. What are the key ventilator settings and what factors affect the patient's oxygen and carbon dioxide levels?

Answer
- Proposed mechanisms of gas transport are:
  - bulk flow (direct flow to alveoli close to large airways)
  - Taylor dispersion (convective flow and diffusion)
  - pendelluft (flow from alveoli with short to longer time constants)
  - asymmetric (coaxial) velocities of gas flow to different areas of lung (central gas moves inwards and peripheral gas flows outwards)
  - cardiogenic mixing (heart beat against adjacent lung affecting gas flow)
  - molecular diffusion (may be facilitated by turbulent flow).
- Important ventilator settings on the SensorMedics™ 3100B include: bias flow, power (delta P), frequency (in Hz), inspiratory time, mean airway pressure (Paw), FiO_2
- Oxygenation may be increased by increasing FiO_2, Paw and using a recruitment manoeuvre (short period of higher Paw); oxygenation may decrease with reductions in FiO_2, Paw and interventions causing derecruitment (e.g. suctioning).
- Increasing delta P, reducing the frequency, reducing the inspiratory time and inducing an endotracheal cuff leak may reduce carbon dioxide levels
- The inspiratory time may affect both oxygenation and ventilation but is less often altered in troubleshooting algorithms.

One way to facilitate learning about equipment is to ensure that any item used at work is viewed as a potential exam topic. In order to assist this process we have constructed an extensive library of items. A common method of description has been used to help obtain, retain and build on knowledge in this area. In general, complications can be considered in terms of those related to the *device itself*, the *insertion* procedure and/ or any *anaesthetic* required for the insertion process. Alternatively, complications can be considered in terms of *immediate*, *early* and *delayed*. These systematic approaches are useful for exams, but for the purposes of keeping the library succinct, only the key/classical problems are listed.

This library has been generally arranged by organ system on the accompanying DVD.

Arrangement of the equipment library
Cardiovascular
- Intravenous equipment
- Monitoring devices
- Cardiac output measuring devices
- Circulatory assist devices
- Pacing equipment
- Defibrillation

- Fluid administration
- Miscellaneous

Respiratory
- Oxygen delivery
- Airway management
- Surgical airways
- Ventilators
- Ventilation circuits
- Gas supply
- Suction devices
- Monitoring devices
- Chest drains

Renal
Gastroenterology
Neurology
Infection control
Other

Each item in these sections is accompanied by an image that serves as an example, and, where relevant, these are labelled to indicate specific features. It should be noted that the items featured reflect the brands and models available to the authors of this book in their workplaces, resulting from a multitude of factors, including cost, hospital contractual arrangements, regional availability and preferences rather than any particular bias. The tables do not claim to be exhaustive of information and aim to provide key information necessary for examinations. Two examples are provided from the cardiovascular devices section.

FIGURE 4.1 Example of a file from the equipment library: a pressure transducer

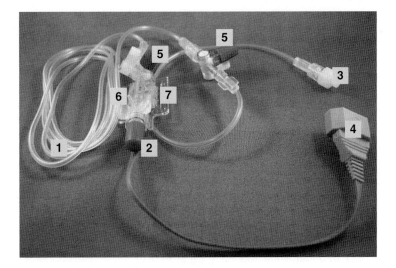

1 Low-compliance tubing
2 Connection to line attached to pressure bag
3 Connection to blood-filled tube (e.g. arterial line)
4 Signal cable for connection to monitor cable
5 Tap-controlled sampling port (also to enable zeroing)
6 Rapid flush device (pull lever)
7 Transducer membrane

1. Item name	Pressure transducer
2. Uses	Allows invasive pressure monitoring in various compartments of the cardiovascular system, including arterial, central venous and right-sided heart pressure. Also used for measuring pressures in other body cavities, i.e. intra-abdominal, intracranial.
3. Description	The components are the in situ catheter (i.e. arterial line), coupled with low-compliance extension tubing, the pressure transducer and the amplifier/monitor. When used for cardiovascular pressures the fluid-filled components are connected to an automatic flush device and inflatable pressure bag.
4. Method of insertion and/ or use	The external end of the catheter is connected to fluid-filled connecting tubing. This fluid transmits the pressure changes at the catheter tip to the pressure transducer (an electromechanical device that converts pressure into an electrical signal). Generally pretested, precalibrated and presterilised disposable transducers are used. All have a pressure-sensitive diaphragm enclosed by a fluid-filled dome and as the patient's pressure pulsations physically strike the diaphragm, this mechanical movement is converted into an electrical signal (via a Wheatstone bridge – a set-up of four resistors and a galvanometer that increase the size of the electrical signal generated), which is processed and displayed by the monitor. The system must be given a zero reference point to establish a standard neutral level for all measurements. This eliminates the effects of atmospheric and hydrostatic pressures. The transducer is exposed to the atmosphere. The monitor should read zero. The system is then levelled to a reference point (e.g. the phlebostatic axis for CVP). Depending on the monitor used, some calibration may be required.
5. Potential complications	Those related to catheter insertion. Inaccuracy related to system set-up. Decision-making based entirely on monitoring information rather than adding this to clinical examination. Bleeding if system disconnected. Accidental drug administration.
6. Other information	**Important associated concepts:** Once the system oscillates from the pulse pressure waveform, further oscillations occur due to the **resonant frequency** of the system (F_0), causing distortion of the recorded waveform. The pressure waveform is a graphical representation of a complex wave, consisting of the summation of mechanical pressure signals at different frequencies. The summation of between 6 and 10 harmonics is required to create an accurate arterial pressure waveform. The longer the fluid-filled tubing, the lower the **natural frequency** of the monitoring system and the greater the chance of signal distortion. 30 Hz is thought to be the minimum desirable natural frequency of an optimally damped monitoring system (1 Hz = 1 cycle/second). **Fundamental frequency** = square of the pulse rate. **Fourier analysis** is the process used to sum the series of waves, which are harmonics of the fundamental frequency. **Damping** is the absorption of oscillatory energy by frictional forces and hence reduces artefacts that can distort the pressure waveform. If the **damping coefficient** (DC) = 1, only the MAP is recorded as there is no resonance at all. **Optimal damping** (DC = 0.6–0.7) is when all

oscillatory forces (of the monitoring system) are diminished such that only the pulse pressure waveform is recorded. Damping is increased by air bubbles, using soft, overly compliant tubing (e.g. as a system length extension), tube narrowings (e.g. clots, partial kinking) and deflated pressure bag, and damping is decreased by using excessive tubing lengths.

Static calibration of a system involves transducer zeroing to a reference point and setting of an appropriate gain for the displayed waveform.

Dynamic calibration is now generally relevant to manufacturers of devices and refers to the use of systems with optimal damping and appropriate resonance frequency for the system. A rough visual assessment may be made with a **fast-flush test** (e.g. for an arterial line, after a rapid flush of fluid from the pressure bag, an obvious square wave will be seen, then one undershoot below the baseline, then a small overshoot above the baseline if the system has acceptable damping. An overdamped system will have no or minimal oscillations and excessive oscillations are seen in an underdamped one.

FIGURE 4.2 Example of a file from the equipment library: Defibrillator

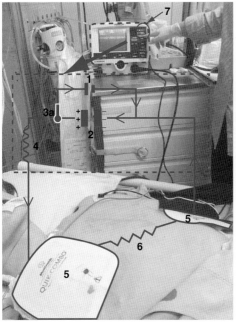 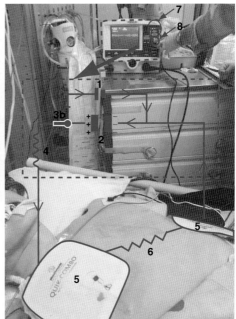

Defibrillator circuit when shock being delivered

Defibrillator circuit when charging

1 Power source with rectifier and transformer
2 Capacitor
3 Gate – 3a position for charging; 3b position for shock delivery
4 Inductor
5 Defibrillator pads
6 Thoracic impedance
7 User interface – on button, energy select, charging
8 Shock delivery button

1. Item name	Defibrillator
2. Uses	Provide electrical shocks of preset energy through the chest wall (expressed in joules) to the heart in an attempt to revert ventricular fibrillation (VF) and pulseless ventricular tachycardia (VT) during cardiac arrest.
	Synchronised shocks (cardioversion) are used in the management of VT with a pulse and other tachyarrhythmias. Some devices also have the capacity to provide transcutaneous pacing.
3. Description	There are various defibrillators available, classified as:
	1. Monophasic defibrillators: these deliver energy in one direction only using a dampened monophasic sinusoidal waveform, which is a single pulse lasting for 3–4 msec. The energy level used should always be set at a maximum in adults (360 J) for defibrillation.
	2. Biphasic defibrillators: these deliver energy in two directions using a variety of waveform technologies. Considered 'gold standard'. These produce bidirectional truncated transthoracic shocks that are much more efficient at lower energies than standard, damped sine-wave shock-defibrillators. This results in less myocardial damage, fewer post-defibrillation ECG abnormalities and more effective first shocks. The energy level set for biphasic defibrillators will depend on the model (e.g. 150–200 J for adults for defibrillation).
	Key features: on/off button, energy select button, charge button, button to deliver a shock, button to dump any charge not needed, how to select the monitoring mode and which lead is the default, how to change from paddle to ECG monitoring; additional pacing features and controls, including rate and output.
	3. Automated external defibrillators (AEDs): have an internal microprocessor that analyses the ECG; if VF/VT are detected it causes the AED to display a warning and then either deliver a shock (automatic) or advise the operator to do so (semi-automatic). AEDS are highly accurate and may reduce the time to the first shock, are simple to learn and use, increasing their availability and application, including for public domains.
4. Method of insertion and/or use	Defibrillation is successful when a critical mass of myocardium is depolarised simultaneously. This means the fibrillation is interrupted and may allow recapture by a single pacemaker. For this to occur the transthoracic impedance must be minimised. Depolarisation of the myocardial cells is accomplished by passage of the electrical current through them. Australian and New Zealand Resuscitation Councils and European Resuscitation Council algorithms/guidelines are used for determining when defibrillation should be used and the number of shocks and energy levels used.
	Pads/paddles are 10–13 cm in size and applied carefully to the skin to ensure good adherence and no interruption to the energy delivered.
	The defibrillator is charged to the required energy and then the operator ensures that everyone has moved away from the patient before discharging. If paddles are used, a pressure of about 5 kg is required and defibrillation should be done in expiration if possible. Shock delivery is confirmed by the patient's motor response and on the defibrillator/cardiac monitor.

Continued

5. Potential complications	Risk of electrical injury to rescuers and the patient in the presence of water, metal fixtures, oxygen, inflammable substances; the 'Stand clear!' command prior to discharge of shocks is essential to ensure safety.
	Paddles should only be charged when resting on the patient's chest. Avoid placement of pads/paddles over ECG leads, GTN patches, lines and implantable devices.
	If defibrillation is unsuccessful: recommence CPR, check paddle/pad position and chest wall contact, consider changing defibrillator pads or changing to the anteroposterior placement and ensure it is set to deliver an unsynchronised shock.
6. Other information	Important associated concepts:
	Charge = quantity of charge passing over a point over 1 sec when a current of 1 A flows past that point (unit C = coulomb).
	Capacitance = the ability of a material to hold an electrical charge (unit F = farad; 1 farad = 1 coulomb/V).
	Capacitor = a device that stores electrical energy (the defibrillator capacitor builds up charge from the mains or battery supply when the charging switch is triggered and it is released when the discharge switch is activated).
	Inductor = a device that stores energy in a magnetic field created when current passes through it; on the defibrillator it controls the nature (waveform characteristics) and duration of the current.
	Rectifier = a device that converts AC to DC voltage (DC is less harmful to myocardium).
	Transformer = a device that transforms electrical energy from one circuit to another in order to increase or decrease the voltage in the second circuit ('steps up' the voltage from mains levels to the much higher level needed for the defibrillator capacitor to charge).
	Impedance = measure of opposition to AC current flow (factors include chest wall thickness, time between shocks and the firmness of the contact of the pad with the chest wall) Stored energy for defibrillation (J) = stored charge (C) x potential (V) (stored energy ranges between devices but may be up to 400 J and the potential is in the order of 5000 V).
	Optimal current is 30–40 A; a shock of 200 J delivers about 30 A to the average patient, but it depends on the thoracic impedance of the individual patient; this may be too little or for others too much. Some newer machines can measure thoracic impedance and adjust the energy delivered accordingly.

It is evident from the examples that, where possible, physics and clinical measurement principles are summarised in conjunction with practical information about equipment items. We have found that the best way to learn and remember the somewhat 'dry' physics concepts is to apply them to understanding the medical devices that you will utilise throughout your career as an intensivist.

Physics and clinical measurement
To further assist candidates with their specific study of physics and clinical measurement, the following items are accompanied by relevant concepts that underpin their function.
Analysis of neural activity
• Depth of anaesthesia monitor; near infrared spectroscopy (NIRS)

Cardiac pacing principles
- Temporary transvenous pacing wire; pulse generator box

Doppler principle
- Oesophageal Doppler; portable ultrasound machine

Electrical concepts
- Defibrillators; electrical safety devices; diathermy

Humidity and its measurement
- Heat and moisture exchanger

Measurement of pressure
- Manometers
  - Non-invasive BP devices
- Intravascular pressure transducers
  - Pressure transducing system

Measurement of cardiac output
- Pulmonary artery catheter; pulse contour analysis for cardiac output measurement; minimally invasive cardiac output measurement

Measurement of gas pressure, volume and flow
- ICU mechanical ventilator; transport ventilator; flow meter; gas cylinders; volatile vapouriser

Measurement of specific gases
- Oxygen
  - ICU mechanical ventilator; pulse oximeter; blood gas machine; metabolic cart
- Carbon dioxide
  - CO_2 detectors; blood gas machine; metabolic cart
- Nitric oxide
  - Nitric oxide delivery system

Measurement of temperature
- Temperature measuring devices; patient-warming systems

Physics of gases and liquids
- Peripheral intravenous cannulae; nebulisers; pulmonary artery catheter; CRRT circuits

Precision and accuracy of measurement
- ECG machine and dots

Resting energy expenditure
- Pulmonary artery catheter; metabolic cart.

References

Bersten AD, Soni N (eds). Oh's Intensive Care Manual. Elsevier; 6th edn: 2009.

Darovic GO. Haemodynamic Monitoring: Invasive and Non-invasive Clinical Application. Saunders; 3rd edn: 2002.

Gwinnutt CL. Clinical Anaesthesia. Blackwell Science: 1996.

Hall J, Schmidt G, Wood L. Principles of Critical Care. McGraw-Hill; 3rd edn: 2005.

Irwin R, Rippe J. Irwin and Rippe's Intensive Care Medicine. Lippincott, Williams & Wilkinson; 6th edn: 2008

Morgan G, Mikhail M, Murray M. Clinical Anesthesiology. McGraw-Hill; 4th edn: 2005.

Prince of Wales Hospital Intensive Care Unit. Nursing Clinical Practice Guidelines.

Sykes M, Vickers M, Hull C. Principles of Clinical Measurement and Monitoring in Anaesthesia and Intensive Care. Blackwell Scientific; 1991.

www.physio_control.com

www.viasyshealthcare.com

Chapter 5

Practical and procedural skills

The ancestor of every action is a thought.
RALPH WALDO EMERSON

Overview

The highest aspiration for those involved in awarding professional credentials in any industry is to deliver an examination process that differentiates between those who are ready to function independently and safely in the 'real-world' and those requiring more education and supervision. An increasing emphasis is being placed on moving beyond tests of knowledge. More complex tasks that evaluate application of knowledge, together with the matching practical skills, are being embraced in healthcare. The use of dedicated task simulators and simulated work environments are increasingly available to add to the fidelity of the examination experience.

In ICM, procedural skills may be readily assessed. Knowledge may be tested in written components of exams. As is discussed in Chapter 7, knowledge about procedures may be discussed and/or directly observed in vivas in any of the exams.

Two of the eight CICM stations in the viva section of the Fellowship exam consistently address practical skills. One station is devoted to communication and the other to a procedure. There is increasing emphasis on using simulated scenarios that assess clinical approaches to patient problems, as well as specific procedural skills.

This chapter will describe the diversity of scenarios that examination candidates can be expected to encounter, both now and, based on current trends, in the future. It contains advice regarding preparation for practical exam components. A library collection of the most pertinent knowledge and individual procedural skills can be found on the accompanying DVD.

Classification of assessment types

Actor stations
These stations revolve around a role-play, where the exam candidate enters a simulated encounter with an individual usually encountered in the course of their work as an intensive care doctor. Classically, the CICM examination contains a communication station where a meeting with a family member is set up to test the communication skills of the doctor in a complex, challenging scenario. For example, breaking bad news to the partner of a patient receiving care in the ICU.

Part task trainers

These stations utilise a simulated patient or body part. Such assessments have been traditionally used in medicine, with a reliance on animal models (e.g. suturing a pig's trotter; performing a cricothyroidotomy on a dog trachea). Sophisticated, realistic, anatomically correct models of human anatomy made of artificial materials are now readily available, making assessment of diverse skills ranging from airway procedures to line insertions easily achievable. They provide an ideal opportunity to simultaneously assess knowledge and skill. For example, a candidate could be asked to demonstrate ultrasound-guided central venous line insertion with discussion regarding the regional anatomy, the Seldinger technique, the physics of transducing a central venous pressure waveform, and the factors influencing the CVP reading.

Full body manikins

Manikins of varying fidelity are now widely available. These may be utilised to test an approach to clinical assessment and/or management of a scenario, with or without associated questions probing into the knowledge of related concepts. Examples include demonstration of brainstem death clinical tests with discussion of preconditions, and troubleshooting the problem of high-peak airway pressures in the context of a ventilated patient.

Hybrids

Possibilities readily exist for combining more than one type of assessment. For example, asking a candidate to demonstrate how they would teach basic life support to a medical student combines the use of an actor with a part task trainer (a simple resuscitation manikin) and enables communication, basic teaching skills and knowledge of ACLS algorithms to be elegantly evaluated.

Advice for approaching procedural skill assessments

Before attempting any exit exam it is imperative to have obtained sufficient experience and proficiency in the range of procedural skills that are expected of a practising intensivist. Logbooks are a useful method of maintaining objective evidence of progress.

Observing and teaching others specific skills is also beneficial. With the wealth of resources now available to improve patient safety and support ethical learning, healthcare is moving away from the 'see one, do one, teach one' paradigm to include where possible a 'sim one' stage of learning.

Some knowledge of educational theory is of benefit when learning (and teaching) clinical procedures. The Dreyfus model postulates five stages of skill acquisition: novice, advanced beginner, competent, proficient and expert. Each stage is a gradual transition from deliberate conscious step-wise thoughts to a final intuitive grasp. It is useful to be able to determine one's own stage of proficiency for each of the skills expected of an intensivist, not only to assist with exam preparation, but also to enable ongoing learning beyond the examination process. Candidates with a low level of proficiency for a specific procedure may best prepare themselves by seeking opportunities to practise that task and benefit greatly from supervision to ensure they learn the appropriate behaviour. Those at a more advanced stage may benefit from supervision to ensure they have not developed inappropriate techniques that could be improved upon. More proficient candidates may also benefit from teaching those with low levels of skill development in order to encourage tacit knowledge to be transformed into specific codified steps that are likely to be rated in examination stations.

Having a consistent personal approach to performing and describing procedures can also be useful, particularly when demonstrating a specific skill on a part task trainer. Table 5.1 provides an example of such an approach.

TABLE 5.1 Approach to a specific procedural skill	
Item	Examples of issues
Patient preparation	Consent, including explanation of risks, review of coagulation parameters, fasting, positioning
Sterile technique	Skin preparations, drapes, gowns/gloves, role of assistant
Anaesthetic technique	Local anaesthetic for infiltration, intravenous sedation or general anaesthesia
Preparation of equipment	Priming lines, preparing transducer system, preparation of procedure tray
Procedural technique	Stepwise description, including reference to anatomic landmarks
Method to confirm satisfactory completion	Transduced pressure trace, chest X-ray, litmus paper test for acid
Potential complications	Acute, subacute, chronic; local and systemic; procedure and anaesthesia related
Other special considerations	Calibration of SvO_2 after pulmonary artery catheter insertion

Performing in an artificial environment can be difficult unless it is practised. Some candidates find it almost impossible to role-play and immerse themselves in simulated scenarios, while others find it second nature. Unfortunately, the exam process does not reward those who are unable to accept the realities of the assessment process presented to them. It is strongly recommended that all those approaching simulated patients approach the tasks presented as they would in real life, accepting the fidelity provided and doing what they normally would with a real patient in the circumstance presented. It is even more important for those who are not naturally comfortable with simulated patient care tasks to practise interacting with manikins and actors sufficiently to obtain a level of comfort that will maximise their performance in the real exam.

It is beneficial to try to anticipate and plan for likely scenarios in each of the assessment types described. Practise with others approaching the exam, practise with an audience and preferably with a mentor and/or examiner. Consider the likely marking schedule for specific tasks. What individual steps in a task would be expected? What questions about knowledge would logically accompany this procedure? Thinking like an examiner will greatly aid one's performance as a candidate. An example of where marks are likely to be allocated is provided in some of the sample scenarios that follow.

Many ICUs have their own supply of educational products, such as part task trainers and training sets of equipment. Nurse educators assigned to the ICU often maintain these and use them for instructing critical care nurses, but are often happy to assist your learning needs by allowing you to use them. Some larger centres have access to a dedicated simulation centre with a wealth of trainers. Actors need not be professionals. The social and pastoral care workers that work in ICU are usually extremely skilled in communication. They are frequently very supportive of ICU trainees and excellent at role-playing difficult patients, relatives, staff members and colleagues who may be encountered in exams. Use all opportunities that arise for you to observe and have your skills observed by senior colleagues. Whenever possible practise scenarios with other candidates.

On the day of the exam ensure that you are clear on what a specific skill assessment is actually asking you to do. Rehearse reading the task descriptions, then performing that task. Clarify what is expected of you if necessary, but try to maintain any fidelity that is presented to you. For example, if you enter a communication role-play with an actor, ask any questions about what you are supposed to be doing from the observing examiner not from the 'family member'. Do not complain about or blame the equipment provided.

Examples of scenarios

The rest of this chapter consists of a collection of procedural skills that demonstrate the range of situations you may encounter to help stimulate you to devise your own examples. Think about the practicalities and appropriateness of assessing certain skills. For example, consistently reproducing a complex, high-fidelity scenario that requires a dedicated simulation centre for vast numbers of candidates is unlikely to be possible due to the logistical implications it would present for examiners. Currently, examining non-technical skills (e.g. crisis management skills) is limited by the lack of availability of a validated tool in ICM. In the future, as emphasis on training and assessing these important qualities increases, it is likely to be examined. A recently developed, self-directed learning package to facilitate learning of these skills is: Foot C, Steel L, Campher D, Medical Crisis Management: Improving Performance Under Pressure, available at www.eruditemedicalbooks.com.

Actor stations

Effective interactions with patients and their families, as well as colleagues both inside the ICU and in other areas of the hospital (medical, nursing, allied health professionals, ward support staff, administration), are frequent and essential. The complexity of the medicine alone mandates that written and verbal communication of treatment plans must be of the highest level. The intensivist should be the leader of a committed and diverse team of people, and be comfortable in dealing with the psychological needs of all who enter the environment of an ICU. This means that a high level of personal self-awareness and interpersonal communication skills are required of the intensivist.

The ICU is a place where intense emotions are encountered, generated by the high acuity of illness and risk of death. Open discussions about many subjects that are not usually approached in general conversation, such as family conflict, end-of-life decision-making and organ donation, are often daily events.

It is therefore not surprising that the CICM consistently assesses these attributes in Fellowship exam candidates. The college's decision to make the Australian Donor Awareness Program Training (ADAPT), which covers issues surrounding brain death, donor management and grief, a mandatory requirement for trainees, also reflects the level of importance it places on effective communication skills.

This component of the exam may be best prepared for through a consistent daily commitment to improved performance as a communicator. This should be a vocational goal that commences from the time candidates enter medical school. It is crucial to observe respected senior colleagues in family conferences and witness a range of approaches to having difficult conversations and breaking 'bad news'. It is invaluable to obtain constructive feedback from individuals (e.g. supervising consultants, senior nurses and social workers) who observe your own interactions, particularly in demanding circumstances.

Role-playing exercises, especially if videotaped, are useful strategies for additional development. The candidate, 'patient' and mentor may assess both verbal and non-verbal communication. Involvement of a professional actor with the creation of possible examination scenarios is offered as a component of some exam training programs.

Regard for ethical principles and knowledge of legal principles concerning end-of-life matters are essential. Specific skills that may be observable in such tasks include empathy, explaining while avoiding the use of medical jargon, active listening, counselling, negotiating and managing difficult emotional issues such as anger, denial and distress.

Some representative cases are provided in Box 5.1. An approach that can be used when preparing for discussions with patients or their surrogates, both in examinations and real life, is provided in Table 5.2. Tackling difficult conversations with other healthcare professionals does not lend itself as easily to a template, although some of the same important steps include ensuring an appropriate setting, defining the meeting purpose and exchanging information. Remaining calm and respectful, finding common ground, listening and negotiating are especially useful skills. An excellent resource containing many examples of cases and strategies is: Corke C, Milne S, Communication for the Intensive Care Specialist, available at www.eruditemedicalbooks.com.

BOX 5.1 Communication stations with actors

Role-plays with a patient's family member

- Discussing end-of-life care with a patient or their surrogate (declining admission, limiting or withdrawing treatment, discussing NFR status, explaining brain stem death).
- Determining appropriateness of ICU admission, including interpretation of advanced health directives (e.g. in the context of someone with an iatrogenic medical complication or someone with a readily reversible disorder) and in situations where no end-of-life decision making has ever been made (e.g. in chronically disabled patients or those with progressive neuromuscular conditions).
- Approaching a family about organ donation (brainstem death or donation after cardiac death).
- Addressing a complaint about care in your ICU.
- Managing special treatment needs (e.g. Jehovah's witness beliefs regarding blood products in the context of life-threatening bleeding).
- Breaking sudden and unexpected bad news.
- Open disclosing about an adverse event that has affected a patient (e.g. life-threatening haemorrhage or hypoxia associated with a percutaneous tracheostomy).
- Discussing a request for an alternative therapy without an evidence basis (e.g. a herbal therapy).

Communication with a member of the healthcare organisation

- Addressing concerns about wellbeing and/or performance with a trainee or colleague.
- Discussing differences in opinion about a therapy or aggressiveness of care with a colleague.
- Managing grief and distress in staff.
- Rationing of resources and bed allocation.
- Exploring allegations regarding sexual harassment or bullying.
- Exploring concerns about an impaired colleague (e.g. where excessive alcohol or drug dependence is suspected).

TABLE 5.2 An approach to communication role-plays	
Item	Comments
1. Setting	Private location. Seated adjacent on same eye level. Tissues available.
2. Introductions	Exchange names, roles/relationships. Define the purpose of the meeting.
3. Gather information	Target to the scenario. Consider issues such as the current level of understanding of the situation, surrogate decision-makers and important people to contact, the patient's actual or probable views on their situation, their baseline level of function, previously expressed wishes regarding end-of-life decisions, attitudes towards quality of life and death.
4. Provide information	Target to the scenario. Consider issues such as the current medical problems, likely prognosis, planned interventions and likely duration of ICU care.
5. Check understanding	Confirm understanding of the most important information.
6. Agree on a plan	Summarise the meeting outcomes. Check agreement.
7. Plan the next meeting	Define the reasons (e.g. review progress).
8. Other issues	Arrange an interpreter if language barriers are identified. Avoid medical jargon and imprecise terms. Document the content of the meeting and key outcomes. If the encounter appears to be going badly try to determine the cause and consider the utility of a break and/or involving colleagues or other family members to assist understanding and resolution of points of conflict. Try to identify and focus on areas of agreement or intent.

Part task trainers

The 'top 20' most important procedures in critical care that can be tested using a part task trainer are summarised on the DVD. It should be noted that variations on how procedures are performed and the equipment utilised will vary between settings. In examinations where differences may be important enough to place an individual candidate at a disadvantage, a variety of relevant devices are generally provided from which the candidate can select (e.g. different percutaneous tracheostomy kits). One approach is provided in this chapter to give readers a basis for preparation in this area. This is NOT intended to be a comprehensive guide to teach procedures to those who need to learn them. It is a guide for those who need to demonstrate their competency at the procedure in an exam setting.

Some considerations relevant for all procedures are:
- explanation to patient or surrogate and consent
- coagulation: consider the need for administering platelets or clotting factors or withholding anticoagulants
- prophylactic antibiotics: consider the need to administer cover (e.g. percutaneous tracheostomy in a patient with mechanical heart valves)
- injuries or medical problems: consider limitations to ideal positioning (e.g. if intracranial pressure is high, then the head-down position should be adopted for as short a duration as possible such as just prior to entering the vein with needle during central line insertion; limited neck extension for tracheostomy in patients with spinal pathology)
- allergies: review before administering any anaesthetic agents
- universal precautions: for operator and assistants
- personnel: ensure sufficient assistance is available

- application of protective layers under/around patient to avoid soiling the patients gown/sheets (e.g. disposable absorptive waterproof sheets)
- monitoring: in an ICU most patients receive continuous monitoring of vital signs with invasive/non-invasive devices. For most procedures a minimum requirement is blood pressure, ECG, heart rate and oxygen saturation. In ventilated patients $ETCO_2$ is also important
- documentation: should follow all procedures, including personnel, technique, as well as complications.

An example of this approach applied to a specific procedure is provided in Table 5.3.

TABLE 5.3 Insertion of intra-aortic balloon pump	
Patient preparation	Position optimally with hip extended and slightly externally rotated. Shave the groin. An assistant may need to retract abdominal folds upwards in obese patients.
Sterile technique	Operator secures hair from face (e.g. under hat), eye protection, face mask, surgical scrub of hands/forearms, then adopts sterile gown and gloves; sterile tray and contents. Application of skin antiseptic to broad area around anatomic site of selected artery (e.g. alcoholic chlorhexidine) – allow to dry; Generous draping of surrounding areas with sterile sheets.
Anaesthetic technique	Infiltrate 3–5 mL of local anaesthetic into subcutaneous tissues over site of planned arterial cannulation with infiltrating needle (e.g. 22G); consider intravenous sedation as adjunct.
Preparation of equipment	Sterile tray with organised lay out of materials – drapes, skin preparation and method of application, local anaesthetic, sterile saline, drawing up and injecting needles, securing method (e.g. suture – inserted with needle holder and scissors), dressings, appropriate sized IABP kit (Fig 5.1). **FIGURE 5.1 IABP being used** It is helpful to use the extensively draped area over the patient's lower limbs and torso as a tray to lay out the kit within the sterile plastic tray it comes in and to use a scrubbed assistant to handle the long tubes and wires. Only open the balloon kit once the sheath is inserted. Ensure a sterile transducer is primed and ready to attach to the balloon and the console assembled with power and helium sources attached.

Continued

TABLE 5.3 Insertion of intra-aortic balloon pump—cont'd

Procedural technique	**Seldinger technique** Fully collapse the balloon by sucking on the drive port with the large syringe in the kit (e.g. 60 mL) to create a vacuum; some kits require that the plunger is completely pulled out to achieve this. Some kits also require that a stylet is removed from the central catheter that can be later used as a measuring device to assist balloon insertion. Insert needle into femoral artery at 45 degrees to the skin until a jet of pulsatile blood flows from the end. Insert J-tip guidewire down needle until estimated distance is in the thoracic aorta. Nick the skin with a scalpel at the skin penetration site. Insert dilator into sheath (many sets are now sheathless). Pass sheath/dilator over wire, then remove dilator. Pass balloon through sheath over guidewire and insert estimated distance – measure from sternal angle to umbilicus then to femoral artery. Remove wire and aspirate 3 mL blood from central lumen, manually flush 3–5 mL of sterile saline, then attach to transducer set and flush. Some kits require removal of a one-way valve and gas lumen insert from drive line; connect pressure line to the catheter extender that fits into the console. Confirm arterial waveform, select timing trigger, then turn on driver and confirm normal balloon trace and appropriate timing in 1:2 augmentation ratio (newer consoles offer algorithms for automatic selection of optimal trigger and adjust timing including during tachyarrhythmias). The ECG can be either slaved from the patient monitor or attached directly to the patient. Secure the device at the sheath with sutures and lower down on the limb using the securing holes on the other end of the sheath once position is confirmed with imaging.
Method to confirm satisfactory completion	Arterial balloon waveform and pressures displayed on console – ensure normal morphology and appropriate timing of inflation and deflation in 1:2 augmentation ratio. Chest X-ray or fluoroscopy confirms radiopaque tip lies in the second intercostal spaces just above the left main bronchus or direct visualisation 1 cm distal to the left subclavian artery with a transoesophageal echo.
Potential complications	Vessel related – arterial dissection, thrombosis, peripheral embolisation and end-organ ischaemia (e.g. limb ischaemia with compartment syndrome), inadvertent femoral vein cannulation, infection, false aneurysm, AV fistula. Haemorrhage after removal – particularly with the sheathed sets; consider surgical repair of insertion sites in sheathed balloons. Balloon related – incorrect positioning with vascular occlusion, perforation, rupture, gas embolisation, thrombocytopenia.

TABLE 5.3 Insertion of intra-aortic balloon pump—cont'd	
Other special considerations	Sites of insertion – femoral artery (rarely other large arteries such as the axillary artery or direct insertion via an incision into the descending aorta).
	Catheter types – balloon size based on height (25–50 cc), sheathed or sheathless kits, new fibre-optic catheters that improve arterial pressure waveform detection and timing.
	Anticoagulation – controversial if routinely required during the first 24 hours but low-dose heparin infusion often prescribed; some units infuse heparinised saline through the transducer set.
	Contraindications – aortic dissection, aortic valve incompetence, severe occlusive atherosclerosis, prosthetic aortic tree grafts.

Anatomy

Figures 5.2–5.10 are included as a reminder of the key regional anatomy that is relevant to procedures covered in this section. Surprisingly, candidates often struggle when asked the major relations to anatomical structures being frequently manipulated.

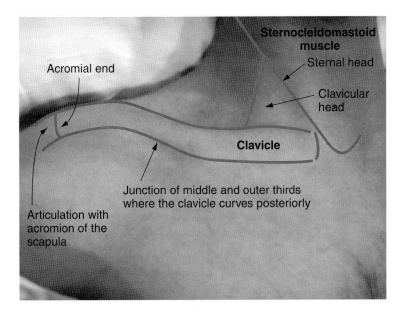

FIGURE 5.2 Neck anatomy relevant to subclavian and internal jugular vein central line insertion

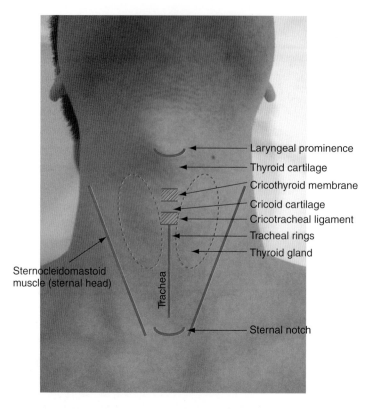

FIGURE 5.3 Neck anatomy relevant to surgical airways

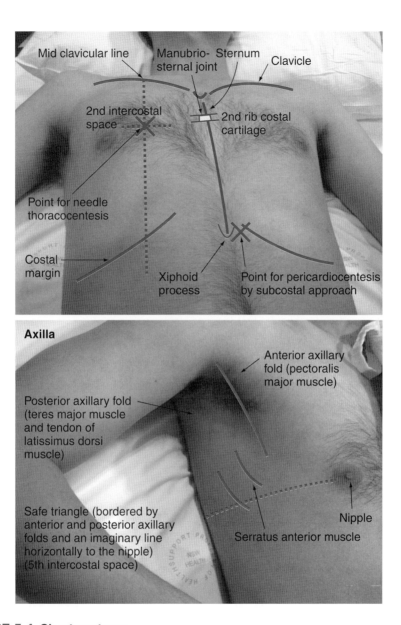

FIGURE 5.4 Chest anatomy

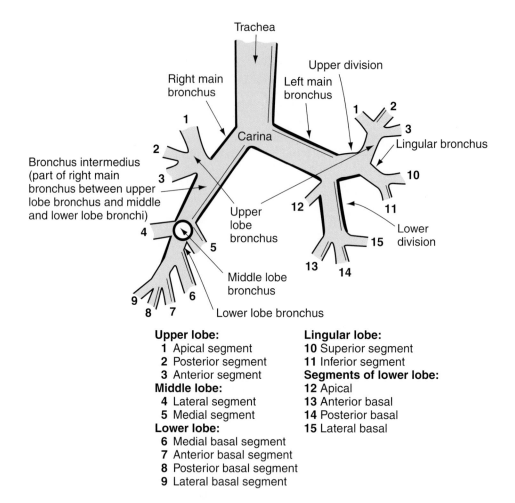

FIGURE 5.5 Bronchial anatomy for bronchoscopy

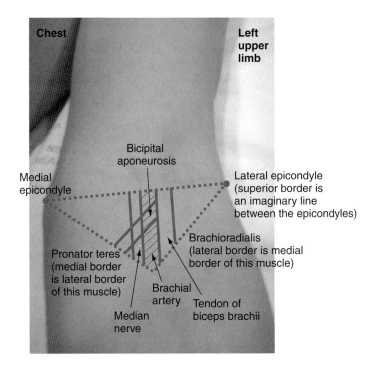

FIGURE 5.6 Cubital fossa anatomy for brachial arterial and venous cannulation, including PICC line insertion

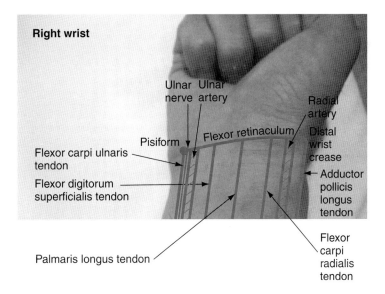

FIGURE 5.7 Wrist anatomy for arterial line insertion

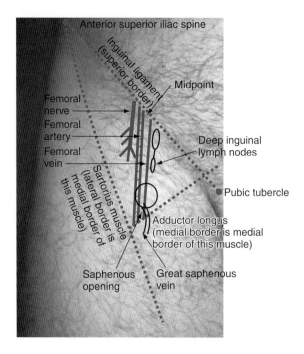

FIGURE 5.8 Femoral triangle for arterial and central venous lines

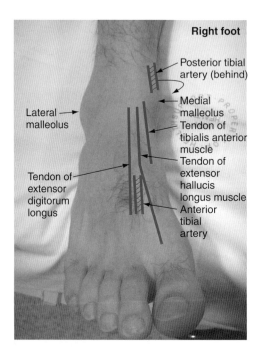

FIGURE 5.9 Foot arterial anatomy

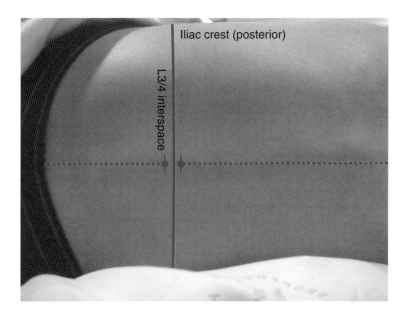

FIGURE 5.10 **Back anatomy for lumbar puncture**

Full body manikins

These manikins range from low-fidelity advanced life support trainers to high-fidelity, lifelike, simulated patients. Lower fidelity manikins are more likely to be utilised for examinations as they are transportable, widely available and can permit multiple simultaneous stations with the same set-up to be run. They may be utilised to assess demonstration of a clinical skill or examination approach or a candidates approach to managing a clinical problem (Table 5.4).

Some examples of these tasks with suggested marking grids are provided to enable a greater understanding of how such scenarios may be presented.

TABLE 5.4 Examples of scenarios using full body manikins	
Demonstration of a clinical skill or assessment	**Approach to managing a clinical problem**
• Basic and advanced cardiac life support – adult, pregnant and paediatric patients, Resuscitation Council guidelines • Measurement and interpretation of intra-abdominal pressure (e.g. intra-vesical pressure) • Demonstration of brain stem death clinical tests with discussion of preconditions • Completion of a tertiary survey for a trauma patient • Testing an epidural catheter anaesthesia block	• High peak airway pressures in a ventilated patient • Undifferentiated shock • Accidental extubation during transport for an imaging procedure • Unexpected difficult airway with failed intubation after rapid sequence induction (can't intubate +/– can't ventilate scenarios) • Uncontrolled intracranial pressure

Questions examining practical and procedural skills in the various exams

Demonstration of brainstem death clinical tests

SAMPLE QUESTION

Demonstrate and discuss how you would clinically test brain-stem function using a simulated patient.

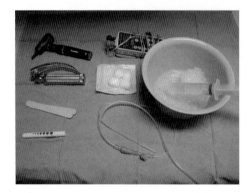

FIGURE 5.11 **Brain death test equipment**

Equipment/setup
- Basic ALS manikin – pupils dilated
- Endotracheal tube in situ
- Nerve stimulator and electrodes
- Cotton wool/tissue for corneal reflex
- Auroscope
- 50 mL syringe
- Kidney dish
- Jug of iced water
- Tongue depressor and Yankeur sucker
- Pen torch
- Green drape
- ETT and 10 mL syringe
- Suction catheter
- Oxygen tubing

Possible approach

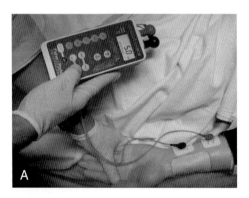

FIGURE 5.12A **Nerve stimulator being used to exclude effects of neuromuscular paralysing drugs**

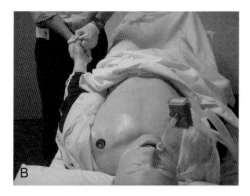
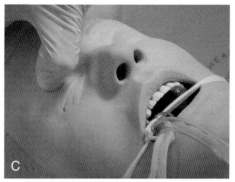

FIGURE 5.12B & C Testing for coma – unresponsiveness to peripheral and centrally applied painful stimuli (nail bed of hand and supraorbital notch)

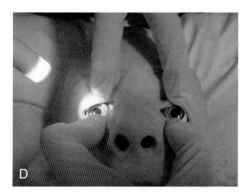
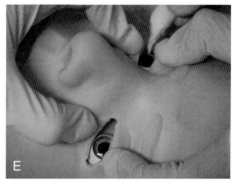

FIGURE 5.12D Testing the pupillary light reflex

FIGURE 5.12E Testing the corneal reflexes

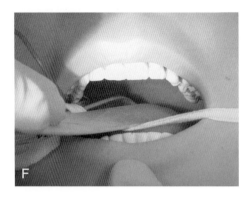

FIGURE 5.12F Testing the gag reflex

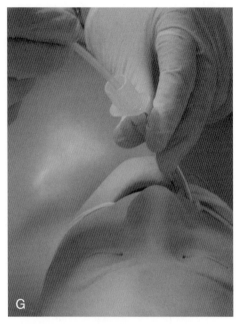

FIGURE 5.12G Testing the cough reflex with tracheal suctioning

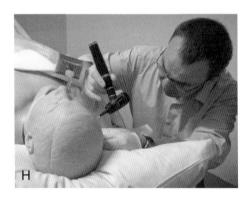

FIGURE 5.12H Examining the ear canal, then preparing to insert ice water for the vestibular–ocular test

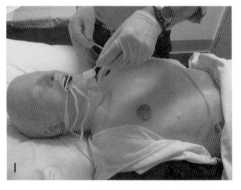

FIGURE 5.12I Performing the apnoea test with 2 L/min oxygen insufflation via a taped suction catheter inserted down the endotracheal tube

Sample marking grid

It should be realised that variations according to local legislation and standard of practice would be incorporated into examinations in different countries. The following scheme reflects ANZICS' recommendations for testing.

TABLE 5.5 Sample marking grid	
Item	**Marks**
Directive: What are the requirements to perform brain-death testing? Minimum 4 hrs observation, two significantly experienced clinicians, independent set of tests; both agree there is: • unresponsiveness • absent brainstem reflexes • apnoea	/2
Directive: What are the preconditions? Evidence of acute brain pathology, normothermia (>35°C) Normotension (MAP >60/SBP >90) Effects of sedatives excluded (possible antagonist test with naloxone/ flumazenil), absence of severe electrolyte, metabolic or endocrine disturbance Intact neuromuscular function Ability to examine reflexes (e.g. at least one eye/ear intact) Ability to perform apnoea testing (e.g. capacity to breathe)	/3
Directive: What do you need to demonstrate? Coma – no response to noxious stimulus to all four limbs, trunk and cranial nerve territory	/1
Pupillary light reflex – absent light response	/1
Corneal reflex – must actually touch the cornea	/1
Reflex response to trigeminal distribution pain (e.g. supraorbital notch pain)	/1
Vestibular–ocular reflex – inspect external auditory canal first; head of bed 30 degrees; instill 50 mL ice-cold water via syringe; hold eyelids open and observe for eye movement for minimum 60 seconds	/1
Gag reflex	/1
Cough/tracheal reflex	/1
Apnoea test Directive: How would you conduct this (preoxygenation, option to ventilate to mild hypercarbia before the test, 2 L/min O_2 via a cannula down the ETT placed above the carina or 100% O_2 via T-piece/CPAP circuit with apnoea alarms off if via a ventilator) Directive: What is the expected rate of rise of $PaCO_2$? (3 mmHg or 0.4 kPa per minute) Directive: What is the target $PaCO_2$ in normocarbic (60 mmHg or 8 kPa) and chronically hypercarbic (+ 20 mmHg or 2.7 kPa) patients? Directive: Why may the $PaCO_2$ fail to rise adequately? (O_2 flow too high via a cannula). Directive: What would you do if hypoxia occurs before CO_2 rises enough (give 1–2 mandatory breaths and/or add CPAP and continue). Directive: What may cause you to think there is spontaneous ventilatory efforts when none are actually present? (autotriggering from cardiac oscillations)	/6
Other questions Directive: 'What is a spinal reflex?' and 'What is the Lazarus sign?' Directive: 'Is having a plantar response or intact deep tendon reflexes consistent with brainstem death?' (yes) Directive: 'Are seizures compatible with brain stem death?' (no)	/2
Total mark	/20

High peak airway pressures in a ventilated patient

SAMPLE QUESTION

A 35-year-old woman with acute urosepsis was admitted to your ICU this morning.

Initial resuscitation measures have included intubation, ventilation, fluids (14 L of crystalloid) and antibiotics (2 g ampicillin and 480 mg gentamicin).

A renal ultrasound suggested that she has an obstructed right ureter, but the images were poor. She is in Radiology awaiting transfer back to the ICU, having just had a CT of her abdomen/renal tracts that was unremarkable.

The nurse has gone to see what is holding up the transfer back to the unit and your registrar has called you as they are 'having problems with the transport ventilator'.

You will be required to assess and manage the simulated patient.

Equipment/set-up
- Basic ALS manikin
- Intubated with size 6 ETT
- Orogastric tube and urinary catheter in situ
- Airway connector attached to HME, ventilator circuit and transport ventilator
- Card with the ventilator settings and readings written on them
- Laminated cards with three states of vital signs and levels of saturation
- Stethoscope.

The examiner provides consistent prompts and ancillary information. They may play a variety of roles, including the junior registrar acting or a separate observer. Consistent questions may be asked, such as: 'What do you think is (are) the cause(s) of the patient's high peak airway pressure?'

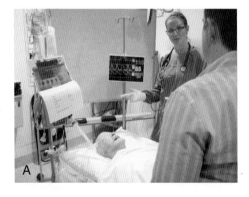

FIGURE 5.13A Set-up of manikin with junior registrar, ventilator settings and vital signs on cards

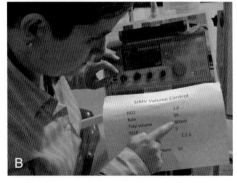

FIGURE 5.13B Candidate reviews ventilator settings

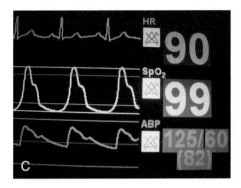 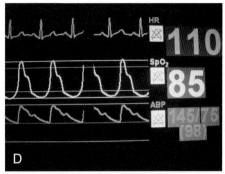

FIGURE 5.13C & D Example of different vital signs that arise during the scenario

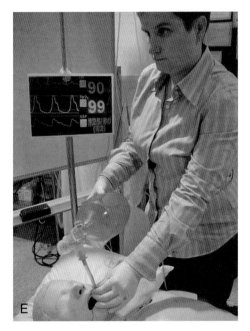

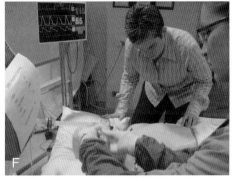

FIGURE 5.13F Candidate suctions the endotracheal tube to detect secretions and exclude a blocked tube (easily simulated with Blu-tak!)

FIGURE 5.13E Candidate disconnects the ventilator and manually ventilates the patient with a self-inflating bag (oxygen saturations improve)

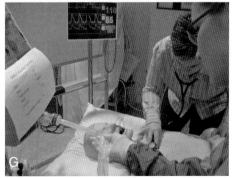

FIGURE 5.13G Candidate auscultates the chest and is told that bilateral coarse crackles are present

Sample marking grid

The task requires the candidate to troubleshoot high peak airway pressures in a patient on a transport ventilator in the radiology department. A systematic approach that considers a broad differential diagnosis, including patient and equipment factors, is expected. The problem is multifactorial, including aggressive fluid loading, ARDS from sepsis, inappropriately high tidal volume setting, and small ETT.

TABLE 5.6 Sample marking grid

Item	Marks
Makes an initial assessment of the ABCs.	/1
Concludes initial situation is safe except for the high peak airway pressure and proceeds to assess further.	/1
Nominates a safe peak airway pressure: 30–35 cmH$_2$0.	/1
Clearly distinguishes patient and equipment factors when approaching causes of high peak airway pressures.	/1
Stops mechanical ventilation and manually ventilates the patient as part of early assessment.	/2 2 marks if done within first 2 minutes No marks if only when desaturates
Recognises that the tidal volume of 800 mL in a 60 kg patient is excessive.	/1
Corrects TV to 6–8 mL/kg (accept 350–500 mL).	/1
Cautiously increases RR after TV reduced.	/1
Increases PEEP until peak pressure is high again – at least 10.	/1
Suctions the airway to ensure endotracheal tube patency.	/1
Recognises the possible contribution of the small endotracheal tube.	/1
Elects not to attempt to change the endotracheal tube to a larger tube while in Radiology.	/1
Administers a bolus of any neuromuscular paralysing agent.	/2 2 marks if extra sedation is attempted first 1 mark if paralysis given
Recognises that fluid overload is a likely problem.	/2 2 marks if also gives a bolus of diuretic 1 mark if only recognises the problem
Recognises that ARDS is a likely problem.	/1
Recognises the importance of returning to the ICU as soon as possible, but only when the ABCs have been stabilised.	/1
Insists on obtaining more help.	/1
Total mark	/20

Hybrids

Actors can be incorporated into scenarios along with part task trainers or full body manikins. Performing procedures using hybrid actors and part task trainers best illustrates this concept. Some examples can be found in Table 5.7.

TABLE 5.7 Examples of hybrid scenarios

Possible question	Notes
Demonstrate how you would insert an arterial line into a patient.	A part task trainer arm is strapped onto a live actor playing a patient, to assess procedural skill and patient communication. The actor can appear anxious and require reassurance and explanation regarding what is happening. Another actor can play a nurse assisting with the procedure to enable interprofessional communication to be simultaneously assessed.
Demonstrate how you would teach basic life support to a medical student allocated for an elective in ICU.	A white board, marker pen, basic ALS manikin and bag-valve mask are provided. It enables testing of knowledge of the algorithm and some basic teaching skills. **FIGURE 5.14A & B A candidate could elect to give a quick tutorial and check understanding, then demonstrate and check skills**

Continued

TABLE 5.7 Examples of hybrid scenarios—cont'd	
Possible question	**Notes**
Please assist a junior ICU registrar to write their first prescription of renal replacement therapy with low-dose heparin as the anticoagulant in a patient with oliguric acute renal failure who has a pH of 7.2, normal serum lactate and mildly increased potassium, and needs the therapy principally for fluid overload. Explain to them the basics of CVVHDF using any of a range of pieces of equipment provided.	An actor plays a junior registrar and a circuit for renal replacement therapy is provided including a heparin infusion, dialysate fluid (with lactate as the buffer). Paper, pens and a basic form for prescribing the therapy are provided.

References

Benner P. Using the Dreyfus model of skill acquisition to describe and interpret skill acquisition and clinical judgment in nursing practice and education. Bulletin of Science, Technology Society, 2004; 24: 188–99.

Bersten AD, Soni N (eds). Oh's Intensive Care Manual. Butterworth-Heinemann; 6th edn: 2008.

Corke C, Milnes S. Communication for the Intensive Care Specialist. Erudite Medical Books; 2008.

Hall J, Schmidt G, Wood L. Principles of Critical Care. McGraw-Hill; 3rd edn: 2005.

Morgan G., Mikhail M, Murray M. Clinical Anesthesology. McGraw-Hill; 4th edn: 2005.

Chapter 6

Data interpretation for intensive care medicine

All truths are easy to understand once they are discovered, the point is to discover them.
GALILEO GALILEI

Overview of data interpretation

Data interpretation is an important component of the EDIC, DICM and FCICM.

In the EDIC data interpretation appears in both Part 1 and 2 of the exam. In Part 1 (the written exam) candidates are often given a series of datasets and are expected to select the response that best interprets the dataset. Typical examples include pressure readings obtained from a pulmonary artery catheter or a set of biochemical abnormalities, such as tumour lysis syndrome. In Part 2 (the oral exam) there is a 15–20 minute viva dedicated to data interpretation where candidates are shown radiology images, ECGs, biochemical and arterial blood gas results. The aim here is for candidates to have a methodical approach to data interpretation, a differential diagnosis and an appropriate management plan.

In the DICM 15 minutes of the clinical viva is currently dedicated to data interpretation (three short cases lasting 5 minutes each), but it may also briefly appear during the long case or viva on general ICU topics. Candidates are expected to confidently interpret ECGs, radiology, arterial blood gases, biochemistry and haematology datasets. Topics that have featured in previous exams include abnormal liver function tests, CT scans showing acute pancreatitis, pulmonary embolus or subdural haemorrhage and chest X-rays of pneumothorax, consolidation or lung collapse. Candidates have also been asked about acid base theory, including the Stewart hypothesis during the general ICU topic viva.

In the FCICM data interpretation is examined mainly in the written paper, along with a whole station dedicated to radiology in the vivas. The stems of the vivas can also include results of investigations and it is not uncommon for investigations to be shown to candidates as part of the clinical cases. In the written exam, generally a clinical-based question is posed and then data is given which has to be applied to the management or diagnostic problem. Common questions include being asked to describe a radiological investigation or ECG, and then using this information in a clinical-based problem. The scope of data and investigations included is very broad, but all are within the scope of everyday practice within intensive care.

An overview of the data types addressed in this chapter is outlined in Box 6.1. The examples presented here should be regarded as a guide only, and are not intended to be a substitute for educational textbooks or journal articles that teach data interpretation.

Additional material, including a summary of microbiology facts relevant to interpreting laboratory microscopy and culture data, is provided on the DVD.

BOX 6.1 Overview of data types

1. Imaging studies
   - Chest X-ray
   - CT chest and neck
   - Abdominal X-ray
   - Abdominal ultrasound
   - CT abdomen
   - CT head
   - Skeletal and soft tissues X-rays
   - Other imaging modalities
2. Electrocardiography
3. Haemodynamic monitoring
   - Central venous pressure waveforms
   - Mixed venous and central venous oxygen saturation
   - Arterial waveforms
   - Intra-aortic balloon pump waveforms
   - Pulmonary artery catheters
   - Other haemodynamic measurement devices
   - Echocardiography
4. Respiratory function tests
   - Spirometry
   - Static lung volumes
   - Diffusion studies
   - Flow volume loops
   - Pressure volume loops
5. Ventilator waveforms
6. Indirect calorimetry
7. Capnography
8. Biochemistry tests
   - Arterial blood gas analysis
   - Biochemistry data sets
   - Other specific investigations (autoimmune markers, short Synacthen tests, thyroid function tests, iron studies, tumour markers and other tests)
9. Haematology tests
   - Blood counts
   - Coagulation studies
10. Analysis of body fluids
    - Urine
    - Pleural fluid
    - Ascitic fluid
    - Cerebrospinal fluid
    - Joint fluid

Imaging studies

A wide range of imaging studies may be examined. Chest and abdominal X-rays, skeletal X-rays, CT scans (plain and contrast studies), ultrasound, and, less often, MR images, have all appeared in the exam. Normal scans should be confidently recognised. The following provides a basic overview of the major modalities and pathologies. A more detailed review of diagnostic imaging in critical care can be found in Joyce et al. (2010).

Knowledge of anatomical structures with reference to vertebral levels may be useful for localisation of structures and lesions when interpreting CT scans, and to a lesser extent plain X-rays. Some helpful levels are presented in Figure 6.1. The boxes and tables that follow provide a summary of each imaging modality.

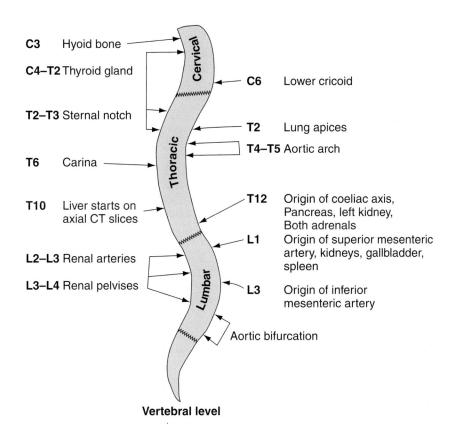

FIGURE 6.1 Anatomical structures relating to vertebral levels

Chest X-rays

Chest X-rays are the most commonly requested imaging investigation, serving as a clinical adjunct to the daily assessment of critically ill patients. Multiple abnormalities are frequently present. These are best elicited with a systematic examination, such as the one presented in Box 6.2.

A summary of the major pathological patterns and problems, encountered on chest X-rays of the critically ill is shown in Table 6.1 on page 115.

BOX 6.2 Systematic assessment of the chest X-ray

1. Technical aspects

- Correct patient/time/date
- Direction of X-ray beam:
  - PA (film placed in front of patient), AP (film placed behind patient) or lateral film
  - Usually designated by a film marker
  - On a PA film the scapulae are laterally located in comparison to the supine AP film, where they are medial.
- Patient position: erect, supine, lateral decubitus:
  - This is usually designated by a film marker; a marker also designates the right or left side of the body on the film.
  - The supine AP film is most commonly obtained in ventilated critically ill patients who are unable to sit up and support a board in front of them.
    - Interpretation differs significantly from an erect PA film by virtue of the differing effects of gravity:
      - Pneumothorax presents as anterior free air with abnormal anterior diaphragmatic lucency and classically the 'deep sulcus sign'.
      - Upper lobe prominence or diversion of the pulmonary vasculature may be normal.
      - Pleural effusion settles posteriorly producing a 'veiling' opacity of the hemithorax rather than a classical meniscus sign.
      - The ratio of the cardiac silhouette to thoracic diameter is less significant.
      - AP films are often taken supine in the critical care unit, full inspiration is often not present and smaller lung volumes appear on the film.
- Rotation: heads of clavicles should be symmetrically positioned in relation to the sternal notch and spinous process of the adjacent thoracic vertebrae.
- Positioning of patient on film: all areas of interest should be clearly visualised.
- Adequate inspiration: at least five anterior ribs should be fully visible.
- Exposure: the lower half of the thoracic vertebral bodies should be just visible behind the heart.

2. Lungs and pleural cavity

- Knowledge of the location of the fissures is the key to localising the lobes (Figs 6.2–6.4)
- Horizontal fissure separates the right upper lobe from the middle lobe. Oriented horizontally, it extends ventrally from the chest wall, and posteriorly to meet the oblique fissure. The horizontal fissure runs at the level of the fourth vertebral body and crosses sixth rib in the mid-axillary line.
- Oblique fissure separates the right upper and middle lobes from the larger right lower lobe. It extends posteriorly and superiorly approximately to the level of the fourth vertebral body. The oblique fissure extends antero-inferiorly, intersecting the diaphragm at the anterior cardiophrenic angle.
- The azygous lobe is a normal variant in the right lung adjacent to the mediastinum. The azygous fissure subdivides the upper lobe in approximately 1% of individuals (Fig 6.4).
- The lobar architecture of the left lung is different from that on the right. There are only two lobes on the left: left upper and lower separated by an oblique fissure, identical to that seen on the right side, although slightly more inferior in location.
- Lungs should be examined for asymmetry between sides:
  - Opacification and mass lesions
  - Hyperlucency

Continued

BOX 6.2 Systematic assessment of the chest X-ray—cont'd

3. Heart and mediastinum

- Cardiothoracic ratio
  - On the PA film, the transverse diameter of the cardiac outline is compared to the widest transverse dimension of the chest.
  - A ratio greater than 50% is suggestive of cardiac enlargement.
- Normal mediastinal contours
  - Right side:
    - Trachea, paratracheal soft tissue stripe and right upper lobe
    - Superior vena cava
    - Right lung hilum is normally 2 cm higher than the left hilum
    - Right atrium
    - Right cardiophrenic angle
  - Left side:
    - Trachea, paratracheal soft tissue stripe and left upper lobe
    - Aortic knuckle
    - Left lung hilum
    - Left atrial appendage
    - Left ventricle
    - Left cardiophrenic angle

4. Bones

- Fractures and lytic lesions should always be looked for.
- The following bones should be inspected:
  - Lower cervical, thoracic and upper lumbar vertebrae
  - Ribs
  - Clavicles
  - Scapulae
  - Sternum
  - Upper humeri

5. Soft tissues

- Diaphragmatic outlines: right side normally higher than left side
- Normal stomach bubble under left hemidiaphragm
- Skin folds
- Breast shadows
- Calcifications: heart valves, costal cartilages, airways, pleura (e.g. asbestosis)

6. Indwelling devices

- All tubes, lines and devices should be identified and their position commented upon.
- Examples include:
  - Endotracheal or tracheostomy tube tips should be at least 2 cm above the carina or located between the clavicular heads.
  - Central venous line tips should be located just above right atrium; note in a left-sided SVC the catheter lies along the left upper mediastinal border.
  - Pulmonary artery catheter tips should not extend lateral to the medial and middle thirds of the diameter of the ipsilateral hemithorax. The balloon should be deflated.
  - Intra-aortic balloon pumps should be placed distal to the left subclavian artery but above the renal arteries. The position of the tip corresponds to just above the left main bronchus or in the third anterior left intercostal space. If an inflated intra-aortic balloon can be seen this indicates diastole in the cardiac cycle.
  - Enteral tubes should project over the stomach or duodenum as appropriate.
  - Chest tubes should be placed anterosuperiorly for air collections and postero-inferiorly for fluid collections. Ensure the most distal side hole of the chest drain is projected inside the ribs.
  - Cardiac pacemakers: atrial and ventricular lead positions should be checked.

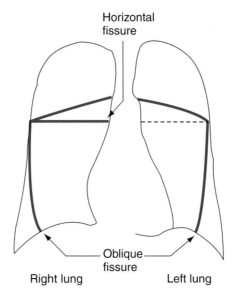

FIGURE 6.2 Location of fissures

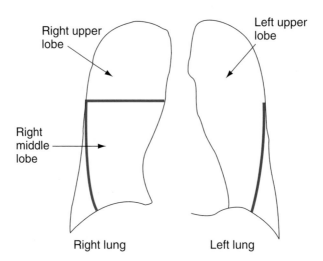

FIGURE 6.3 Location of upper lobes and right middle lobe of the lungs

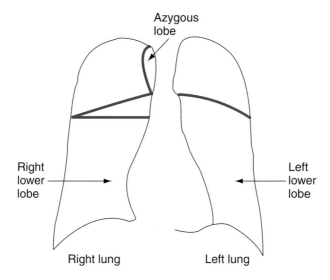

FIGURE 6.4 Location of lower lobes and azygous lobe of the lungs

TABLE 6.1 Abnormalities seen on chest X-rays		
Abnormality	**Findings**	**Causes**
Pulmonary and pleural pathology		
Collapse	Look for shift in the position of normal structures (e.g. movement in the location of the fissures, trachea) towards the collapsed area of lung	• Tumour: primary, secondary, benign or malignant • Bulky lymph nodes • Inhaled foreign body (e.g. peanuts) • Infection: bacterial, TB, fungi or parasites • Inflammation: sarcoid, rheumatoid nodules • Sputum plug
Alveolar opacification	Alveoli and small airways fill with dense material. Sparing of larger airways, causes presence of air bronchograms	• Cardiogenic pulmonary oedema • Non-cardiogenic pulmonary oedema • Pulmonary haemorrhage • Pneumonia • Primary alveolar proteinosis • Alveolar cell carcinoma (classically more localised)

Interstitial opacification	Reticular, nodular and/or reticulonodular opacities	• Cardiac failure (in cardiac failure there are frequently prominent septal lines:
		  ○ Kerley A lines: radiate from the periphery to the hilar areas in the mid and upper zones
		  ○ Kerley B lines: most often seen in the costophrenic regions running <2 cm from the edge of the lung at right angles to the pleura)
		• Interstitial lung disease
		• Infection
		• Lymphangitis carcinomatosis

Continued

TABLE 6.1 Abnormalities seen on chest X-rays—cont'd

Abnormality	Findings	Causes
Pleural fluid	At least 75 mL of pleural fluid must be present in order to blunt the costophrenic angle on the lateral chest X-ray, and 200 mL on the PA chest X-ray. Pleural effusions typically have a meniscus visible on an erect chest X-ray, but loculated effusions (as occur with an empyema) may have a lenticular shape. On the supine AP film in ICU this is often seen as a 'veiling' appearance	• Transudates or exudates • Haemothorax • Chylothorax • Empyema
Hyperlucency of a lung field	Hyperlucent hemithorax indicates a decrease in the radiographic density of the thorax Can be caused by intra- or extrapulmonary diseases. Comparison should be made with the contralateral hemithorax	• Pneumothorax • Compensatory hyperinflation • Air trapping (e.g. obstructive lung disease) • Vascular oligaemia (e.g. pulmonary embolism, tetralogy of Fallot or pulmonary atresia) • Mastectomy
Obstructive lung disease	Hyperinflation (>6 anterior ribs), peribronchial thickening, signs of barotrauma (localised air cysts, pneumothorax, pneumomediastinum)	• Asthma • Chronic obstructive airways disease: emphysematous bullae • Bronchiectasis: 'tram-track' appearance with bronchial dilatation
White-out of a hemithorax	Hemithorax is completely opacified. To establish presence of volume loss, observe position of the trachea, mediastinum and diaphragm	• Collapse: trachea classically deviates to side of pathology • Consolidation: look for air bronchograms • Pleural fluid: trachea classically deviates away from side of pathology • Pneumonectomy: look for surgical clips/staples • Tumour
Localised Pulmonary opacities	Single 'coin lesion' or multiple nodules	• Tumour: primary or secondary, benign or malignant • Foreign body • Infection: bacterial, TB, fungi, viruses or parasites • Inflammation: sarcoid, rheumatoid nodules, Wegener's granulomatosis • Infarction: septic embolism • Congenital anomalies: sequestered segment, arteriovenous malformations • Loculated pleural collection

Continued

TABLE 6.1 Abnormalities seen on chest X-rays—cont'd

Abnormality	Findings	Causes
Mediastinal pathology		
Mediastinal mass	Lateral chest X-ray (+CT scan) helps determine whether mass is present in anterior, middle or posterior mediastium	• Anterior mediastinum: (4Ts) thyroid masses, thymomas, teratomas, terrible lymphomas • Middle mediastinum: lymphadenopathy, lymphoma, aortic aneurysm • Posterior mediastinum: aneurysm of descending aorta, oesophageal masses, hiatus hernia
Aortic dissection	Widened mediastinum, blunted aortic knob, left apical cap, tracheal deviation, depressed left main stem bronchus, oesophageal deviation, loss of paratracheal stripe, left pleural effusion. For CT findings see Table 6.3.	• Spontaneous (e.g. hypertension and cystic medial necrosis) • Traumatic injury
Myocardial pathology		
Cardiomegaly	Cardiothoracic ratio >50% on full inspiration PA views Cardiothoracic ratio >50% may not be abnormal but represent poor inspiratory effort (e.g. obese, pregnant) or structural abnormalities (e.g. pectus excavatum)	• Congestive cardiac failure • Ischaemic heart disease • Valvular heart disease • Congenital heart disorders • Cardiomyopathy
Dextrocardia	Myocardium on right side of chest. Look for presence of stomach bubble on right (situs inversus) and bronchiectasis (Kartagener's syndrome)	• Situs inversus • Kartagener's syndrome (autosomal recessive disorder caused by a defect in the action of cilia lining the respiratory tract)
Pericardial effusion	Enlarged globular heart	• Infection: viruses (e.g. coxsackie), bacteria, fungi • Myocardial infarction • Uraemia • Trauma • Malignancy • Radiotherapy • Rheumatoid arthritis • SLE
Left atrial enlargement	Often associated with prominent pulmonary arteries	• Mitral valve disease
Diaphragmatic pathology		
Abnormal free air under the diaphragm	Appears as a dark crescent of gas under diaphragm on erect chest radiograph. Free gas is best seen on the right side above the dome-shaped outline of the liver.	• Perforated viscus • Surgical pneumoperitoneum • Peritoneal dialysis • Penetrating abdominal injury

Continued

TABLE 6.1 Abnormalities seen on chest X-rays—cont'd

Abnormality	Findings	Causes
Abnormal unilaterally elevated hemidiaphragm	Right hemidiaphragm should be 2–3 cm higher than left	• Phrenic nerve palsy • Sub-pulmonic collection • Hepatomegaly
Soft tissue abnormalities		
	Variable	• Surgical emphysema • Foreign bodies (e.g. wound shrapnel) • Breast shadows including prominent nipples, nipple piercing, implants • Calcified heart valves or pericardium • Prosthetic heart valves • External monitoring leads (e.g. ECG, oximetry cables) • Defibrillator pads • Oxygen tubing or ventilation devices (e.g. corrugated tubing, HME, CPAP mask) • Surgical clips and drains • Sternal wires • Pacemakers, implantable cardioverter-defibrillators • Ventricular assist devices • Ventriculoperitoneal shunt tubing
Bone abnormalities		
		• Fractures • Lytic lesions • Rib notching: co-arctation of the aorta. If a chest X-ray looks normal in the exam, always double check for this • Thoracic kyphosis, scoliosis: look for fractures causing the deformity • Previous distortion of bony thorax from surgical management of upper lobe pulmonary tuberculosis
Indwelling devices		
		The presence and confirmation of appropriate positioning should be made for: • Central venous lines • Pulmonary artery catheters • Endotracheal or tracheostomy tubes (commonly right endobronchial intubation with variable collapse of right upper lobe and left lung) • Intercostal/intrapleural catheters • Enteral tubes (nasogastric, gastrostomy) • Intra-aortic balloon pumps

A number of commonly encountered chest X-ray examples are shown in Figures 6.5–6.10.

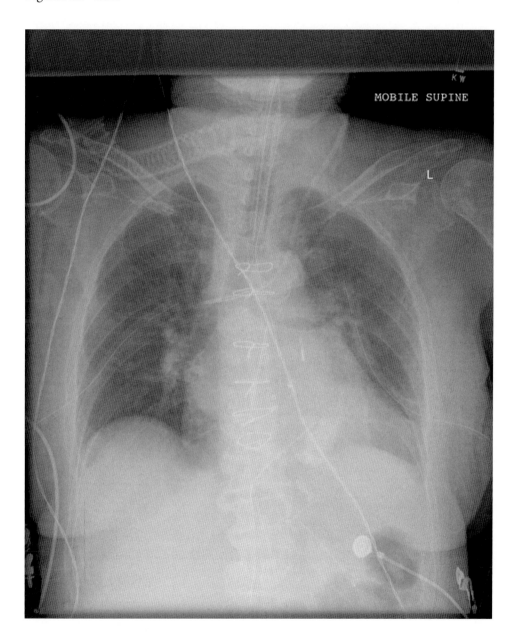

FIGURE 6.5 Multiple medical devices
Note the endotracheal tube, left internal jugular central venous line, two chest drains and a mediastinal drain, a low-lying intra-aortic balloon pump, a nasogastric tube, sternal wires, superimposed monitoring leads and ventilator tubing, and the radio-opaque components of an aortic valve bioprosthesis.

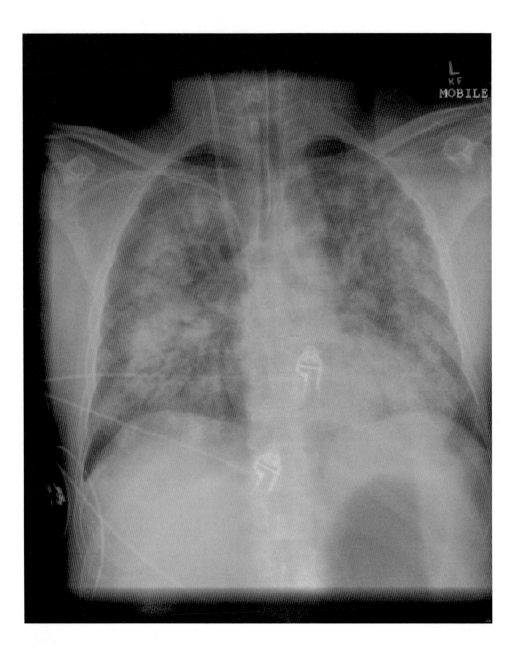

FIGURE 6.6 Alveolar opacification
There are fluffy infiltrates involving both lung fields. A right subclavian central line, a dialysis catheter, an endotracheal tube, a nasogastric tube and overlying monitoring leads are present.

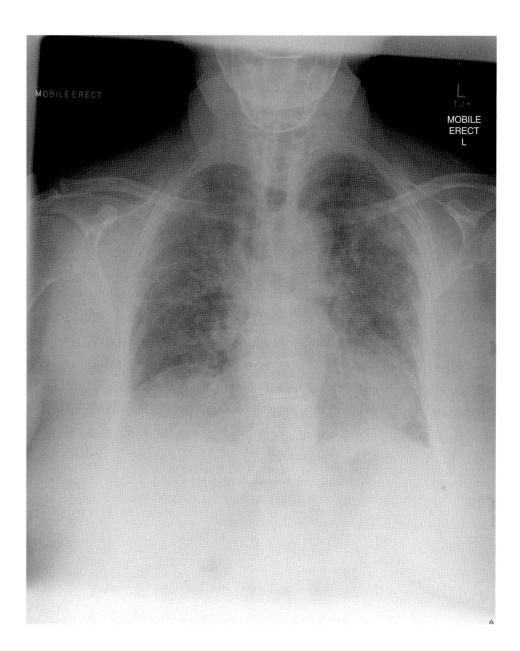

FIGURE 6.7 Interstitial infiltration
There are linear reticular and small nodular opacities affecting both lung fields. The right hemidiaphragm is also elevated.

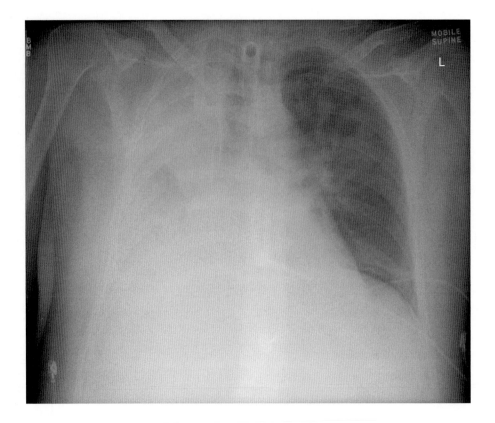

FIGURE 6.8 White-out of hemithorax
There is opacification of the right hemithorax with shift of the trachea (which contains a tracheostomy tube) to the right. There is some aeration of lung in the right lower zone. The patient had collapse of the right lung with associated pleural effusion. Other findings include a right internal jugular and left subclavian central line, monitoring leads and increased markings of the left lung.

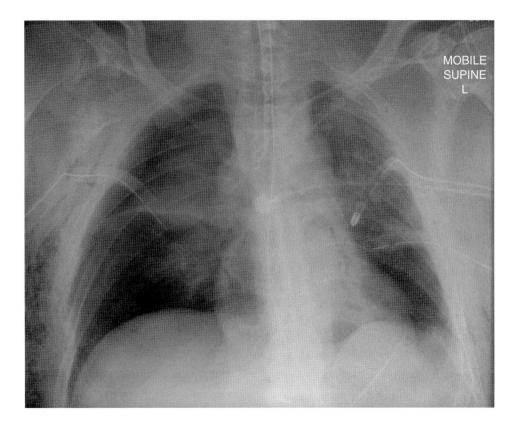

FIGURE 6.9 Chest trauma
There is a right-sided pneumothorax with a visible lung edge and deep sulcus sign. A right-sided chest drain looks kinked in the chest wall, where there is subcutaneous emphysema. There is a well-positioned endotracheal tube, left-sided central venous line, and gastric drainage tube and overlying monitoring leads.

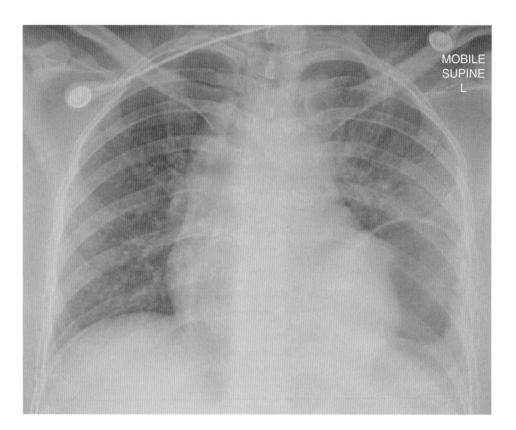

FIGURE 6.10 Ruptured left hemidiaphragm
The left hemidiaphragm is abnormally elevated with gas bubbles representing the stomach and/or intestine. The ipsilateral lung markings are congested, suggesting an element of collapse.

CT scans – chest and neck

A number of thoracic pathologies are best diagnosed with CT scanning. Table 6.2 outlines the key findings in some common conditions. Examples are also provided (Figs 6.11–6.16).

TABLE 6.2 Abnormalities seen on CT scans of the chest and neck	
Pathology	**Findings**
Pulmonary embolism	• Central (pulmonary trunk or main pulmonary arteries to the segmental arteries) or peripherally located emboli (segmental and subsegmental arteries) • Single or multiple lesions • Acute emboli are centrally located within arteries, causing a contrast filling defect or a vessel 'cut-off' sign if it occludes the lumen, classically with distension of the involved vessel • Features suggesting chronic emboli are lesions eccentric and contiguous with the vessel or with recanalisation
Aortic dissection	• Location of intimal tear, extent of the disease, evaluation of the true and false lumens • Flaps in the ascending aorta are easily missed • Stanford classification: A – Ascending aorta B – Distal to the left subclavian
Retrosternal masses	• Retrosternal masses include goitres, lymphadenopathy, thymoma, teratoma and thoracic aortic aneurysm • The airway should be assessed for compression and reduced diameter
Ruptured oesophagus	• Extraluminal air in the mediastinum and surrounding the oesophagus • Mediastinal inflammation with obliteration of mediastinal fat planes • Mediastinal and peri-oesophageal fluid • Oesophageal thickening • Pleural effusions (usually unilateral) • Mediastinal abscess with air-fluid levels • Extravasation of oral contrast into the peri-oesophageal tissues • Rarely a tract at the site of the tear
ARDS	• Early parenchymal consolidation with air bronchograms and ground glass attenuation in the dependent areas; variable pleural effusions, pneumatocoeles or pneumothoraces • Late fibrosis, traction bronchiectasis, lobular distortion and honeycombing
Bronchiectasis	• Bronchial wall thickening • Internal bronchial diameter greater than the adjacent artery • Lack of bronchial tapering, bronchi within 1 cm of the pleura, clusters of cystic spaces • Fluid-filled bronchi • Mediastinal lymphadenopathy

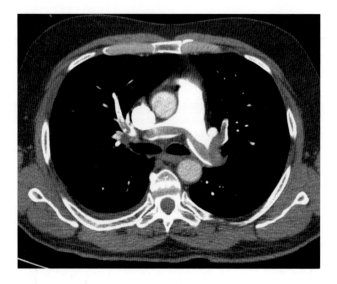

FIGURE 6.11 Saddle pulmonary embolism
This CT pulmonary angiogram shows a tubular clot curled around the pulmonary artery bifurcation.

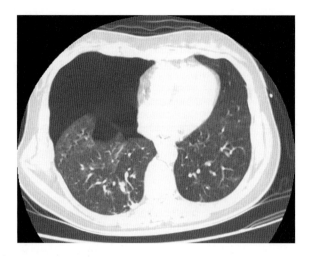

FIGURE 6.12 Pneumothorax
There is a pneumothorax involving the right hemithorax with collapse of the underlying lung. The patient has been scanned in the supine position and so the pneumothorax is located anteriorly. The CXR findings of a pneumothorax are seen in Figure 6.9.

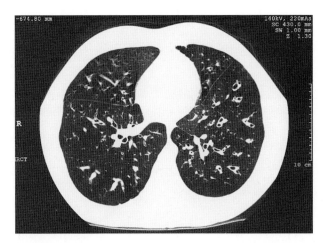

FIGURE 6.13 Bronchiectasis
There are dilated, thickened airways diffusely distributed throughout both lungs.
There is dilatation of airspaces from fibrosis-related traction injury, which is best seen anteriorly.

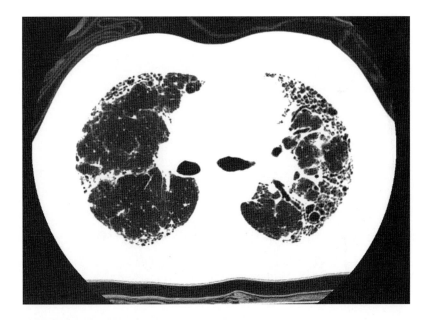

FIGURE 6.14 Severe interstitial lung disease
There are thickened interstitial markings with areas of destruction resulting in a 'honeycomb' appearance, particularly in the left lung.

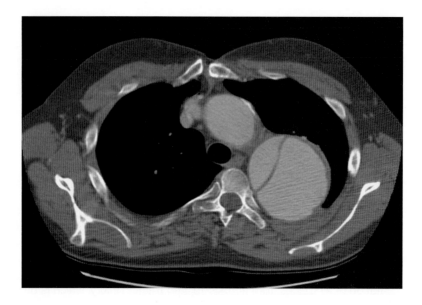

FIGURE 6.15 Aortic dissection with flow in both lumens
There is a markedly dilated descending aorta with a dissection partition. Blood appears to be flowing on both sides of this. The ascending aorta also appears dilated.

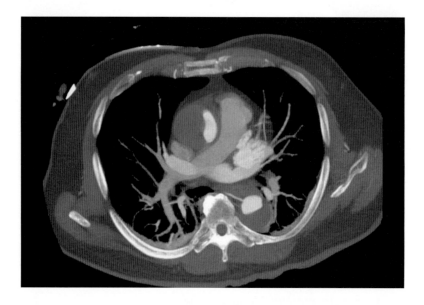

FIGURE 6.16 Aortic dissection with no flow in false lumen
The ascending aorta is dilated and both the ascending and descending aorta have a dissection partition. There is a narrowed lumen with blood flow, compressed by the second lumen, which is most likely filled with clotted blood. Contrast extravastion is seen near the left pulmonary artery, suggesting luminal rupture has occurred.

Abdominal X-rays

CT scans have become the major imaging modality for most intra-abdominal pathology. However, a basic knowledge of plain abdominal films is still required, because they are often used as a screening study in patients unable to be easily transported to a radiology department for more definitive studies. Table 6.3 is a summary of the main abnormalities that may be detected on a plain abdominal X-ray, followed by a number of examples (Figs 6.17–6.19).

TABLE 6.3 Abnormalities seen on abdominal X-rays	
Pathology	Findings
Bowel obstruction	Small bowel: loops dilated >3 cm diameter, centrally located, mucosal valvulae conniventes cross the bowel wall • Number of loops and air-fluid levels increase with more distal levels of obstruction • Multiple air-fluid levels create a 'ladder' appearance • 'Sentinel loops' are limited sections of dilated small bowel adjacent to inflammatory lesions (e.g. pancreatitis, appendicitis) Large bowel: loops dilated >5 cm; caecum >9 cm; peripherally located, mucosal haustrations only partially cross the bowel wall; gas contained within large bowel if the ileo-caecal valve is competent. In mechanical obstruction, may see a 'cut-off' sign with the presence of faeces distal to the point of obstruction, an interface between air-filled colon and solid matter is apparent. Faecal material has a mottled appearance
Volvulus (twisting of bowel around its mesentery)	• Sigmoid: single, large, ovoid, dilated large bowel loop fills the lower abdomen • Caecal: single, large, dilated large bowel loop fills the left upper quadrant, creating an 'empty caecum' sign
Toxic megacolon (inflammatory bowel disease)	Grossly dilated large bowel (>8 cm diameter), usually transverse colon; oedematous bowel wall produces an indented mucosal appearance – 'thumbprint' sign
Duodenal obstruction	'Double-bubble' sign due to air seen in the stomach proximal to the pylorus, then in the duodenum between the pylorus and point of obstruction
Gastric dilatation	Distended air-filled stomach seen with any cause of gastroparesis
Extra-luminal air	• Free gas Crescent-shaped air collection under the diaphragm or in non-dependent location on lateral decubitus films. This is best seen on the right where it is not obscured by stomach gas Rigler's sign (gas on both sides of the bowel wall making the serosal surfaces of the bowel easy to see) Falciform-ligament sign (thin straight line from right upper quadrant to umbilicus, outlined by air) Causes of extra-luminal air: • Post-laparotomy or laparoscopy • Perforated viscus – duodenal ulcer, appendicitis, diverticulitis • Subphrenic abscess – circumscribed air collection above the liver which may have an air-fluid level

Continued

TABLE 6.3 Abnormalities seen on abdominal X-rays—cont'd

Pathology	Findings
	• Gas in biliary tree – branching frond-like streaks of air Normal after sphincterotomy or after biliary surgery; abnormal causes are fistula between biliary tree and bowel, ascending cholangitis • Portal venous gas – similar appearance to gas in biliary tree. Seen with ischaemic bowel, including toxic megacolon and necrotising enterocolitis • Pneumotosis coli – gas within the bowel wall; can progress to pneumoperitoneum; poorly understood and may be benign
Calcification	• Renal tract – from large, complex staghorn calculi in the renal pelvis to single or multiple stones along the line of the ureter (along transverse processes, crossing the sacro-iliac joints to run medial to ischial spines) and in the bladder • Renal parenchymal calcification – renal tubular acidosis, hyperparathyroidism, medullary sponge kidney • Atherosclerotic vessels • Porcelain gallbladder • Pancreatic speckling in chronic pancreatitis • Uterine fibroid
Ascites	Diffuse, hazy appearance to whole film with loss of clarity of structures
Abdominal aortic aneurysm	'Egg-shell' outline of a calcified aorta can permit a rough estimation of the aortic diameter – increased risk of rupture if >4 cm Cannot diagnose rupture on an abdominal X-ray
Gallstone ileus	• Biliary tree gas • Small bowel obstruction • Gallstone – usually large stones which fail to pass beyond the ileo-caecal valve
Organomegaly	Liver – displacement of bowel gas away from the right upper quadrant Spleen – displacement of bowel gas away from left upper quadrant Kidneys – renal outline (between T12 and L2) enlarged (e.g. polycystic kidneys)
Bony abnormalities	• Lytic lesions • Paget's disease • Fractures – spinal fractures are easily missed if you are not systematic in looking for them
Indwelling devices	• Nasogastric, transpyloric and percutaneous enterogastrostomy tubes • Femoral venous lines • IVC filters • Vascular stents • Tenckhoff catheters • TIPS – transjugular intrahepatic portosystemic shunt • Surgical clips • Stoma rings • IUCD – intrauterine contraceptive device • Vaginal pessaries

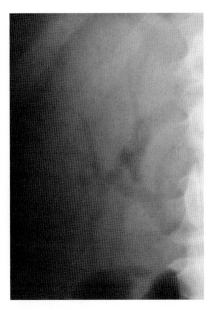

FIGURE 6.17 Air in the biliary tree
This magnification of the right upper quadrant of a plain abdominal X-ray
demonstrates gas outlining the biliary tree.

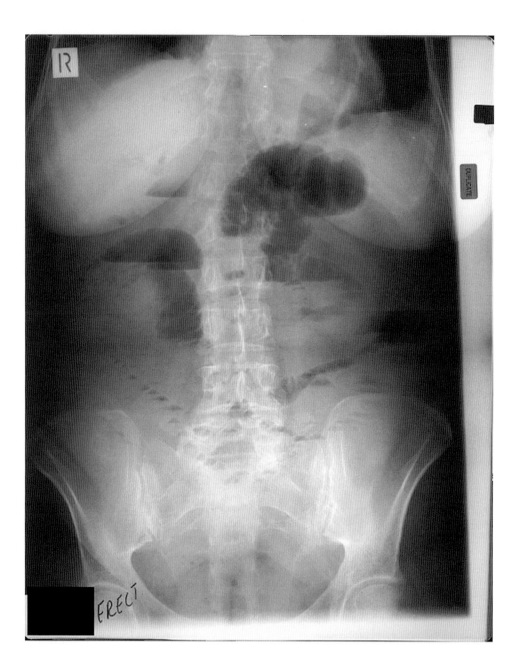

FIGURE 6.18 Small bowel obstruction – erect

This erect abdominal X-ray shows central dilated loops of bowel, many of which have air–fluid levels. The appearances are those of a small bowel obstruction (the linear markings – plicae circulares – extend completely across the lumen). There is no gas visible in the large bowel.

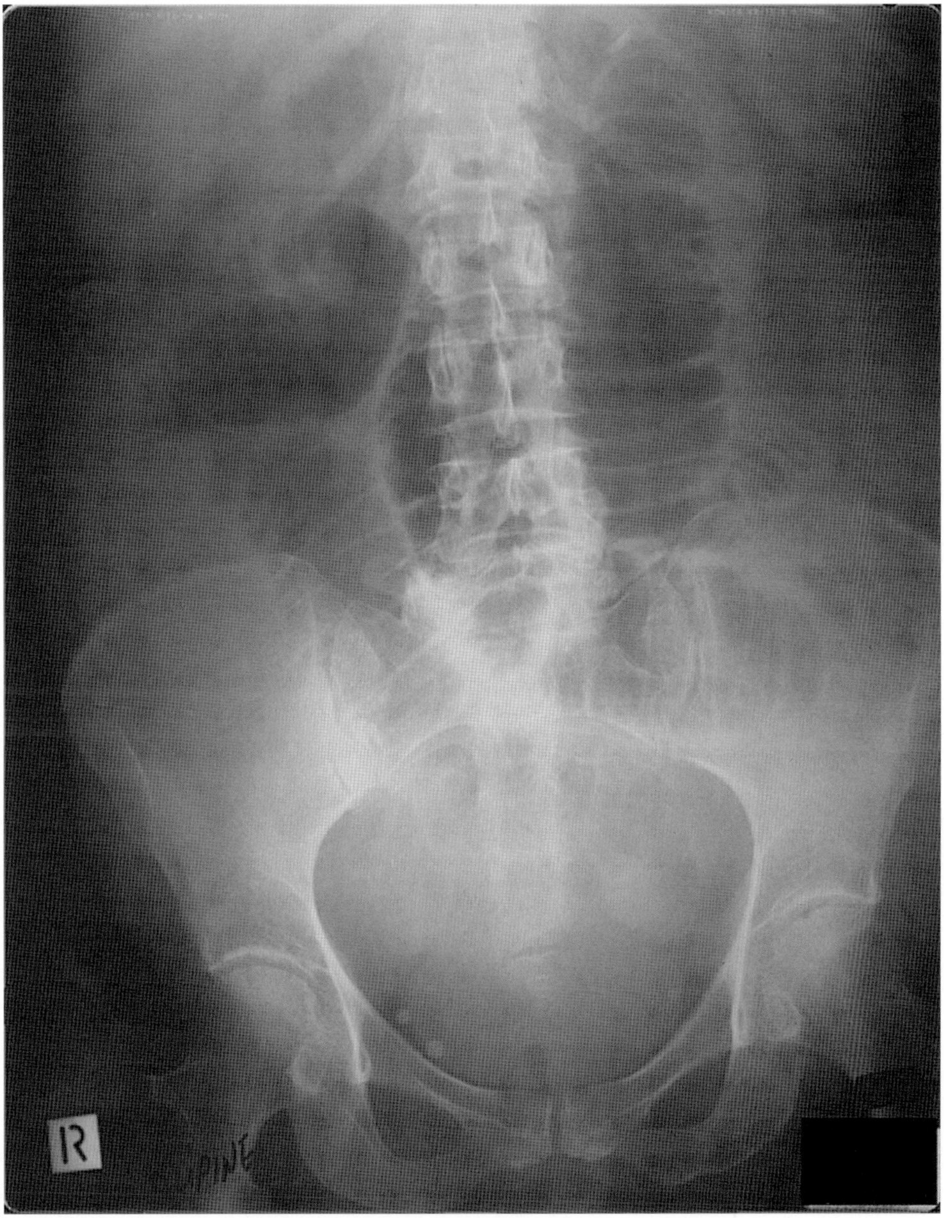

FIGURE 6.19 Small bowel obstruction – supine
This supine film also shows central dilated bowel loops with plicae circulares, but there are no air–fluid levels as the intra-luminal fluid has layered in a dependent fashion posteriorly and therefore cannot be visualised. Phleboliths can be seen within the pelvis.

Abdominal ultrasound

In certain circumstances ultrasound examination of the abdomen may be the most efficient and practical imaging modality. Tables 6.4 and 6.5 provides a number of such examples.

TABLE 6.4 Abnormalities seen on abdominal ultrasound	
Pathology	**Findings**
Cholecystitis	• Acalculous cholecystitis: gallbladder wall thickening >3 mm in a non-collapsed gallbladder; striated gallbladder secondary to wall oedema; sonographic Murphy's sign (localised gallbladder tenderness); pericholecystic fluid (without generalised ascites); mucosal sloughing; intramural gas; echogenic bile (sludge); gallbladder distension (>5 cm transverse diameter) • Calculous cholecystitis: same features plus echogenic gallstones which may be impacted in the gallbladder neck
Obstructed renal tract	• Should be routinely performed in the presence of acute renal failure. • Unilateral or bilateral • Dilated caliceal system, renal distortion and perinephric oedema, hydronephrosis with ureteric dilatation • Obstructing masses or calculi • Obstruction occasionally may not produce hydronephrosis
Abdominal aortic aneurysm	• May diagnose aortic dilatation • Poor sensitivity for detection of rupture (ileus often accompanies rupture and the gas degrades images, leading to false negative diagnoses)

TABLE 6.5 Specific ultrasound scans	
Scan type	**Findings**
FAST (Focused Abdominal Sonography for Trauma)	Controversial role in blunt trauma victims with haemodynamic instability (alternative to diagnostic peritoneal lavage (DPL) or exploratory laparotomy)
	Screens for free fluid (usually dark and anechoic in appearance), gross solid organ injury and pericardial tamponade
	Four views: • perihepatic – Morison's (hepatorenal) pouch • perisplenic – splenorenal recess • pelvic – pouch of Douglas (female) or rectovesical pouch (male) • pericardial – subxiphoid and parasternal views
Duplex scan kidneys	May demonstrate: • renal artery stenosis • renal artery obstruction (e.g. arterioembolism, aortic dissection) • renal vein thrombosis (e.g. procoagulant states, renal cell carcinoma)
Post liver transplant duplex ultrasound	May demonstrate: • fluid collections (may indicate ongoing bleeding, bile leakage, infection or ascites) • portal vein thrombosis or stenosis • hepatic artery thrombosis, stenosis, pseudoaneurysm • IVC stenosis or thrombosis • bile duct strictures – anastomotic or non-anastomotic

CT scans – abdomen

A number of abdominal pathologies are best diagnosed with CT scanning. Table 6.6 outlines the key findings in some common conditions. Some examples are also provided (Figs 6.20–6.24).

TABLE 6.6 Abnormalities seen on CT scans of the abdomen	
Pathology	Findings
Abdominal trauma	Solid organ injury: • Spleen, liver and renal injuries, ranging from subcapsular haematomas and lacerations to major parenchymal disruption; hilar devascularisation, intraperitoneal bleeding; associated lower rib fractures Hollow organ injury: • Stomach, duodenal, bowel and mesenteric injuries may be missed, especially on early scans Bladder and urethral injuries are better imaged with retrograde urethrography Other injuries: • Pancreatic injury associated with liver, spleen and duodenal (including common bile duct) injury • Diaphragmatic injury may be missed, especially with positive pressure ventilation • Retroperitoneal haematoma – may be due to injury to the lumbar spine, bony pelvis, kidney, intraperitoneal bladder or colon, pancreas, duodenum or major vascular injury
Acute pancreatitis	Gold standard, non-invasive method of diagnosing pancreatic necrosis is multiphase contrast-enhanced abdominal CT scanning. Non-viable tissue fails to enhance due to the abnormal microvasculature. Ideally performed 72 hours after the onset of symptoms. Grades of peripancreatic inflammation (as per Balthazar) are as follows: A Normal pancreas B Focal or diffuse pancreatic enlargement C Pancreatic gland abnormalities associated with peripancreatic inflammation D Single fluid collection E Two or more fluid collections and/or gas present in or adjacent to the pancreas
Adrenal haemorrhage	• Hyperdense mass-like lesion enlarging the adrenal gland • May be spontaneous (e.g. Waterhouse-Friderichsen syndrome in meningococcal sepsis) or secondary to an underlying adrenal abnormality (e.g. tumour or infection)
Psoas abscess	• Enlarged swollen psoas muscle(s) with hypodense centres and contrast enhancement • Associated causes – lumbar vertebral abscess, renal abscess, bowel perforation, metastatic infection (e.g. staphylococcal sepsis), TB and clostridial infections
Ruptured abdominal aortic aneurysm	• High-attenuation extravasated blood in acute rupture – iso- and low-attenuation appearance with subacute and chronic rupture • 'Crescent' sign – enhancement within the mural thrombus of the aneurysm is a sign of impending rupture • Peri-aortic fat stranding is commonly seen in contained or imminent rupture • Peri-aortic fibrosis outside subintimal calcification is a feature of an inflammatory aneurysm • Soft tissue inflammatory changes outside, but adjacent to the aorta may occur with inflammatory processes in adjacent organs

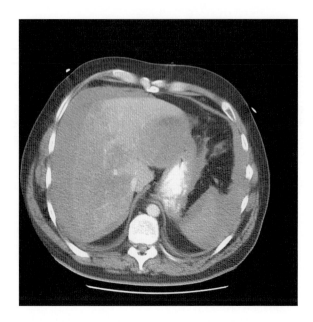

FIGURE 6.20 Traumatic liver injury
There are multiple, low-density hypoperfused areas throughout the left and right lobes of the liver with a separate low-density cresenteric area surrounding the right lobe. The appearances are consistent with multifocal liver haemorrhage with a right subcapsular haematoma. Similar changes are seen around the spleen.

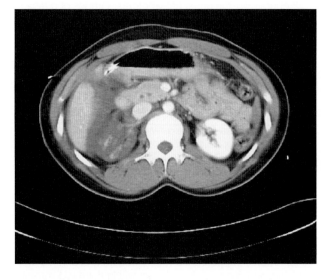

FIGURE 6.21 Traumatic renal injury
The right kidney is enlarged, irregular and poorly enhancing. There is evidence of a perinephric collection extending to the right lobe of the liver. The appearances are consistent with a traumatic renal vascular injury and/or renal parenchymal injury. Note the contrast in the IVC – a distended IVC suggests adequate volume status – and the presence of a NG tube in the stomach.

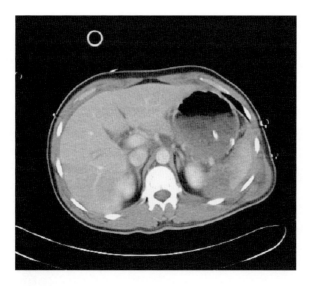

FIGURE 6.22 Traumatic rupture of the spleen
The normal architecture of the spleen has been grossly disrupted. Adjacent soft tissue
swelling is also noted.

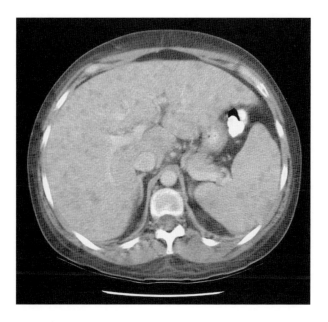

FIGURE 6.23 Metastatic lymphoma
In addition to hepatosplenomegaly, there are innumerable focal hypodensities within
the liver and spleen.

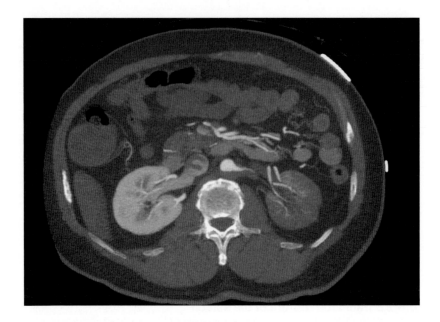

FIGURE 6.24 Impaired renal perfusion
This contrast study shows normal right renal perfusion, although there appears to be a filling defect in the right renal artery. The left kidney has grossly reduced perfusion and a more well-defined filling defect obstructing flow into the left renal artery.

CT scans – head

In Table 6.7 the findings of common pathologies that may appear on CT head scans are presented. This is followed by a review of normal basic neuroanatomy (Fig 6.25) which may be readily identified, complemented by some classical abnormalities (Figs 6.26–6.31).

TABLE 6.7 Abnormalities seen on CT scans of the head	
Pathology	Findings
Features suggesting raised intracranial pressure	• Effacement of basal cisterns • Loss of grey–white differentiation • Loss of sulcal-gyral clarity • Midline shift • Herniation of cerebellar tonsils into foramen magnum • Uncal herniation: shift of brainstem and distortion of adjacent cisterns, dilation of contralateral temporal horn, posterior cerebral artery compression with infarction of this vascular territory
Traumatic brain injury	• Coup and contrecoup injuries • Skull fractures: base of skull or vault; closed or open with intracranial air; opacification of the sinuses from blood • Contusions • Haemorrhages: extradural, subdural, subarachnoid, intracerebral • Diffuse axonal injury with punctate white matter haemorrhages
Cerebral infarction	• Anterior cerebral artery distribution • Middle cerebral artery distribution • Posterior cerebral artery distribution • Watershed distribution (hypotensive injury) • Basal ganglia (hypoxic injury)
Cerebral haemorrhage (high-density signal with acute bleeding)	• Extradural (lens-shaped, convex, confined within the suture lines) • Subdural (follows contour of brain surface, concave, blood passes across a suture line) • Subarachnoid (within CSF spaces) • Intracerebral
Non-traumatic subarachnoid haemorrhage	• Blood outlining the brain surface, Sylvian fissure and in the CSF spaces (lateral ventricles, third ventricle, fourth ventricle, aqueduct, interventricular foramen, cisterns – pontine, quadrigeminal, ambient, supra-sellar) • Non-obstructive hydrocephalus • Component of intracerebral haemorrhage or infarction in a vascular distribution (most commonly an anterior cerebral artery distribution complicating a ruptured anterior communicating artery aneurysm) • Calcified berry aneurysm or arteriovenous malformation
Mass lesions	• Tumours: secondary deposits are most common in adults; glioblastoma multiforme is usually a complex lesion with loss of architecture and necrosis • Cerebral abscess: ring of contrast enhancement; single or multiple lesions; complex partitioning seen with hydatid cysts

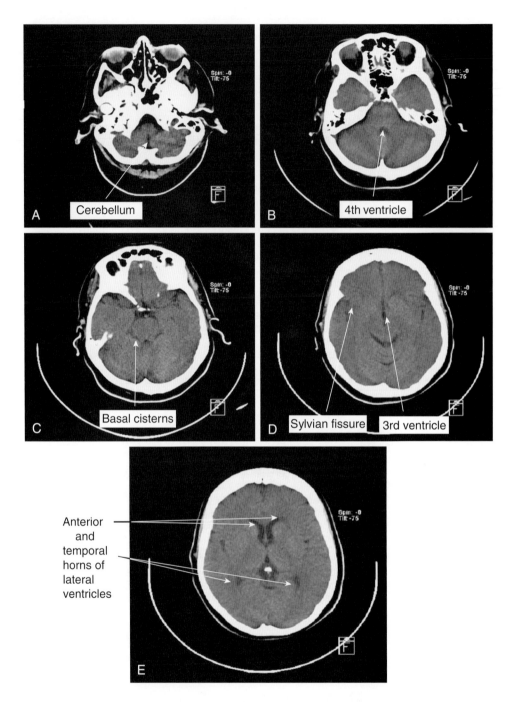

FIGURE 6.25A–E Normal basic neuroanatomy seen on CT scan from the cerebellum progressively upwards
Candidates should possess a rapid means of assessing the CT scan. To do this it is useful to develop 'pattern recognition' of the normal anatomical features, which are then contrasted with abnormal scans.

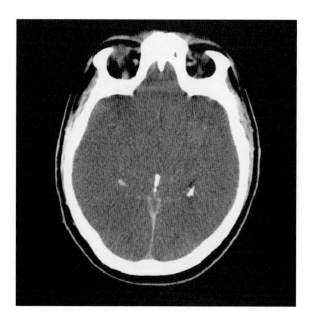

FIGURE 6.26 Diffuse cerebral oedema
There is loss of grey–white differentiation and obliteration of the ventricular system.

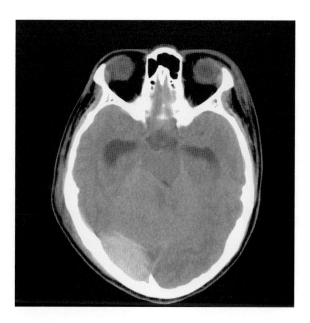

FIGURE 6.27 Extradural haematoma
There is a lens-shaped opacity compressing the right occipital lobe with associated cerebral oedema causing distortion of the midbrain and obliteration of the quadrigemminal cistern. The blood is confined within the suture lines. The temporal horns are dilated.

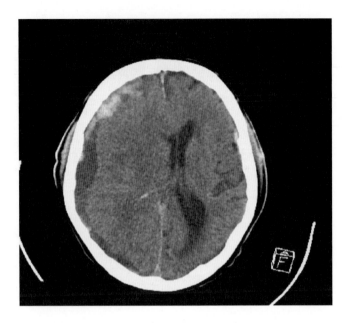

FIGURE 6.28 Acute on chronic subdural haematoma
There is abnormal space occupying material that has collected over the surface of the brain on the right, consistent with subdural haematoma. The blood passes across the suture lines. The high-density opacification represents acute bleeding and intermingles with hypodense chronic bleeding. There is massive midline shift to the left with compression of the right ventricular system.

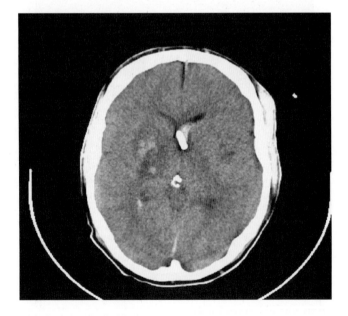

FIGURE 6.29 Diffuse axonal injury
There are foci of haemorrhage in the region of the right internal capsule, with acute blood in the anterior horn of the left lateral ventricle. There is loss of grey–white differentiation and an external ventricular drain is in situ.

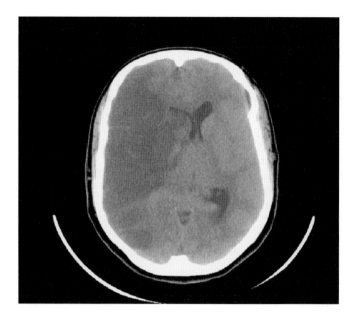

FIGURE 6.30 Right middle cerebral artery territory infarct
Extensive hypodensity of cerebral tissue in the middle cerebral artery territory is
present with predominant involvement of the parietal lobe. There is associated diffuse
cerebral oedema with midline shift and loss of grey–white differentiation.

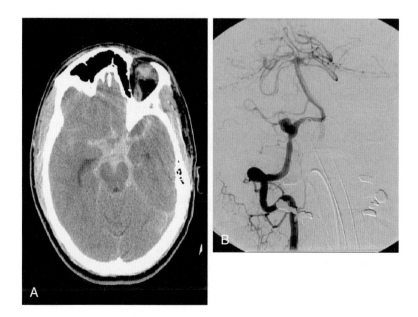

FIGURE 6.31A & B Subarachnoid haemorrhage
A) The CSF spaces are outlined diffusely by high-density fluid representing acute
bleeding in the subarachnoid space. B) The cerebral angiogram shows a berry
aneurysm of the right middle cerebral artery.

Skeletal and soft tissue imaging

Fractures and dislocations appearing on axial and peripheral skeletal films are common. Lesions are described by the structure(s) involved. Dislocation and subluxation are described with reference to the normal anatomical position. Fractures may be transverse, oblique, spiral or comminuted.

Interpretation of some major pathology involving facial bones is provided in Figure 6.32.

The normal cervical spine is shown in Figure 6.33. It is supplemented with a number of examples of pathologies (Figs 6.34–6.38). Important types of fractures that should be readily identifiable on spinal imaging are shown in Figure 6.39.

An approach to assessing pelvic X-rays is shown in Figures 6.40–6.41. There are a number of radiologic classification systems for pelvic fractures. Arguably the Tile classification is the most simple and widely known.

Other pathologies are reviewed in Table 6.8 and an example is given in Figure 6.42.

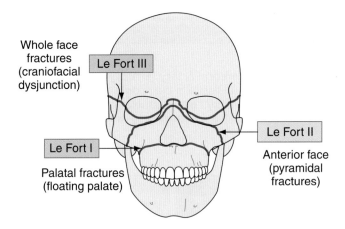

FIGURE 6.32 Le Fort classification of facial fractures
A range of facial injuries (involving both the mandible and cranium) may threaten the airway. The Le Fort classification is often used to classify craniofacial injuries, with fractures classified on each half of the face separately.

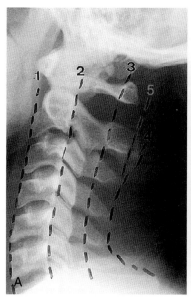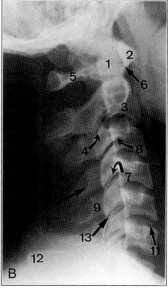

FIGURE 6.33A & B Cervical spine X-rays
The entire cervical spine must be imaged from the craniocervical junction to the T1 vertebral body. A systematic method of examination is essential in order to adequately assess for injuries.

A After ensuring that all vertebrae of interest are present, the 5 'lines' should be traced, with any loss of the smooth outlines raising suspicion about injury.
   • Line 1 = anterior vertebral line
   • Line 2 = posterior vertebral body line
   • Line 3 = spinolaminal line
   • Line 4 = line along the tip of the spinous processes
   • Line 5 = the line along the base of the spinous processes of C1–C3. This should be a straight line ± 1 mm
The interspinous distances gradually reduce from C3 to T1.
Soft tissues should also be inspected, with abnormally increased diameters raising concerns about occult injury.
Useful 'normal values' for prevertebral soft tissue diameters are:
   • Odontoid peg to C1 level = 3 mm for an adult and 5 mm for a child
   • At C2 = less than half the same level vertebral body width
   • At C3–4 = less than 40% of the same level vertebral body width
   • C5–7 = on inspiration should be no greater than 14 mm for children and 22 mm for adults
B Key anatomical features should then be inspected closely. These are numbered as follows:

   1. Odontoid peg
   2. Anterior arch of C1
   3. C2 body
   4. Superior articular process
   5. Posterior arch of C1
   6. Atlantodental space
   7. Inferior articular process
   8. Pedicle
   9. Lamina
   10. Base of spinous process
   11. C5–6 disc space
   12. C7 spinous process (vertebra prominens)
   13. C5–6 joint

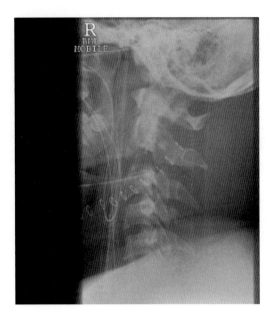

FIGURE 6.34 C2 fracture

There is a 'tear drop' fracture of the inferior corner of C2 vertebral body. There is associated facet dislocation with abnormal widening of the C2–3 intervertebral space. A nasogastric tube is curled back on itself in the pharynx. The film is an inadequate lateral as only the C5–6 interspace level is seen.

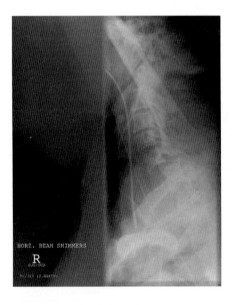

FIGURE 6.35 Swimmer's view with dislocation

There is a 50% C5 on C6 anterior dislocation. This view was used extensively in the past before CT became more available and rapid to help visualise all cervical vertebrae in patients with inadequate standard lateral views.

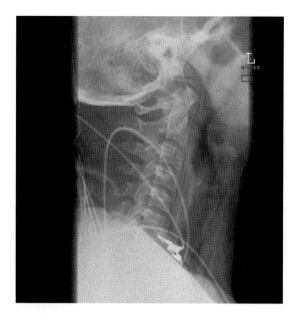

FIGURE 6.36 Subcutaneous emphysema
The soft tissue planes of the anterior neck are outlined by linear streaks of air.
This patient was in a motorbike accident and sustained a bronchial injury with a
bronchopleural fistula.

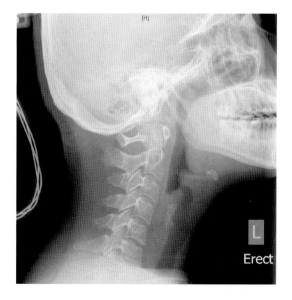

FIGURE 6.37 Epiglottitis
The epiglottis is swollen resembling a thumb in profile rather than a linear flap –
termed the 'thumbprint' or 'thumb sign'.

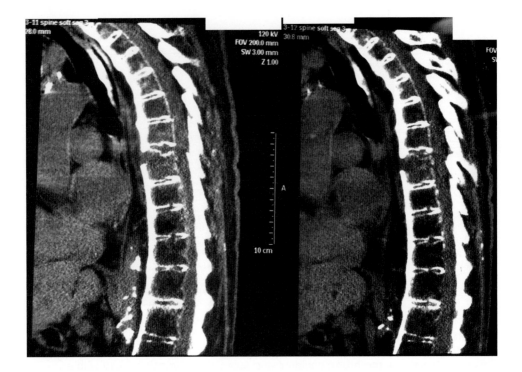

FIGURE 6.38 Ankylosing spondylitis with fracture
There are syndesmophyles present throughout all levels displayed, most prominent anteriorly. The vertebral bodies are abnormally squared, the natural curvature lost and there is a fracture involving the mid thoracic region.

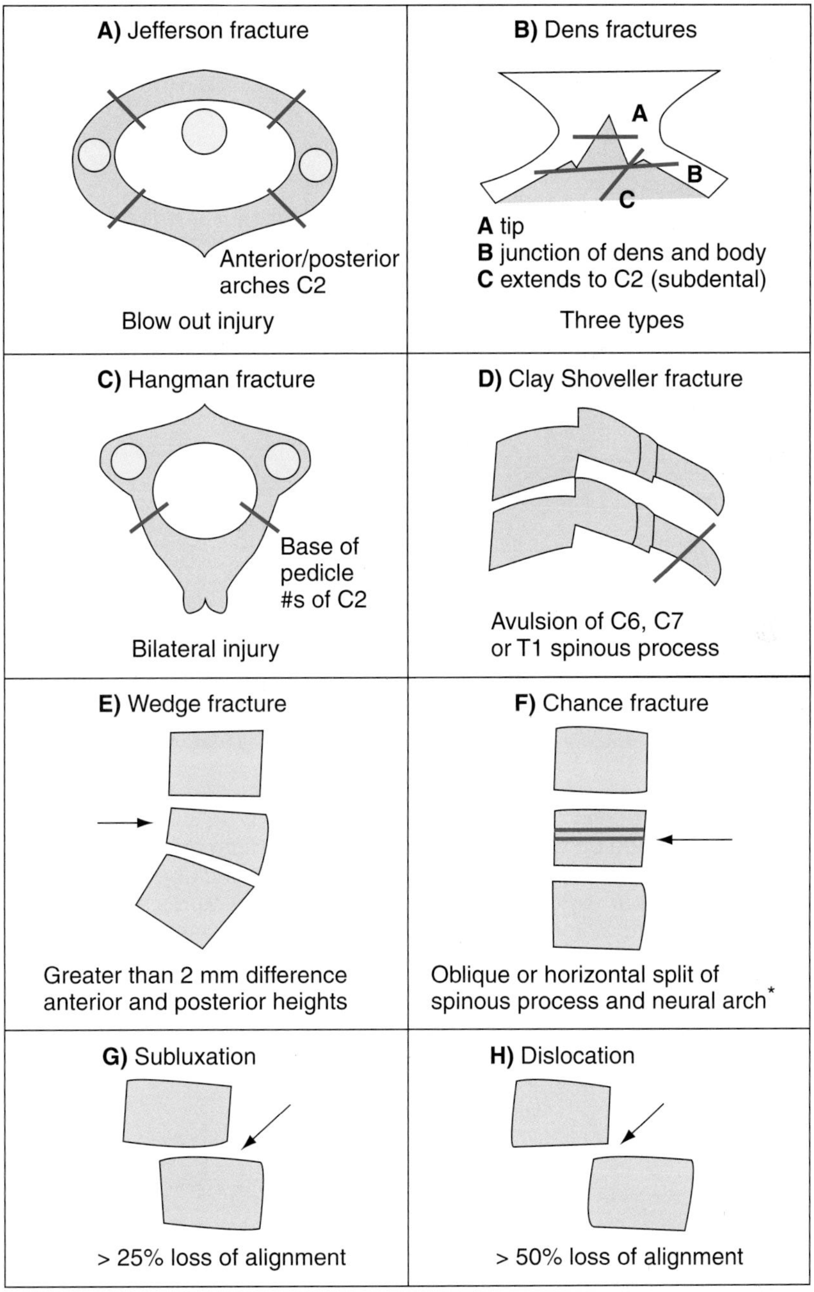

A) Jefferson fracture	B) Dens fractures
Anterior/posterior arches C2	A tip B junction of dens and body C extends to C2 (subdental)
Blow out injury	Three types
C) Hangman fracture	D) Clay Shoveller fracture
Base of pedicle #s of C2	
Bilateral injury	Avulsion of C6, C7 or T1 spinous process
E) Wedge fracture	F) Chance fracture
Greater than 2 mm difference anterior and posterior heights	Oblique or horizontal split of spinous process and neural arch*
G) Subluxation	H) Dislocation
> 25% loss of alignment	> 50% loss of alignment

*Called horizontal fissure fracture if it extends to anterior vertebral body.

FIGURE 6.39A–H Spinal fractures

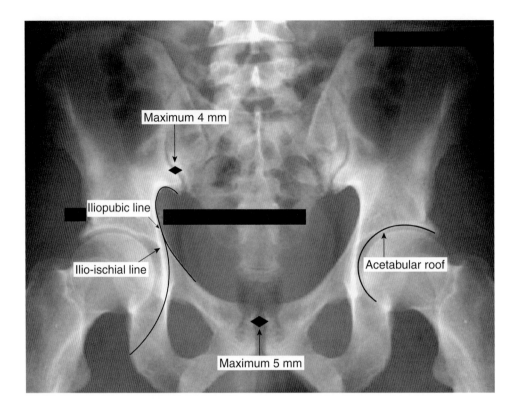

FIGURE 6.40 X-ray pelvis
Each hemipelvis is made up of the fusion of the ilium, ischium and pubis. The articulations with the sacrum and femoral heads should be included on films. The femurs and lower lumbar vertebrae should be inspected. Fractures should also be suspected if the smooth outlines of the iliopubic and ilioischial lines are lost. Pathological increases in the normal iliosacral and pubic joint lucencies must be appreciated as markers of instability.

A)   Tile A fractures – stable

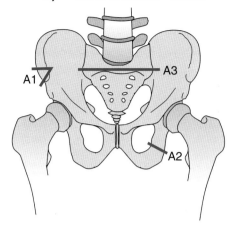

— Fracture line

A1 Avulsion injury not
involving the pelvic ring

A2 Minimally displaced
stable isolated ring
fracture

A3 Transverse sacral
fractures

B)   Tile B fractures – vertically stable, rotationally unstable

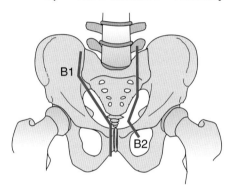

— Fracture line

B1 Unilateral rotationally unstable fracture
complex

B2 Lateral compression injury with internal
rotational instability

B3 Bilateral injuries

C)   Tile C fractures – rotationally and vertically unstable

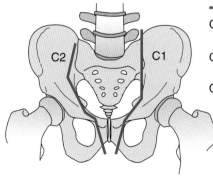

— Fracture line

C1 Unilaterally vertical unstable fracture
(complete loss of integrity of sacroiliac joint)

C2 Bilateral injury—one side is vertically
unstable but the other side is a B injury

C3 Bilateral C1 injuries

FIGURE 6.41A, B & C Tile classification of pelvic fractures

TABLE 6.8 Other skeletal and soft tissue abnormalities seen on X-ray

Pathology	Findings
Arthritis	Osteoarthritis • Subchondral sclerosis and cysts, joint space narrowing, osteophytes Rheumatoid arthritis • Soft tissue swelling and erosions with cartilage and bone destruction, evidence of associated osteoporosis • Deformity with subluxations and dislocations – classic ulnar deviation of wrists and radial deviation of fingers; Z, Swan-neck and Boutonnière digital deformities • Cervical spine disease with odontoid peg erosion and atlanto-axial subluxation Gout • Great toe metacarpophalangeal joint most common site • Intra- and extra-articular tophaceous deposits • Relative sparing of articular cartilage
Ankylosing spondylitis	Syndesmophytes – ossification of the outer layers of the annulus fibrosis (Sharpey's fibres), 'bamboo spine', squaring of vertebrae, loss of the normal lumbar lordosis and thoracic kyphosis, obliteration of sacroiliac joints
DISH (Diffuse Idiopathic Skeletal Hyperostosis)	• Ossification of anterior longitudinal ligament • Large bony excrescences along the spine • Associated with heterotopic calcification at surgical sites (e.g. after joint replacements)
Osteomyelitis	• Soft tissue swelling • Periosteal elevation • Cortical and medullary lucencies • Sequestrum and involucrum
Bone lesions	Osteolytic (radiolucent lesions): • Metastases (e.g. non-small cell lung cancer, melanoma, non-Hodgkin's lymphoma, squamous cell carcinoma of the aerodigestive tract, renal cell carcinoma, thyroid carcinoma) • Multiple myeloma – classic punched out lesions with a 'pepper-pot' skull Primary bone tumours (e.g. giant cell tumour, osteoblastoma, chondroblastoma, fibroma, Ewing's sarcoma) • Brown tumour – hyperparathyroidism Osteoblastic (radiosclerotic lesions): • Metastases (e.g. prostate, carcinoid, Hodgkin's lymphoma, small cell carcinoma of the lung) Mixed osteolytic and osteosclerotic lesions: • Metastases (e.g. breast and squamous cell carcinomas) • Primary bone tumours (e.g. osteoma, osteosarcoma) • Paget's disease • Hyperparathyroidism • Avascular necrosis • Osteopetrosis • Stress fractures

Continued

TABLE 6.8 Other skeletal and soft tissue abnormalities seen on X-ray —cont'd

Pathology	Findings
Paget's disease	Lytic and sclerotic phases Skull – large lytic lesions, especially of frontal and occipital bones described as 'osteoporosis circumscripta' Vertebral bodies – sclerotic or enlarged with prominent cortices, causing a 'picture-frame' appearance Pelvis – early thickening of the ileo-pectineal line, varied degrees of lucency and sclerosis, protrusion acetabuli from weakened acetabular bone Long bones – areas of lysis, thickening and sclerosis with bowing – classic 'sabre tibia' (differential diagnosis of sabre tibia includes rickets, syphilis, yaws and leprosy)
Spinal deformity	Scoliosis (side bend) Kyphosis (forward bend) Spondylolisthesis (forward shift) – pars interarticularis defect with 'scottie dog' collar appearance
Soft tissue calcification	Dystrophic calcification – small to large deposits in damaged tissues Metastatic calcification (causes calciphylaxis) – finely speckled calcification (e.g. lower limbs, blood vessels, kidneys, lungs, gastric mucosa) Osteosarcoma – Codman's triangle – subperiosteal elevation and thickening with surrounding 'sun-ray' spiculation
Epiglottitis	Lateral soft tissues of the neck – classic 'thumbprint' sign

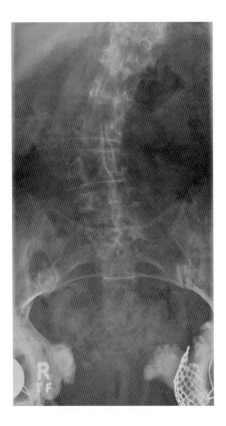

FIGURE 6.42 Scoliosis
There is a notable lumbar region scoliosis with a convexity to the right. There are associated degenerative changes with loss of the normal intervertebral joint spaces. Incidental bilateral hip joint prostheses with cement in the acetabular regions.

Other imaging modalities

A complex description of how MR images are generated is not practical in this book and readers are again directed to the radiology text, Joyce et al., Diagnostic Imaging in Critical Care. All images carry details of the type of sequences used and a single study may use multiple modalities. Detailed interpretation of MR images is beyond the scope of what is expected of examination candidates. Gross pathologies should be recognised, and could include epidural abscesses and herpes simplex encephalitis (Table 6.9).

Nuclear medicine imaging is infrequently utilised in the critical care setting. However, HIDA scans to diagnose acalculous cholecystitis, white cell scans to help localise occult inflammatory foci, and red cell scans to pinpoint the source of gastrointestinal bleeding may be helpful in select patients.

Angiography is helpful in certain circumstances, particularly for the detection and anatomical definition of aneurysms, arteriovenous malformations and vascular disruptions involving central and peripheral structures (e.g. cerebral, aortic and peripheral vascular structures). It is therefore possible that classical overt images of these types could be included in examinations. An example is provided in Figure 6.43.

TABLE 6.9 MRI	
Pathology	Findings
Epidural abscess	Homogeneous enhancement of the affected area during the early inflammatory phase Later there is formation of a liquefying abscess, surrounded by inflammatory tissue which shows varying degrees of peripheral enhancement with gadolinium
Herpes simplex encephalitis	T2 MRI reveals hyperintensity in oedematous temporal lobes (especially medially), inferior frontal lobes and insula, usually sparing the basal ganglia Foci of haemorrhage Patchy parenchymal or gyral enhancement

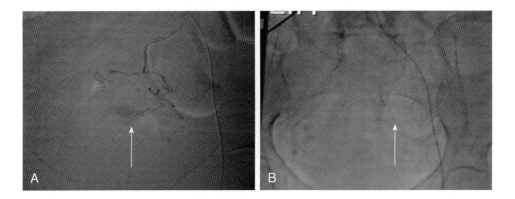

FIGURE 6.43A & B Brisk PR bleeding
A CT angiogram of the abdomen suggested this patient had an actively bleeding vessel in the rectum. Selective angiography was performed and a catheter inserted into the rectal branches of the inferior mesenteric artery (A). When contrast was injected, a 'blush' of extravasation confirmed the site of bleeding and embolisation was performed (B).

Electrocardiographs

Those experienced in reading ECGs will rapidly identify major abnormalities. An ECG that appears normal on first glance will need to be subjected to a rigorous systematic assessment. Items such as T-wave flattening in hypokalaemia, or a bifid P wave suggesting mitral valve disease, will otherwise be missed. A systematic approach to ECG interpretation is vital. One useful approach is to assess rate, rhythm, axis, P wave, P–R interval, QRS complex, QT interval duration, ST segment heights and T wave.

A broad range of potentially and previously examined ECG abnormalities is provided in Table 6.10, supplemented by simple and important findings that may be used to make the diagnosis. Common causes, as well as the treatment of these pathologies should be known.

TABLE 6.10 Common ECG patterns and abnormalities

Problem	Findings
Acute myocardial infarction	Convex ST elevation with reciprocal ST segment depression Variable Q waves, T-wave peaking or inversion and disturbances of rate and rhythm • Anterior – elevation in V2–4 • Lateral – elevation in V3–5, I, aVL • Inferior – elevation in II, III, aVF • Posterior – Dominant R in V1 without features of RV hypertrophy, ST depression V1–3
Pericarditis	Diffuse concave 'saddle-shaped' ST segment elevation across all leads, PR segment depression Causes: myocardial infarction, uraemia, rheumatoid arthritis, SLE, trauma, surgery, Dressler's syndrome, viruses (e.g. coxsackie), bacteria (e.g. TB, rheumatic fever), malignancy, radiotherapy
Electrical alternans	Alternating axis with each beat due to swinging of the heart within a fluid-filled pericardium
Conduction blocks	• Right bundle branch block – broad complex QRS with RSR1 pattern in V1s Causes: normal variant, atrial septal defect, pulmonary embolus • Left bundle branch block – broad complex QRS with 'M' pattern of QRS complex in lateral leads Causes: hypertension, ischaemic heart disease, cardiomyopathy • Left anterior hemiblock – left axis deviation associated with other evidence of conduction delay • Left posterior hemiblock – right axis deviation with other evidence of conduction delay • First-degree heart block – prolonged PR interval (>0.2 secs) • Second degree heart block Mobitz type 1 (Wenckebach) – cyclical progressive PR interval lengthening, then failure to conduct a beat Mobitz type 2 – normal AV conduction then complete loss of conduction with a P wave without a QRS Causes of first/second-degree heart block: normal variant, myocardial ischaemia, sick sinus syndrome, athletes, drugs (e.g. AV-nodal, beta-adrenergic, and calcium channel blocking agents) • Third-degree (complete) heart block – complete loss of relationship of P waves with QRS complexes; broad complex ventricular 'escape' rhythm Causes of complete heart block: congenital, myocardial ischaemia, drugs (e.g. AV-nodal, beta-adrenergic, and calcium channel blocking agents), cardiac surgery, myocardial trauma, cardiomyopathy (e.g. Lyme carditis, acute rheumatic fever, *Trypanosoma cruzi* infection) • Bifascicular and trifascicular block – evidence of two or three types of block on the same trace (e.g. Mobitz type 2 plus axis deviation of a hemiblock and/or a bundle branch block). Remember that LBBB is a bifasicular block
Sinus arrhythmia	Beat-to-beat variation in the interval between the QRS complexes with a regular pattern of increasing, then slowing the rate. Reflects the normal increase in heart rate on inspiration. More accentuated in children than adults

Continued

TABLE 6.10 Common ECG patterns and abnormalities—cont'd

Problem	Findings
Significant axis deviation	• Right axis (+90 to +180 degrees) – predominant downward QRS deflection in I Causes: right ventricular hypertrophy, pulmonary embolus, anterolateral myocardial infarction, Wolff-Parkinson-White (WPW), left posterior hemiblock, atrial septal defect, ventricular septal defect • Left axis (–30 to –90 degrees) – predominant downward QRS deflection in II Causes: left anterior hemiblock, inferior myocardial infarction, WPW, emphysema, ostium primum atrial septal defect, tricuspid atresia
Chamber hypertrophy	• Right atrial – peaked P waves with 'shark-fin' appearance (called P pulmonale), most obvious in inferior leads • Left atrial – bifid P waves (called P mitrale), best seen in lateral leads • Right ventricular – right axis deviation, dominant R in V1, T wave inversion in V1–3, deep S wave V6 • Left ventricular – deep S in V2 and tall R in V5 (sum of S and R wave is >35 mm)
Atrial fibrillation	Irregularly irregular rhythm with narrow QRS complexes, unless a bundle branch block co-exists; P waves of varying morphology may be seen within the baseline, blurring with T waves
Atrial flutter	Narrow complex regular tachycardia with 'saw-tooth' appearance of the baseline Regular or variable rate of ventricular conduction (commonly 2:1 conduction with a ventricular rate of 150/min)
Wandering pacemaker	Multiple P wave morphologies with normal nodal conduction and narrow regular QRS complexes
Atrial tachycardia	Narrow complex regular tachycardia with inverted P waves, best seen in the inferior leads
Accessory pathways	• WPW syndrome – short PR interval with delta waves (slurred upstroke of QRS), tall R in V1–3 in type A; predominant deflection downwards V1–3 in type B • Lown-Ganong-Levine syndrome – short PR interval without delta waves Both are associated with very rapidly conducted atrial arrhythmias; drugs that block the AV node (e.g. adenosine, verapramil, diltiazem, beta-blockers) are contraindicated as they increase conduction down the aberrant pathway
Junctional rhythm	Narrow complex regular tachycardia without P waves
Ventricular tachycardia	• Monomorphic – regular broad complex tachycardia • Polymorphic (Torsades de pointes) – broad complex tachycardia with cyclical complexes that vary about an isoelectric axis
Broad complex tachycardia	Classical diagnostic issue of differentiating VT from SVT with aberrant conduction VT favoured on the ECG if there is a QRS width greater than 140 ms, AV dissociation, fusion or capture beats, QRS complexes inconsistent with a bundle branch morphology or significant axis deviation

Continued

TABLE 6.10 Common ECG patterns and abnormalities—cont'd

Problem	Findings
Ventricular fibrillation	Broad complex, irregularly irregular tachycardia with a random axis
Paced rhythms	• Atrial pacing – pacing 'spikes' followed by P waves; narrow QRS complexes if conduction subsequently via AV node • Ventricular pacing – pacing spikes followed by broad QRS complexes. Classically left bundle branch pattern (LBBB) • Dual chamber pacing – atrial and ventricular pacing spikes with variable evidence of native atrial and ventricular conduction activity
Long QT (>0.44 secs)	QT interval varies with rate. Corrected QT interval: $QT_C = (QT)/\sqrt{(R-R)}$. Prolonged QT interval may progress to polymorphic VT Causes: drugs (erythromycin, sotalol, quinidine, procanamide, amiodarone, cisapride, domperidone, antihistamines, tricyclic antidepressants, phenothiazines); electrolyte abnormalities (hypokalaemia, hypomagnesaemia, hypocalaemia); myocardial ischaemia, hypothermia, head injury and congenital syndromes (Jervell-Lange and Nielsen, Romano-Ward)
Brugada syndrome	RSR pattern with downward-sloping ST elevation in V1–2; predisposes to ventricular arrhythmias
Digoxin effect	ST segment depression appearing like a 'reverse tick'
Hypertrophic obstructive cardiomyopathy	Left ventricular hypertrophy with marked, diffuse, deep anterolateral T wave inversion
Small QRS complex	Causes include non-standard gain on ECG machine, thick chest wall, pericardial effusion, severe hypothyroidism
Electrolyte disturbances	• Hyperkalaemia – peaked T waves, small P waves, prolonged QRS progressing to sine wave morphology • Hypokalaemia – U waves, T wave flattening and inversion, prolonged PR interval • Hypocalcaemia – prolonged QT interval • Hypercalcaemia – short QT interval
Pulmonary embolism	Range of findings, including sinus tachycardia, supraventricular arrhythmias, right axis deviation, P pulmonale, 'S1 Q3 T3', right ventricular strain, RBBB
Causes of a tall R in V1	WPW type A; dextrocardia; right ventricular hypertrophy; posterior infarction
Hypothermia	Osborne or 'J' waves deforming the downstroke of the QRS complexes; slow atrial fibrillation is common, with ventricular arrhythmias upon rewarming
Dextrocardia	Right axis deviation, inverted P wave in I, dominant R in aVR, lack of R wave progression across chest leads with V6 still showing a right ventricular pattern

Haemodynamic monitoring

Central venous lines, arterial lines, pulmonary artery catheters, oesophageal Doppler and pulse contour analysis methods (e.g. PiCCO, LiDCO and FloTrac/Vigileo) are important sources of data, which, when appropriately interpreted, may provide useful information that can guide patient management.

Central venous pressure waveforms

A normal waveform that should be visualised after insertion of a central venous line is presented in Figure 6.44. Table 6.11 outlines some abnormalities and their significance. Catheters, such as the Edwards PreSep™ oximetry catheter, are capable of measuring central venous oxygen saturation ($ScvO_2$) continuously.

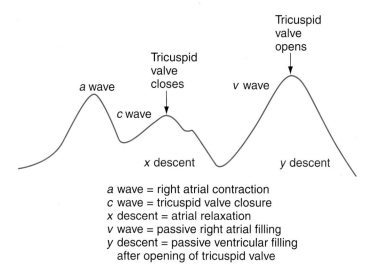

a wave = right atrial contraction
c wave = tricuspid valve closure
x descent = atrial relaxation
v wave = passive right atrial filling
y descent = passive ventricular filling
  after opening of tricuspid valve

FIGURE 6.44 Normal central venous pressure waveform

TABLE 6.11 CVP waveform analysis	
Characteristic	**Significance**
Dominant *a* wave	Pulmonary hypertension, tricuspid and pulmonary stenosis
Cannon *a* wave	Occurs with atrioventricular dissociation Causes: Complete heart block, single chamber ventricular pacing, nodal rhythm
Dominant *v* wave (common)	Tricuspid regurgitation
Absent *x* descent	Atrial fibrillation with tricuspid regurgitation
Exaggerated *x* descent	Pericardial tamponade, constrictive pericarditis
Sharp *y* descent	Severe tricuspid regurgitation, constrictive pericarditis
Slow *y* descent	Tricuspid stenosis, right atrial myxoma

Mixed venous oxygen saturation (SvO₂) and central venous oxygen saturation (ScvO₂)

SvO_2 and $ScvO_2$ measure the relationship between oxygen consumption and oxygen delivery. Measurement of SvO_2 requires the insertion of a pulmonary artery catheter, whereas measurement of $ScvO_2$ uses a central venous catheter. In health the SvO_2 is generally higher than the $ScvO_2$, because the upper body extracts more oxygen than the lower. This relationship changes in shock states. Although the values of SvO_2 and $ScvO_2$ may differ, the trend is similar. The differential diagnosis for major deviations of $ScvO_2$ and SvO_2 is provided in Figure 6.45.

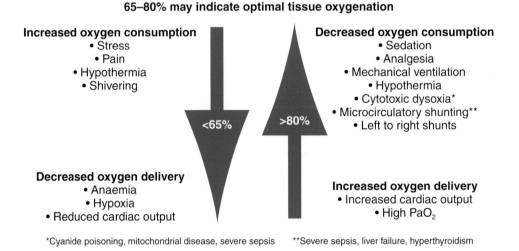

65–80% may indicate optimal tissue oxygenation

Increased oxygen consumption
- Stress
- Pain
- Hypothermia
- Shivering

Decreased oxygen consumption
- Sedation
- Analgesia
- Mechanical ventilation
- Hypothermia
- Cytotoxic dysoxia*
- Microcirculatory shunting**
- Left to right shunts

<65%   >80%

Decreased oxygen delivery
- Anaemia
- Hypoxia
- Reduced cardiac output

Increased oxygen delivery
- Increased cardiac output
- High PaO₂

*Cyanide poisoning, mitochondrial disease, severe sepsis   **Severe sepsis, liver failure, hyperthyroidism

FIGURE 6.45 Interpretation of SvO₂ and ScvO₂

Arterial waveforms

The characteristics of a normal arterial waveform are shown in Figure 6.46, and a summary of the important variations in Table 6.12.

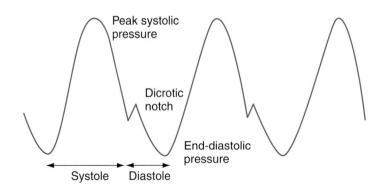

Peak systolic pressure

Dicrotic notch

End-diastolic pressure

Systole   Diastole

FIGURE 6.46 Normal arterial waveform

TABLE 6.12 Arterial waveform analysis

Characteristic	Significance
Pulsus paradoxus (>10 mmHg reduction in systolic pressure during inspiration in the spontaneously breathing patient and expiration in the positively pressure ventilated patient)	Reduced left ventricular preload, pericardial tamponade, severe bronchospasm
Pulsus alternans (alternating beats of higher systolic pressure)	Pericardial effusion or severe left ventricular failure
Pulse deficit (every QRS complex is not accompanied by a transmitted beat)	Atrial fibrillation, ectopic atrial or ventricular beats
Slow upstroke	Severe aortic stenosis or reduced myocardial contractility
Wide pulse pressure	Aortic regurgitation
Narrow pulse pressure	Elevated systemic vascular resistance
Location of dicrotic notch (should be at least one-third of the height of the systolic peak)	Low dicrotic notch suggests low systemic vascular resistance

Intra-aortic balloon pump waveforms

Knowledge of a normal, well-timed balloon trace (Figure 6.47) is essential in order to understand and recognise the features of poorly timed balloon inflation and deflation (Figs 6.48–6.51).

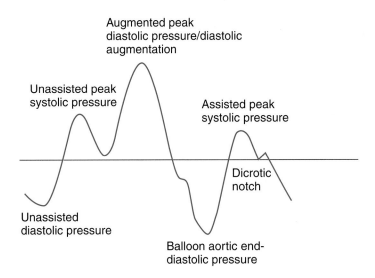

FIGURE 6.47 Normal waveform with 2:1 balloon inflation

Key features visible on a well-timed balloon trace are:
- Inflation just prior to the dicrotic notch
- Balloon aortic end diastolic pressure less than the patient aortic end-diastolic pressure
- Assisted peak systolic pressure less than the unassisted peak systolic pressure

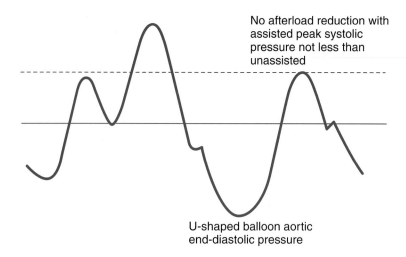

No afterload reduction with assisted peak systolic pressure not less than unassisted

U-shaped balloon aortic end-diastolic pressure

FIGURE 6.48 Early balloon deflation

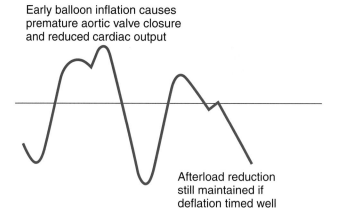

Early balloon inflation causes premature aortic valve closure and reduced cardiac output

Afterload reduction still maintained if deflation timed well

FIGURE 6.49 Early balloon inflation

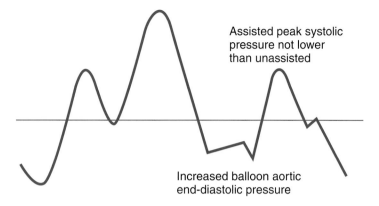

Assisted peak systolic
pressure not lower
than unassisted

Increased balloon aortic
end-diastolic pressure

FIGURE 6.50 Late balloon deflation

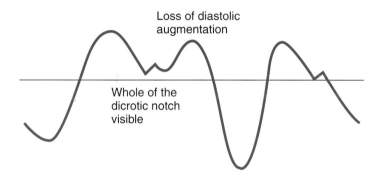

Loss of diastolic
augmentation

Whole of the
dicrotic notch
visible

FIGURE 6.51 Late balloon inflation

Pulmonary artery catheters

Normal waveforms that should be identified during the insertion of a PA catheter can be seen in Figure 6.52. Candidates have been asked to draw this in previous exams. Conventionally, the 'wedge' value or occlusion pressure is measured at the end of expiration and provides a surrogate estimate of left atrial pressure. Candidates should be able to readily calculate parameters such as systemic vascular and pulmonary vascular resistance. Normal values are provided in Table 6.13. Figure 6.53 illustrates some classical patterns of data and the likely causes of these scenarios.

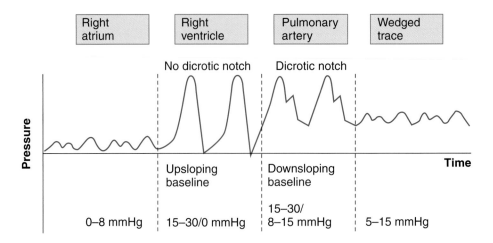

FIGURE 6.52 Pulmonary artery catheter waveforms

TABLE 6.13 Normal haemodynamic parameters obtained from pulmonary artery catheters	
Variable	**Normal range**
Mean arterial pressure (MAP)	90 mmHg (65–85 mmHg acceptable in a ventilated patient)
Central venous pressure (CVP)	0–5 (rises to 8–15 mmHg in a ventilated patient)
Right ventricular pressure	Systolic 15–25 mmHg/Diastolic 0–8 mmHg
Pulmonary artery pressure	Systolic 15–25 mmHg/Diastolic 8–15 mmHg
Mean pulmonary artery pressure (MPAP)	10–20 mmHg
Pulmonary artery occlusion pressure (PAOP)	10–20 mmHg
Cardiac output/index	3.0-5.0 L/min/2.5–4.5L/min/m^2
Systemic vascular resistance/index (SVR/I) = (MAP–CVP)/CO or CI	770–1500 dyne-s/cm^5 – 1760–2600 dyne-s/cm^5/m^2
Pulmonary vascular resistance/index (PVR/I) (MPAP–PAOP)/CO or CI	20–120 dyne-s/cm^5 – 44–225dyne-s/cm^5/m^2
Stroke volume	1 mL/kg

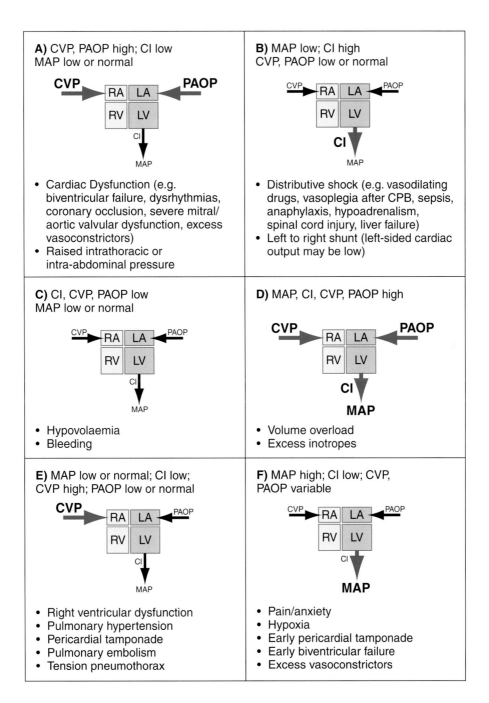

FIGURE 6.53A–F Interpretation of pulmonary artery catheter data

Newer haemodynamic measurement devices

In recent years less invasive devices have become available that permit measurement of haemodynamic values, such as the PiCCO, LiDCO, FloTrac/Vigileo, which use continuous pulse contour analysis. The role and accuracy of these devices is still the subject of considerable debate. An overview of how PiCCO data can be interpreted, both at the bedside and when encountered in examinations, is provided (Table 6.14).

TABLE 6.14 Interpretation of PiCCO data			
ITBVI	**Cardiac index**	**EVLWI**	**Interventions to consider**
Low	Normal or high	High	Diurese for improved pulmonary function
Low	Normal or high	Low	Volume load for improved tissue perfusion
Low	Low	High	Cautious volume loading in conjunction with vasoactive drugs – vasoconstrictor/dilator and inotrope balance based on SVR and effect of chosen therapy
Low	Low	Low	Fluid load
High	Normal or high	High	Volume restrict and consider diuresis for improved pulmonary function
High	Normal or high	Low	Observe
High	Low	High	Cautious diuresis in conjunction with vasoactive drugs – vasoconstrictor/dilator and inotrope balance based on SVR and effect of chosen therapy
High	Low	Low	Vasoactive drugs – vasoconstrictor/dilator and inotrope balance based on SVR and effect of chosen therapy

The PiCCO, LiDCO and Flotrac/Vigileo pulse contour analysis methods also enable stroke volume variation (SVV) or pulse pressure variation (PPV) to be calculated in patients receiving controlled mechanical ventilation. Patients with values less than 10% are considered to be unlikely to improve their cardiac output with fluid loading.

Oesophageal Doppler

The oesophageal Doppler technique is minimally invasive and provides real-time continuous cardiac output monitoring. Spectral analysis of the Doppler shift obtained from the oesophageal Doppler gives velocity time waveforms (Fig 6.54). Candidates may be asked to comment on measured variables and different waveforms.

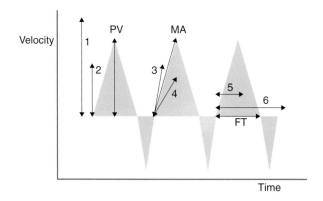

FIGURE 6.54 Oesophageal Doppler waveforms
PV = peak velocity (normally 70–100 cm/s)
   1. Increased velocity (e.g. inotropes)
   2. Decreased velocity (e.g. LV failure)
MA = mean acceleration
   3. Increased slope (e.g. increased contractility state)
   4. Decreased slope (e.g. decreased contractility state)
FT = flow time (normally 330–360 ms)
   5. Decreased time (e.g. hypovolaemia, vasoconstrictors)
   6. Increased time (e.g. vasodilatation)
Area under the velocity vs time curve is proportional to stroke volume (SV)
CO = SV × HR

Echocardiography

Ultrasound examination of the heart is a widely available investigation that may provide useful morphologic and haemodynamic information about critically ill patients. Transthoracic (TTE) and transoesophageal echocardiography (TOE) are complementary investigations. A range of factors, including equipment availability, patient body habitus and the cardiac structure that needs to be visualised, determine preference for one over the other. Intensive care specialists should be proficient in understanding the role of two-dimensional, M-mode and Doppler techniques, and be able to recognise common and important abnormalities. In some centres echocardiography has become the dominant modality used to characterise the nature of major haemodynamic disturbances. Basic interpretation of 2-D images or echo reports are considered reasonable exam questions, whereas full reporting of echo images would be well beyond the scope of the exam requirement at this time. Therefore this section aims to serve as a reference source.

Understanding the anatomy of structures visualised with common transthoracic windows is the key to interpreting pathologies. Figure 6.55A and 6.55B illustrate some of the most useful views.

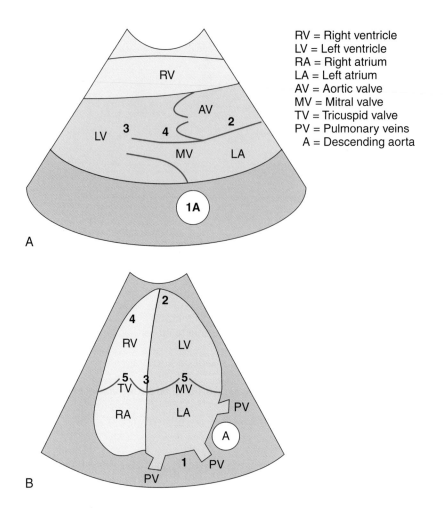

RV = Right ventricle
LV = Left ventricle
RA = Right atrium
LA = Left atrium
AV = Aortic valve
MV = Mitral valve
TV = Tricuspid valve
PV = Pulmonary veins
A = Descending aorta

FIGURE 6.55A Parasternal long-axis window
1. Descending aorta – this structure is used to differentiate pleural from pericardial effusions, with pericardial fluid localising anterior and pleural fluid posterior to this vessel.
2. The aortic root and left atrium in cross-section should be a similar diameter in this view or one of these structures may be abnormally dilated.
3. A cursor placed as a fixed reference point in the middle of this chamber may be used to assess the contractility of ventricular wall segments.
4. Both the aortic and mitral valve opening and closing may be visualised.

FIGURE 6.55B Apical four-chamber window
1. This view may readily detect pericardial effusions that classically spare the bare area around the left atrium where the pulmonary veins enter.
2. In a true four-chamber view the left ventricle should appear at its most elongated.
3. A distinct cross appearance is seen at the centre of the image.
4. The right ventricle is often well visualised and major changes, such as dilatation and reduced contractility, may be identifiable.
5. Both the mitral and tricuspid valve opening and closing may be visualised.

Abnormalities to look for
Pericardial effusion and tamponade
- Effusion may appear as a variable amount of poorly echo-reflective 'black' fluid in the pericardial space – circumferential or localised (e.g. over the right heart) and possibly with echo-dense fibrin strands.
- Pericardial tamponade is suspected when right atrial and/or ventricular diastolic collapse is seen.

Aortic dissection
- TOE is superior to TTE because it allows visualisation of ascending and descending aortic defects.
- TOE can detect and localise a dissection intimal flap, true and false lumens and proportionate flow-down lumens (e.g. spontaneous echo contrast in lumen with sluggish flow); in type A dissections aortic regurgitation, pericardial effusion and tamponade and region wall motion abnormalities heralding coronary artery occlusion may also be seen.

Abnormal left ventricular wall thickness
- Left ventricular hypertrophy: >1.5 cm systolic wall thickness.
- Left ventricular thinning (e.g. infarct scarring, dilated cardiomyopathy): <0.6 cm systolic wall thickness.

Left ventricular systolic dysfunction
- Visual assessment of regional and global function gives a good estimate if the operator is experienced.
- M-mode can assess LV cavity dimensions, wall motion and thickness throughout the cardiac cycle and can be used to calculate:

Fractional shortening = percentage change in LV internal dimensions between systole and diastole (normally 30–45%)

Ejection fraction = percentage change in LV volume between systole and diastole (normally 50–85%); can also be assessed with 2-D echo using Simpson's method.

Other useful measures:

Stroke volume = LV diastolic volume – LV systolic volume

Cardiac output = stroke volume × heart rate

Left ventricular diastolic dysfunction
- Also known as preserved ejection fraction heart failure.
- Evidence of abnormal LV stiffness and impaired relaxation may be seen alone or in combination with systolic dysfunction.
- M-mode 'slow relaxation' diastolic changes in the motion of the anterior mitral valve leaflet; sensitive (but not specific) markers:
  - reduced leaflet excursion during passive atrial filling (small E wave)
  - increased contribution of atrial systole (prominent A wave)
  - reduced E:A ratio (normally the E wave is greater than the A wave)
  - prolonged acceleration time of the E wave (time from start of diastole until the peak of the E wave).
- May also see abnormalities associated with diastolic dysfunction – LV hypertrophy, myocardial infiltration, ischaemic changes.

Aortic stenosis
- Obstruction may be supravalvular, valvular or subvalvular, but valvular is the most common (e.g. bicuspid valve, calcific degeneration).
- Continuous Doppler permits estimation of the peak velocity and therefore pressure gradient across the valve using the Bernoulli equation:

$$\text{pressure gradient} = 4 \times \text{peak velocity across the narrowing}^2$$

A normal peak gradient is <10 mmHg and in severe disease this may be >60 mmHg; >70 mmHg is considered 'critical'.
- Valve area is calculated using the continuity equation:
  - a normal area is 2.5–5.5cm^2 and in 'critical' disease this may be <0.75 cm^2; this is a better marker of severity in the presence of LV dysfunction, as velocity calculations may be misleading in low flow states.
- Abnormal cusp number, thickening, calcification and movement may be seen.
- Complications such as LV hypertrophy, LV dilatation, systolic and diastolic dysfunction and post-stenotic aortic dilatation should be noted.

Mitral stenosis
- Rheumatic valve disease accounts for most cases.
- Note thickened, calcified leaflets, which are strongly echogenic but indistinct. The anterior mitral leaflet has a characteristic 'hockey-stick' appearance from fusion and reduced mobility at the tip, but intact cusp mobility with long-axis views. A tight 'fish-mouth' appearance is seen on short-axis views.
- Classic M-mode pattern of abnormal mitral valve leaflet opening and closure from restricted, fused leaflets, posterior leaflet is pulled towards the anterior leaflet and the A wave is often lost because atrial fibrillation is usually present.
- LA dilatation may be massive.
- Features of severity include:
  - valve area <1 cm^2 (normally 4–6 cm^2) – determined from pressure half time – the time taken for the pressure gradient to reach half its peak value which is equivalent to the time taken for the peak blood velocity to reach 0.7 of its value (valve area = 220/pressure half time)
  - pressure gradient >10 mmHg
  - pulmonary hypertension.

Aortic regurgitation
- Colour Doppler shows site and size of the regurgitant jet during diastole.
- Features of severity in chronic AR include:
  - LV dilatation (e.g. LV end-systolic diameter >5.5 cm)
  - large jet size filling the LV (e.g. a jet extending to the LV apex)
  - a large regurgitant orifice (e.g. >60% of the aortic width at the cusps)
  - reversal of diastolic flow in the aortic arch
  - pressure half time <300 ms – time taken for the maximum pressure gradient across the aortic valve to drop to half its normal value – determined from the fall in velocity measured with continuous wave Doppler.
- The underlying cause may be evident (e.g. bicuspid valve, thickened leaflets of a connective tissue disorder, endocarditis, aortic root dilatation, aortic dissection).

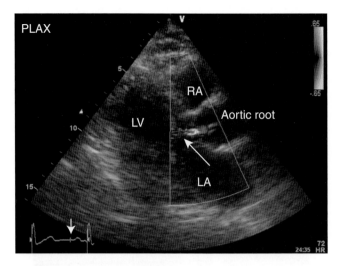

FIGURE 6.56 Aortic valve regurgitation
At early to mid diastole, there is a regurgitant jet of blood flowing backwards into the outflow tract. (The timing in the cardiac cycle is critical to diagnosis of valve jets – see arrows.)

Mitral regurgitation
- Colour Doppler shows site and size of the regurgitant jet during systole.
- Features of severity in chronic MR include:
  - a large regurgitant orifice – wide jet measured at the leaflet tips
  - large jet size filling the LA
  - reversal of systolic flow in the pulmonary veins
  - pulmonary hypertension
  - dilated LV and LA.
- The underlying cause may be evident (e.g. dilated LV with regional wall motion abnormalities and functional MR, rheumatic leaflets, endocarditis, ruptured chordae or papillary muscle, HOCM with SAM).

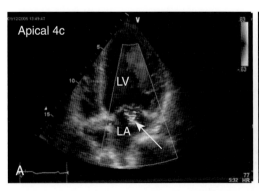
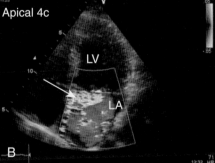

FIGURE 6.57A & B Mitral valve regurgitation
A The LV appears dilated and there is a small regurgitant jet of MR. The leaflets appear normal and the MR related to dilatation of the valve ring.
B There is a large jet of MR associated with marked LA dilatation. This patient had moderately severe MR when this was quantified.

Endocarditis (Fig 6.58)
- TOE is superior to TTE.
- Vegetations, most often attached to valves, of varying size – usually mobile echo-reflective masses.
- Native, diseased (e.g. calcific, rheumatic) or prosthetic valves.
- Tricuspid valves, especially in intravenous drug abusers.
- Complications, including valve obstruction or regurgitation, leaflet perforation, spread of vegetation to adjacent structures and abscess formation.

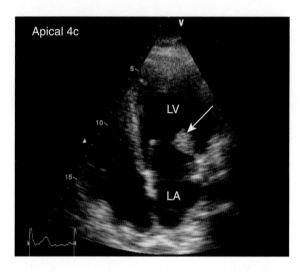

FIGURE 6.58 Mitral valve endocarditis
There is a large globular abnormal mass attached to the anterior mitral valve leaflet. Vegetations are generally attached to the ventricular side of valve leaflets.

Dilated cardiomyopathy
- Dilated chambers, especially involving the left ventricle with thinning and reduced contractility (ejection fraction and fractional shortening) of the ventricle walls – classically a global pattern.
- 'Spontaneous echo contrast' and thrombi.

Restrictive cardiomyopathy
- Normal or mildly increased chamber sizes.
- Impaired ventricular contractility (ejection fraction and fractional shortening).
- Impaired diastolic function with a restrictive filling pattern – abnormal motion of the anterior mitral valve leaflet with M-mode:
  - very tall E wave
  - small A wave
  - short deceleration time of the E wave (time from the E wave peak until where the deceleration slope meets the baseline)
- May see evidence of infiltration (e.g. amyloid) – thickening of the walls with patches of high-intensity 'speckling' ('starry sky').

Hypertrophic obstructive cardiomyopathy
- Asymmetrical left ventricular hypertrophy – septum involved more than the free wall (ratio >1.5:1), variable right ventricular hypertrophy (>0.5 cm wall thickness) and diastolic dysfunction.

- Systolic anterior movement (SAM) of the mitral valve apparatus.
- Dynamic outflow tract obstruction with an increased peak pressure gradient below the aortic valve with continuous wave Doppler (>50 mmHg).
- Mid-systolic mitral valve closure.

Takotsubo cardiomyopathy (transient apical ballooning syndrome) (Fig 6.59)
- Bulging of the left ventricular apex.
- Hypercontractile base.

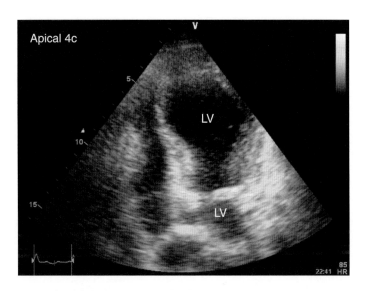

FIGURE 6.59 Takotsubo cardiomyopathy
At the end of systole the LV has a balloon-like appearance with contraction of the basal segments, but dilatation of the apical region (the 'octopus pot' of Takotsubo syndrome).

Acute myocardial infarction
- Can detect wall motion and wall-thickening abnormalities of ischaemic/infarcted myocardium – can assess distribution and predict the likely culprit: the coronary artery.
- May demonstrate complications – systolic and diastolic dysfunction, acute MR (papillary muscle infarction or ruptured chordae tendinae), VSD, pericardial effusion and tamponade (free wall rupture), mural thrombus, ventricular aneurysm and pseudoaneurysm.

Right ventricular dysfunction
- RV dilatation is obvious if RV is the same size or larger than the LV. May see gross RV dilatation with bulging of the interventricular septum and a compressed LV with diastolic dysfunction. Hypokinesis of varying severity is usually graded as mild, moderate or severe. The apex is classically spared in pulmonary embolism (McConnell's sign).
- Should also look for features of pulmonary hypertension.

Pulmonary hypertension
- Pulmonary artery systolic pressure >30 mmHg or mean >20 mmHg at rest.
- TOE superior to TTE, especially if associated lung disease (e.g. COPD).

- Can diagnose and detect severity – most often Doppler can approximate pulmonary artery systolic pressure (PASP) using tricuspid valve velocity (V_{TR}), the estimated JVP (or measured CVP) and the Bernoulli equation:

$$PASP = RVSP = 4V_{TR}^2 + CVP$$

- May see a dilated PA (greater than the aortic diameter), RA dilatation, RV dilatation and/or hypertrophy or a possible predisposing cause (e.g. LV failure, mitral or aortic valve disease, shunts, pulmonary embolism).

Shunts
- Atrial septal defect – patent foramen ovale common (approximately 30% of the general population) (Fig 6.60A); ostium secundum defects more common than ostium primum lesions; TOE superior to TTE.
- Ventricular septal defect – most often congenital or infarct-related; usually involves upper membranous or lower muscular septum.
- Bubble contrast study ± Valsalva manoeuvre (e.g. agitated saline is rapidly injected into a vein) – bubbles are seen crossing a shunt which may otherwise be missed.
- Left to right shunt commonly seen with colour Doppler and flow velocity calculated with continuous wave Doppler (Fig 6.60B).
- High-pressure gradients correlate with smaller shunts.
- If irreversible pulmonary hypertension occurs causing shunt reversal – termed Eisenmenger syndrome.

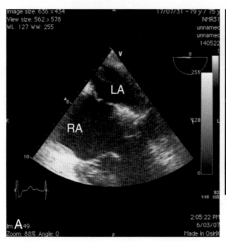
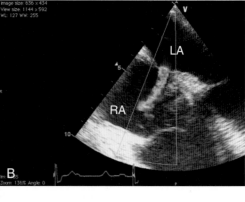

FIGURE 6.60A & B **Patent foramen ovale**
A   A TOE image (mid-oesophageal with probe at 0 degrees). The RA is dilated and there appears to be a defect in the thin-walled interatrial septum.
B   Colour Doppler confirms an abnormal jet of flow from LA to RA consistent with a PFO.

Intracardiac masses
- Mural thrombus – may be seen in dilated atria (especially atrial appendages) or ventricles (e.g. over thinned scarred dilated chambers):
  ○ unlike myocardium, thrombus does not thicken during systole
  ○ sluggish blood flow is marked by 'spontaneous echo contrast', which looks like wisps of smoke.

- Tumours — appear as echo-dense masses most often attached to chamber walls (atrial myxomas are classically attached to the interatrial septum). Secondary tumours (e.g. with primary pulmonary neoplasms) are more common than primary lesions (e.g. benign atrial myxomas, malignant sarcomas).
  - may interfere with valvular function or contractile function if infiltrating.

Hardware
- Prosthetic valves – varying appearances dependent on type; complications such as endocarditis, dehiscence and paravalvular leaks may be seen.
- Pacing wires.

Respiratory function tests

The following tests may feature in exams, although increasingly the emphasis is on those studies that are performed in ICU, particularly analysis of the ventilator data.

Spirometry
Forced expiratory volume in one second (FEV_1), forced vital capacity (FVC) and the ratio of FEV_1/FVC are the primary measurements. This test is very effort and technique dependent. Normal and classical patterns are graphically represented in Figure 6.61. Spirometry can identify acute and chronic deteriorations in lung function. There are two classical patterns – obstructive lung disease such as COPD and asthma, and restrictive disease seen in pathological conditions that reduce total lung capacity, e.g. kyphoscoliosis or fibrosing lung disease.

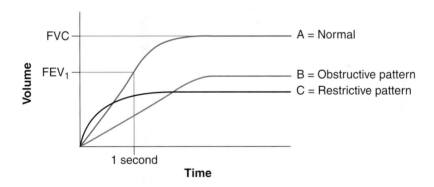

FIGURE 6.61 Key spirometry patterns

DLCO
Results of studies performed prior to ICU admission, such as formal static lung volume testing and DLCO, may facilitate diagnosis in an individual patient. Of particular relevance is DLCO. The diffusing capacity of carbon monoxide (DLCO) is used to assess the transfer of gas by diffusion from the alveoli to the pulmonary capillaries. A low concentration of CO (e.g. 0.3%) is inspired and the breath held for 10 seconds. Expired CO concentration is measured and the difference between the inspired and expired concentrations is used to calculate DLCO. Causes of increased and decreased DLCO are listed in Table 6.15. This test is often used to evaluate a patient with undifferentiated dyspnoea.

TABLE 6.15 Abnormalities of DLCO	
Causes of increased DLCO	**Causes of decreased DLCO**
Pulmonary haemorrhage Polycythaemia Asthma Early congestive cardiac failure Left to right intra-cardiac shunt Severe obesity High altitude Exercise just prior to the session Hyperthyroidism	Interstitial lung diseases Emphysema Congestive cardiac failure Pulmonary vascular diseases (e.g. emboli) Severe anaemia Increased carboxyhaemoglobin Hypothyroidism Hypothermia

Flow–volume loops

Flow–volume tracings allow visual assessment of the relationships between flow rates and volumes. Candidates should be able to recognise the following patterns:

- Lower airway obstruction (e.g. asthma, Fig 6.62)
  - the shape of the expiratory flow curve may also vary between disease processes, with asthma producing a 'smooth' concave trace as obstruction is more fixed, compared to chronic obstructive airways disease (COAD), where there is sometimes an 'angled' appearance due to a more sudden forceful end expiratory collapse.
- Fixed upper airway obstruction, (e.g. tracheal stenosis, Fig 6.63).
- Variable extrathoracic upper airway obstruction (e.g. vocal cord paralysis, Fig 6.64)
  - normal expiratory flow with a constant reduction in inspiratory flow.
- Variable intrathoracic upper airway obstruction (e.g. tumour in lower trachea, Fig 6.65)
  - normal inspiratory flow with a constant reduction in expiratory flow.
- Restrictive lung disease (e.g. pulmonary fibrosis, Fig 6.66)
  - total lung capacity and functional residual capacity are both reduced and the expiratory part of the loop has a steep upslope.

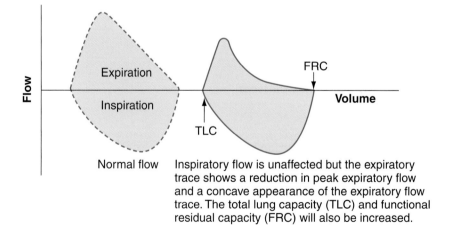

Normal flow   Inspiratory flow is unaffected but the expiratory trace shows a reduction in peak expiratory flow and a concave appearance of the expiratory flow trace. The total lung capacity (TLC) and functional residual capacity (FRC) will also be increased.

FIGURE 6.62 Lower airway obstruction

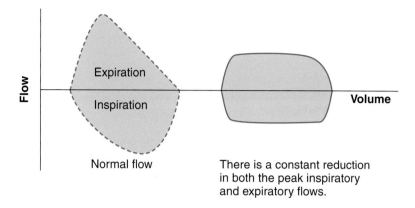

FIGURE 6.63 **Fixed upper airway obstruction**

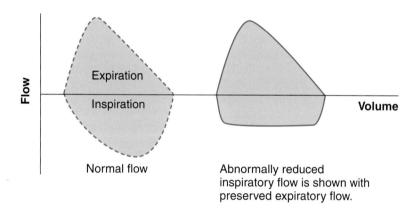

FIGURE 6.64 **Variable extrathoracic upper airway obstruction**

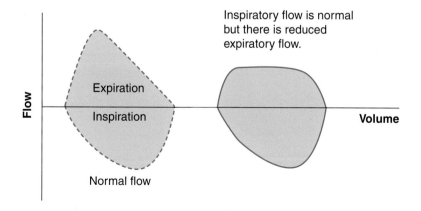

FIGURE 6.65 **Variable intrathoracic upper airway obstruction**

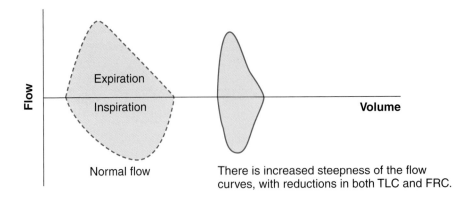

FIGURE 6.66 Restrictive lung disease

Pressure–volume loops

Pressure–volume loops are a graphical representation of the relationships between pressure and volume during both inspiration and expiration. The slope of an imaginary line drawn between the start of inspiration and expiration represents lung compliance. The curve is shifted to the right with conditions causing reduced lung compliance (e.g. ARDS), and to the left with increased lung compliance (e.g. emphysema, Fig 6.67). A lower inflection point may be recognisable as a point on the inspiratory limb of the loop where the compliance suddenly increases. A 'beak-like' appearance to the junction between the end of inspiration and start of expiration represents over-distension as too much volume is delivered.

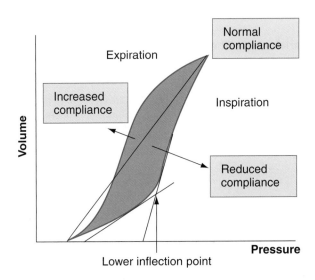

FIGURE 6.67 Pressure–volume loop showing normal lung compliance, increased lung compliance (e.g. in emphysema) and decreased lung compliance (e.g. in ARDS)

Ventilator waveforms

Analysis of waveforms reflecting pressure, flow or volume plotted against time may yield important information about the interaction between the patient and ventilator. Candidates should be able to confidently discuss the differences in waveforms seen in volume and pressure controlled modes (Figs 6.68–6.70), as intensivists frequently use this information to tailor their ventilatory strategy. The examples provided are modelled on the modes used in the Draegar™ Evita XL ventilator.

Examples of some abnormalities of pressure-time waveforms that could be presented in the exam include:

- autoPEEP (Fig 6.71) – expiratory flow does not return to baseline before the next inspiration commences. Interventions to manage this problem include reducing the respiratory rate and prolonging the I:E ratio
- patient ventilator asynchrony – failure of synchronisation between patient and ventilator. May be as a result of inadequate gas flow, incorrect trigger settings, premature or delayed breath termination and autoPEEP. Leads to patient discomfort and increased work of breathing. Analysis of ventilator waveforms can be used to determine underlying mechanism for asynchrony

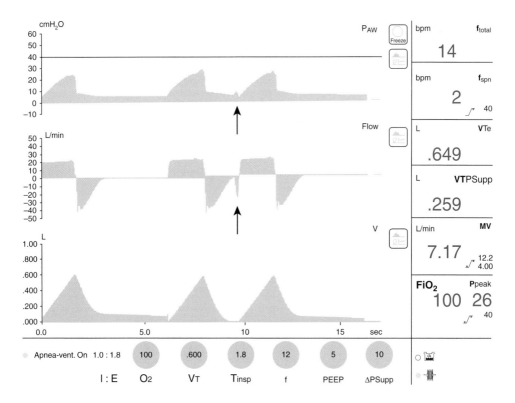

FIGURE 6.68 SIMV volume control with pressure support
The square 'constant flow' waveform is commonly used for delivering breaths in volume-controlled modes. The arrows indicate a synchronised breath that has a characteristic negative flow deflection representing the patient's triggering. If this was a pressure-supported breath there would most likely be a descending ramp 'decelerating flow' waveform classically seen with pressure-controlled breaths.

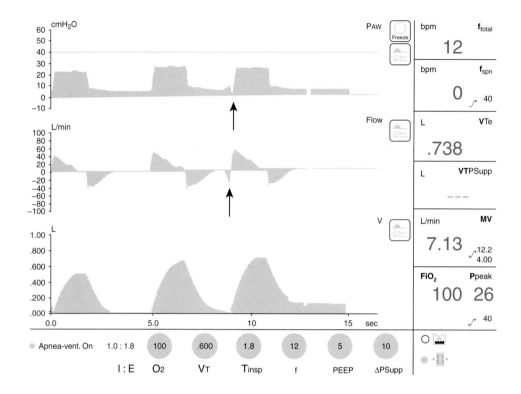

FIGURE 6.69 SIMV with autoflow and pressure support
The settings look the same as in Figure 6.68, but there is now a descending ramp flow pattern classic for pressure control modes. This is a special setting called SIMV autoflow, a method of allowing 'pressure regulated volume control'. The arrow indicates a synchronised breath. The waveform would be similar if this was a pressure-supported breath. The fspn rate is 0 and VTPsupp, suggesting that this is not a pressure-supported breath.

- circuit leaks – the baseline of the pressure–time waveform drifts downwards
- cardiac oscillations – the baseline of the pressure–time waveform shows slight up and down movement with the heartbeat; these may be initiate triggering of synchronised breaths
- inadequate inspiratory flow rate – on the pressure–time waveform there will be a 'scooped-out' appearance to synchronised breaths.

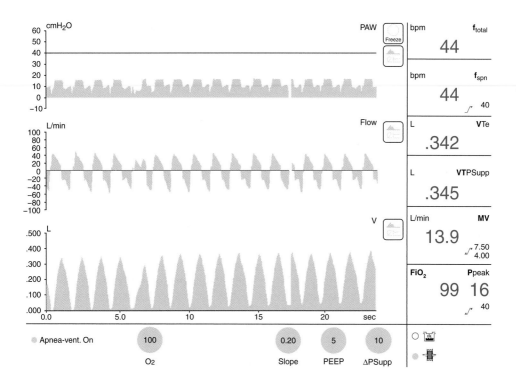

FIGURE 6.70 Pressure support with PEEP
This mode is also known as CPAP/ASB (continuous positive airway pressure/assist support breaths). All of the breaths are triggered by the patient and there are no mandatory breaths. The respiratory rate is very fast and the tidal volumes, although the patient's weight is unclear, seem low for an adult.

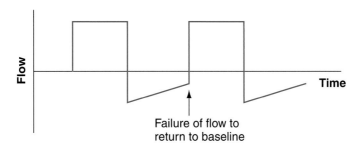

FIGURE 6.71 Flow–time waveform with autoPEEP
Auto PEEP is caused by trapping of gas in the airways at end-expiration, which generates a positive pressure. This is reflected as a failure of expiratory flow to return to basline prior to onset of the next breath.

Indirect calorimetry

Candidates may be asked to comment on results of indirect calorimetry, derived from measurements of oxygen consumption and carbon dioxide production in ventilated patients. Some intensivists use serial respiratory quotient ($RQ = VCO_2/VO_2$) measurements to tailor their feeding regimens.

In the examination a high or low RQ may be provided. A RQ <0.85 may indicate underfeeding and RQ >1 overfeeding, although these findings are not sensitive or specific and these numbers may be physiological in some individuals. The RQ for fat is 0.7, protein 0.8 and carbohydrate 1.0.

Candidates could be asked to comment on a feeding regimen in the context of knowing the RQ with indirect calorimetry. Classically, patients failing to wean from ventilation have high RQs and are receiving feeds high in carbohydrate content. They may theoretically benefit from feeds with a lower RQ, such as those with a higher ratio of fat to carbohydrate. It should be realised that indirect calorimetry readings are subject to a host of potential errors, for example: measurements taken when the patient is not in a steady state (e.g. after an acute stressor); when high FiO_2 is required; in the setting of high respiratory rates; if an air leak is present (circuit, endotracheal tube cuff, pneumothorax with intercostal catheters); if there is water in the circuit from humidifier rain-out.

Capnography

The graphical representation of expired CO_2 during the respiratory cycle may provide useful information. A normal capnography trace is provided in Figure 6.72. Common and important patterns are described in Table 6.16.

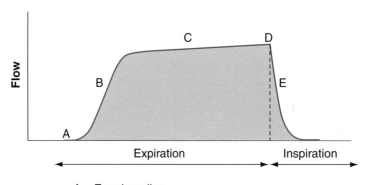

A = Zero baseline
B = Rapid sharp rise at start of expiration
C = Alveolar plateau
D = End-tidal CO_2 value
E = Rapid sharp downstroke with inspiration

FIGURE 6.72 Normal capnography waveform

TABLE 6.16 Capnography traces	
Waveform characteristic	**Significance**
Sudden drop in $ETCO_2$ to zero or near zero	Circuit disconnection Dislodged, occluded or kinked endotracheal tube Oesophageal intubation Massive CO_2 embolism during laparoscopy Cardiac arrest
Sudden decrease in $ETCO_2$ with normal plateaus	Reduced pulmonary blood flow – pulmonary embolism (clot, fat, air), profound hypotension, sudden cardiac arrest with active CPR
Persistent low $ETCO_2$ with normal plateaus	Hypothermia Hyperventilation Deep anaesthesia/sedation Increased dead-space ventilation
Increase in $ETCO_2$ with normal plateaus	Hypoventilation Increased CO_2 production, e.g. hyperthermia, malignant hyperpyrexia Absorption of CO_2 from peritoneal insufflation
Increase in $ETCO_2$ with failure to return to zero baseline	CO_2 rebreathing
Slanting and prolonged phase B and upward sloping phase C (loss of plateau)	Incomplete expiration related to partial airway occlusion, bronchospasm or mucus plugging
Curare cleft in phase C plateau	Wearing off of neuromuscular blockade
Cardiogenic oscillations in phases C to E	Caused by beating of heart against lungs

Biochemistry tests

Arterial blood gas analysis

Blood gas analysis is frequently examined. A wealth of information, including an understanding of acid–base abnormalities and an assessment of gas exchange, may be gleaned from this single, commonly performed investigation.

Clinical acid–base abnormalities have traditionally been explained using the approach that the pH is maintained and regulated by the renal and respiratory systems and explained mathematically by the Henderson-Hasselbalch equation.

There are a number of useful rules based on this traditional theory that facilitate calculation of primary correction of an acid–base disturbance and give information as to whether a mixed acid–base disturbance is present (Table 6.17). The differential diagnosis for these acid–base disturbances is outlined in Table 6.18. The exam candidate should be versed in the calculation and significance of the various 'gaps' that assist blood gas interpretation (Table 6.19).

The Stewart theory is an alternative perspective based on the law of electroneutrality where the total number of cations must equal the anions and that only certain independent variables can change the acid–base status. These are carbon dioxide (pCO_2), strong ions (electrolytes such as Na, K, Mg, Ca, Cl and strong organic acids such as lactate and urate), which dissociate completely in solutions and total weak acids (so-called A_{TOT}, principally composed of albumin and phosphate). Based on

TABLE 6.17 Some simple rules for blood gas interpretation		
Acid-base disorder	Rule (kPa)	Rule (mmHg)*
Primary acute respiratory acidosis	HCO_3 increases 1 mmol/L per 1.3 kPa rise in $PaCO_2$ above 5 kPa (up to 30 mmol/L)	HCO_3 increases 1 mmol/L per 10 mmHg rise in $PaCO_2$ above 40 mmHg (up to 30 mmol/L)
Primary chronic respiratory acidosis	HCO_3 increases 4 mmol/L per 1.3 rise in $PaCO_2$ above 5 kPa (up to 36 mmol/L)	HCO_3 increases 4mmol/L per 10 mmHg rise in $PaCO_2$ above 40 mmHg (up to 36 mmol/L)
Primary acute respiratory alkalosis	HCO_3 decreases 2 mmol/L per 1.3 fall in $PaCO_2$ below 5 kPa	HCO_3 decreases 2 mmol/L per 10 mmHg fall in $PaCO_2$ below 40 mmHg
Chronic respiratory alkalosis	HCO_3 decreases 5 mmol/L per 1.3 kPa fall in $PaCO_2$ below 5kPa	HCO_3 decreases 5 mmol/L per 10 mmHg fall in $PaCO_2$ below 40 mmHg
Primary metabolic acidosis	$PaCO_2$ (kPa) = 0.2(HCO_3) + 1	$PaCO_2$ should be within 5 mmHg of the number denoted after the decimal point in the pH (down to a $paCO_2$ 10) e.g. pH 7.10 – $PaCO_2$ should be 10 With a pure metabolic acidosis the $PaCO_2$ (mmHg) = 1.5(HCO_3) + 8
Primary metabolic alkalosis	$PaCO_2$ (kPa) = 0.12(HCO_3) + 1.2	$PaCO_2$ should be within 5 mmHg of the number denoted after the decimal point in the pH (up to a $paCO2$ 60) e.g. pH 7.6 – $PaCO_2$ should be 60 With a pure metabolic alkalosis the $PaCO_2$ (mmHg) = 0.9(HCO_3) + 9

HCO_3 = bicarbonate ion
*Assume normal $paCO_2$ = 40 mmHg (5kPa) and HCO_3 = 24

this theory, some intensivists use two simplified equations related to the Stewart equation to help determine the cause of acid–base disturbance, which blend with the traditional concept:

Strong ion difference (SID) = $[HCO_3] + A^-$ (where normal is approximately 42)

Strong ion gap (SIG) = anion gap $- A^-$ (where normal is approximately 0)

where $A^- = 0.28 \times$ albumin (g/L) $+ 2.14 \times$ phosphate (mmol/L)

For example, when considering the causes of a metabolic acidosis:
- If low SID with high SIG – the differential diagnosis is as per causes of increased anion gap metabolic acidosis.
- If low SID with low or normal SIG – the differential diagnosis is as per causes of normal anion gap metabolic acidosis.

Calculation of the A–a gradient should also be performed routinely. This is the calculated alveolar O_2 concentration (PaO_2 using the alveolar gas equation shown in

TABLE 6.18 Differential diagnosis for major acid–base abnormalities

Metabolic alkalosis	Loss of hydrogen ions: • Gastrointestinal – vomiting, nasogastric tube drainage, villous adenoma • Renal – Conn and Cushing syndromes, drugs (e.g. corticosteroids, liquorice, loop and thiazide diuretics), post-hypercapnoea syndromes (Bartter, Liddle, Gitelman) Gain of bicarbonate ions: • Sodium bicarbonate (NaHCO$_3$) infusions or dialysate buffer • Metabolic conversion of citrate (e.g. regional anticoagulation), acetate and lactate (e.g. dialysate buffers) Factors tending to maintain an alkalosis: • Hypokalaemia, hypochloraemia, hypomagnesaemia, renal failure, intravascular dehydration, chronic hypercapnoea

Metabolic acidosis	Normal anion gap:
	• Loss of bicarbonate ions
	• Lower gastrointestinal tract – diarrhoea, ascites, cholestyramine, fistulae (pancreatic, small bowel, biliary), ureteroenterostomy
	• Renal – renal tubular acidosis, carbonic anhydrase inhibitors (acetazolamide), hypoaldosteronism, prolonged uncorrected ketoacidosis
	• Hyperchloraemia (e.g. normal saline fluid resuscitation)
	• Acid absorption/administration (e.g. HCl, HF)
	Increased anion gap:
	• Ketoacidosis – diabetic, alcoholic, starvation
	• Lactic acidosis – increased production or reduced clearance
	  ○ L-lactate (common type) – tissue hypoxia, dialysate buffer, liver failure, sympathomimetics, drugs and toxins (e.g. metformin, paracetamol, cyanide, salicylates), inborn errors of metabolism, thiamine deficiency, malignancies
	  ○ D-lactate (e.g. jejuno-ileal bypass, short bowel syndrome)
	• Renal failure
	• Toxic alcohols (e.g. methanol, ethanol, ethylene glycol)
	• Pyroglutamic acidosis

Respiratory alkalosis	• Hypoxia • Early sepsis • Respiratory centre stimulation – progesterone in pregnancy, theophylline, salicylates, amphetamines • Brainstem dysfunction • Hepatic encephalopathy • Anxiety, pain and fear • Exercise • Mechanical hyperventilation
Respiratory acidosis	Consider an anatomical classification of causes of hypoventilation and impaired gas exchange – CNS, spinal cord, peripheral nerve, neuromuscular junction, chest wall, pleural space, pulmonary, airway diseases Increased dead space and mechanical hypoventilation

Box 6.3) minus the measured arterial O_2 concentration (PaO_2 on an arterial blood gas). A normal A–a gradient is <2 kPa (<15 mmHg) and increases with age to 4 kPa (30 mmHg). An abnormally increased A–a gradient suggests a V/Q mismatch, diffusion defect (e.g. interstitial lung disease) or right-to-left shunt.

TABLE 6.19 Important 'gaps'

Gap	Calculation	Significance
Anion	Na+ – (HCO$_3$+Cl) Normal range 6–15 mmol/L	Assists the clarification of the aetiology of metabolic acidosis – increased versus non-anion gap (see causes of metabolic acidosis) A reduced anion gap may be seen with: • Hypermagnesaemia • Hypercalcaemia • Lithium toxicity • Excess immunoglobulins (multiple myeloma, intragam infusion) • Hypoalbuminaemia
Anion gap corrected for hypoalbuminaemia	AG$_c$= AG + 0.25 x (44 – observed albumin in g/L)	More accurate estimate of AG in patients with low albumin – most critically ill patients
Osmolar	Measured osmolality* – calculated osmolality* Calculated osmolality* = 2(Na+K) + urea* + glucose* Normal is <10 mmol/L Measured osmolality is calculated via the depression in the freezing point of sample	Increased osmolar gap seen with: • alcohols • mannitol • glycine (e.g. TURP syndrome) • radiocontrast media • sorbitol • maltose (e.g. intragam – immunoglobulin)
Delta	Delta anion gap – delta HCO$_3$ The difference between the rise in AG and the fall in bicarbonate (compared to normal)	Assists the clarification of mixed acid–base disorders: • If > +6 mmol/L, then a metabolic alkalosis co-exists with an increased anion gap metabolic acidosis • If < –6 mmol/L, then a normal anion gap and increased anion gap metabolic acidosis co-exist
Lactate	Bedside lactate (lactate oxidase method) – laboratory lactate (lactate dehydrogenase method)	Seen with ethylene glycol toxicity – due to interference with the bedside (blood gas machine) assay but not the laboratory test
Oxygen saturation	SpO$_2$ (pulse oximetry) – Co-oximetry SaO$_2$	A saturation gap arises in the presence of abnormal haemoglobins, which are only detected with co-oximetry: • carboxyhaemoglobin (normally <2%)** • methaemoglobin (normally <2%) • sulfhaemoglobin (normally undetectable)***

*Units are mmol/L
**Endogenous CO is produced by heme oxygenase breaking down heme (to biliverdin and CO)
***Older co-oximeters may confuse this with methaemoglobin because of similarities in the spectral absorbance profile of these substances

BOX 6.3 Alveolar gas equation

$$PAO_2 = FiO_2(P_B - P_{H_2O}) - PaCO_2/R$$

where:

FiO_2 is the fraction of inspired oxygen

P_B is the barometric pressure (101.3 kPa or 760 mmHg at sea level)

PH_2O is the saturated water vapour pressure (6.3 kPa or 47 mmHg at 37°C)

$PaCO_2$ is the measured arterial carbon dioxide concentration on a blood gas

R is the respiratory quotient – approximately 0.8 for most patients

Biochemistry data sets

Multiple abnormalities, which, when observed together, should prompt consideration of a specific pathological process, diagnosis or differential diagnosis, lend themselves well to the exam. There are a number of classical patterns in critical care (Table 6.20). Causes of other abnormalities are presented in Tables 6.21–6.22 and in Figure 6.73.

TABLE 6.20 Classic exam biochemistry data sets	
Diabetic ketoacidosis (DKA)	• Increased anion gap (ketoacids, lactate) and normal anion gap (HCO_3 wasting) metabolic acidosis • Variable serum potassium, though total body potassium is depleted • Increased urea and variable creatinine (some assays for creatinine cross-react with ketone bodies) • Elevated glucose with increased osmolality and hyponatraemia (correct for glucose – serum Na decreases 1 mmol/L for every 3 mmol/L rise in glucose) • Assays for creatinine using a colorometric method are subject to artefactual elevation of the result, in the presence of acetoacetate
Hyperosmolar non-ketotic coma (HONK)*	• Markedly increased glucose (often >40 mmol/L) • Increased serum and urine osmolality • Variable sodium – often high • Lactic acidosis • Low level or absent ketones • Increased urea and creatinine
Diabetes insipidus (DI)	• Neurogenic DI (idiopathic, head injury, brain tumour, neurosurgery or radiotherapy) due to lack of vasopressin secretion by the posterior pituitary or hypothalamus • Nephrogenic DI (hereditary, amyloid, polycystic kidney disease, post-obstruction, pyelonephritis, amyloid, myeloma, chronic hypercalaemia, chronic hypokalaemia, drugs including lithium, amphotericin B, gentamicin, glibenclamide, demeclocycline) due to lack of renal response to vasopressin • Rule of 2: Urine output >200 mL for 2 hours, increased plasma osmolality and low urine osmolality <200 mosmol/kg • Low urine specific gravity • Desmopressin stimulation test differentiates between neurogenic (symptomatic and biochemical improvement) and nephrogenic DI (no change)
Syndrome of inappropriate ADH secretion (SIADH)	• Ectopic ADH production: central nervous system disorders (subarachnoid haemorrhage, meningitis, brain tumours, brain abscesses), pulmonary disorders (pneumonia, small cell lung cancer, lung abscesses) and drugs (chlorpropamide, clofibrate, phenothiazine, cyclophosphamide, carbamazepine, SSRIs)

Continued

TABLE 6.20 Classic exam biochemistry data sets—cont'd	
	• Hypo-osmolar hyponatraemia • Increased urinary Na (>20 mmol/L) with hypertonic urine relative to serum • Normal renal, adrenal, thyroid, pituitary and cardiac function in the absence of stimulating drugs or physiologic stimuli for ADH secretion
Hypoadrenalism	• Hypo-osmolar hyponatraemia • Hyperkalaemia • Hypoglycaemia • Mildly increased urea • Mild metabolic acidosis • Hypercalcaemia • Eosinophilia
Refeeding syndrome	Occurs when normal caloric intake is resumed after a period of starvation. The glucose levels are restored and insulin secreted with cellular uptake of phosphate, potassium and magnesium with depletion of ATP. Profound hypophosphataemia, hypokalaemia and hypomagnesaemia can result. Thiamine deficiency may be unmasked. Manifests as cardiorespiratory failure, paraesthesias and seizures
Pyloric stenosis	• Infants, usually male, aged 2–8 weeks, present with non-bilious vomiting and a palpable 'olive' in the epigastrium • Hypokalaemic, hypochloraemic, metabolic alkalosis • Increased urea and variable creatinine • Ketones in urine
Rhabdomyolysis	• Caused by trauma, compartment syndromes, toxins, drugs, seizures, inflammatory myopathies, thermal injury, sepsis, severe hypokalaemia • Hyperkalaemia • Hyperphosphataemia and hypocalcaemia • Increased urea and creatinine (with reduced urea to creatinine ratio) • Increased CK, AST and LDH • Myoglobinuria • Metabolic acidosis
Acute pancreatitis	• Hypocalcaemia • Hyperglycaemia • Hypophosphataemia • Increased urea and variable creatinine • Increased amylase and lipase
Tumour lysis syndrome	Hyperkalaemia (real and/or pseudohyerkalaemia from potassium release from tumour cells in vitro), hyperphosphataemia, hypocalcaemia, increased urea and creatinine (with increased urea to creatinine ratio), hyperuricaemia, metabolic acidosis
Beta-adrenergic stimulation	Lactic acidosis with hypokalaemia
Myxoedema	• Hyponatraemia • Hypoglycaemia • Hypercholesterolaemia and hypertriglyceridaemia
Plasma exchange	• Reduced plasma proteins and enzymes – globulin, antithrombin, protein C, plasma cholinesterase • Albumin may not be significantly low if human albumin has been used as the replacement fluid
Immunoglobulin therapy	• IgG can produce a negative anion gap • Manifests as metabolic alkalosis + negative anion gap

*Also called diabetic hyperglycaemic hyperosmolar syndrome

TABLE 6.21 Disorders of electrolytes

Hyponatraemia (<130 mmol/L)	Classified according to:
	• Hyperosmolar (plasma osmolality >290 mosmol/L): causes include hyperglycaemia (correct for glucose – serum Na decreases 1 mmol/L for every 3 mmol/L rise in glucose), mannitol, ethanol and ethylene glycol
	• Iso-osmolar (plasma osmolality 270–290 mosmol/L): causes include hyperlipidaemia (triglycerides >50 mmol/L) and hyperproteinaemia e.g. multiple myeloma
	• Hypo-osmolar: (plasma osmolality <270 mosmol/L): can be further divided into:
	  ○ Hypovolaemic – due to Na+ loss in excess of water loss. Causes include Addison's disease, polyuric renal failure, diuretics, burns, gastrointestinal losses
	  ○ Hypervolaemic – due to water excess. Causes include excessive 5% dextrose infusions, congestive cardiac failure, cirrhosis, nephrotic syndrome, renal failure
	  ○ Normovolaemic. Causes include psychogenic polydipsia, SIADH, hypothyroidism, acute adrenal insufficiency

Hypernatraemia (>145 mmol/L)	Hyperosmolar and classified according to: • Hypovolaemic (water loss in excess of Na+ loss). Causes include diuretics, glycosuria, renal failure, gastrointestinal losses, skin losses, burns, fever, and thyrotoxicosis • Normovolaemic (pure water loss) diabetes insipidus (can become hypovolaemic) • Hypervolaemic (Na+ gain in excess of water gain)–0.9% saline infusions, sodium bicarbonate infusions ($NaHCO_3$), feeding formulae, parenteral nutrition, mineralocorticoid excess, Conn's and Cushing's syndromes To calculate water deficit: $$\text{Water deficit} = \text{TBW} \times \left[\left(\frac{\text{Serum Na}}{140}\right) - 1\right] \text{ (in L)}$$ where TBW = total body water = 0.6 × body weight (in kg)
Hypokalaemia (<3 mmol/L)	Intracellular shift: alkalaemia, catecholamines, salbutamol, insulin, refeeding syndrome, hypomagnesaemia Reduced intake: starvation Increased losses: diuretics, mannitol, acetazolamide, steroids, ampotericin, lithium, renal tubular acidosis Type 1 and 2, gastro-intestinal losses, ureterosigmoidostomy, fistulae, skin losses
Hyperkalaemia (>5 mmol/L)	Artefact: drip arm specimen, haemolysed specimen Extracellular shift: acidosis, tissue breakdown, rhabdomyolysis, haemolysis, ischaemia, reperfusion, tumour lysis syndrome, leukaemia, suxamethonium, DKA (normokalaemia with DKA is associated with a marked total body K+ deficit) Increased intake: direct IV/oral, transfusion Reduced clearance: acute renal failure, hypoaldosteronism, Type 4 renal tubular acidosis, potassium-sparing diuretics, spironolactone, amiloride

Continued

TABLE 6.21 Disorders of electrolytes—cont'd	
Hypomagnesaemia (<0.65 mmol/L)	Excess losses: malabsorption syndromes, gastrointestinal tract fistulas, short bowel syndrome, diarrhoea, pancreatitis, prolonged nasogastric suction, renal tubular acidosis, Reduced intake: alcoholism, parenteral nutrition Redistribution: hypokalaemia with hypocalcaemia Others: hyperparathyroidism, hyperthyroidism, diabetes, hyperaldosteronism, drugs (aminogylcosides, amphotericin, diuretics, cyclosporin, cisplatinum)
Hypermagnesaemia (>1.05 mmol/L)	Excessive administration of magnesium salts, laxatives, parenteral nutrition, renal failure
Hypophosphataemia (<0.81 mmol/L)	Hyperparathyroidism, osteomalacia, hypomagnesaemia, acute alkalosis, haemodialysis, ketoacidosis, parenteral nutrition, refeeding syndrome, chronic alcoholism
Hyperphosphataemia (>1.45 mmol/L)	• Artifact: haemolysis • Increased intake: excess vitamin D excess replacement • Increased release from cells/bone: rhabdomyolysis, malignancy, starvation, diabetes, tumour lysis syndrome • Decreased excretion: hypoparathyroidism, renal failure
Hypocalcaemia (<2.1 mmol/L)	About 40% of plasma calcium is bound to albumin. Total plasma calcium is usually measured, but it is the unbound, ionised portion that is important. The adjusted (ionised) calcium may be reported, or calculated using the formula: adjusted calcium = measured total calcium + [(40 − serum albumin) × 0.02] Causes: • decreased parathyroid activity: hypoparathyroidism • decreased vitamin D activity: chronic renal failure, intestinal malabsorption, poor diet, liver disease • increased calcium loss: chelating agents • decreased ionised calcium: alkalosis Others: hypomagnesaemia, pancreatitis, rhabdomyolysis, hyperphosphataemia
Hypercalcaemia (>2.6 mmol/L)	Primary or tertiary hyperparathyroidism, malignancy (myeloma, bone metastasis), sarcoidosis, vitamin D intoxication, hyperthyroidism, milk-alkali syndrome, immobilisation, thiazide diuretics
Hypokalemic alkalosis	• Diuretics (loop, thiazide) • Excess mineralocorticoid (Cushing and Conn syndromes) • Vomiting, diarrhoea and laxatives • Villous adenoma of the rectum
Hyponatraemia with hyperkalaemia	• Hypoadrenalism • Potassium-sparing diuretics • Renal failure (salt-losing nephropathy) • Diabetic ketoacidosis (beware of the pseudohyponatraemia)
Hypocalcaemia with metabolic acidosis	• Acute renal failure • Tumour lysis syndrome • Rhabdomyolysis • Pancreatitis • Ethylene glycol poisoning • Hydrofluoric acid intoxication
Hypoglycaemia with metabolic acidosis	• Fulminant hepatic failure • Septic shock • Salicylate poisoning

TABLE 6.22 Liver function tests

Bilirubin	Knowing the fraction of unconjugated vs conjugated hyperbilirubinaemia helps to distinguish between the pre-, intra- and post-hepatic causes of jaundice Unconjugated/indirect bilirubin: physiological (neonatal), Gilbert syndrome (glucuronyl transferase deficiency), haemolysis, resorption of haematoma Conjugated/direct bilirubin: 'ICU jaundice': part of multiple organ dysfunction syndrome related to cytokines, drugs causing cholestasis (e.g. flucloxacillin, chlorpromazine, prochlorperazine), parenteral nutrition, cirrhosis, heart failure including pericardial tamponade, hepatitis (ischaemic, toxins, drugs, infections), tumour (metastases, hepatoma), obstructed biliary tree (gallstones, sludge, pancreatic or bile duct tumour, sclerosing cholangitis, porta hepatis lymph nodes, choledochal cyst, biliary atresia, post-surgical strictures)
Transaminases	Aspartate aminotransferase (AST): released from liver, heart (e.g. myocardial infarction), skeletal muscle (e.g. rhabdomyolysis) and brain Alanine aminotransferase (ALT): released from liver and muscle. Massive increases in transaminases seen with ischaemic and toxic hepatitis Alcoholic hepatitis: AST is 1.5–2 times greater than ALT (reverse ratio in other causes of hepatitis); levels rarely >500 U/L. GGT/AlkP may be elevated first early in the insult Transaminases may be minimally elevated in cirrhosis
Gamma glutamyl transpeptidase (GGT)	Released from liver (in bile), pancreas, kidneys Increased with cholestasis, but also any type of liver injury Isolated increases may reflect moderate alcohol consumption (e.g. 3–4 standard drinks per day)
Alkaline phosphatase (AlkP)	Released from liver (in bile) and bone Isolated increases seen with late pregnancy, Paget's disease, bone growth or injury (including metastatic malignancies) and in primary biliary cirrhosis
Lactate dehydrogenase (LDH)	Increased levels, which may be massively elevated, reflect ischaemic/necrotic tissue in any part of the body (ischaemic liver injury, ischaemic bowel, haemolysis, pneumonias, myocardial infarction, rhabdomyolysis)
Albumin	Reduced in acute and chronic inflammatory states, nephrotic syndrome, severe malnutrition and liver disease, protein-losing enteropathies and normal pregnancy (dilution) If no other liver markers are abnormal then suspect extra-hepatic disease
Blood ammonia	Variable increase in hepatic encephalopathy May aid in diagnosis of altered conscious state of unclear cause Increases in urea cycle disorders

Dehydration
Gastrointestinal bleeding
High protein diet
Corticosteroids
Severe catabolic state

Urea: Creatinine

Low protein diet
Malnutrition
Severe liver dysfunction
Pregnancy
SIADH
Rhabdomyolysis

FIGURE 6.73 Urea-to-creatinine ratios

Autoimmune markers

These tests may be used for diagnosis of rare conditions that require ICU admission (Table 6.23).

TABLE 6.23 Autoimmune markers	
ANA	SLE, other autoimmune diseases, can be normal in low titre, especially with increased age or if drug induced (low specificity)
Rheumatoid factor (IgG vs IgM)	Rheumatoid arthritis, mixed cryoglobulinaemia, subacute bacterial endocarditis, any cause of chronic antigenic stimulation (low specificity)
Anticardiolipin	Antiphospholipid syndrome, SLE, other autoimmune diseases, viral illnesses Increased significance if lupus anticoagulant and anti-phospholipid antibodies also present (low specificity)
Anti-DNA	SLE
Anti-Smith	SLE
Anti-Ro and La	SLE with congenital heart block, Sjögren's syndrome
Anti-centromere	Limited cutaneous scleroderma (CREST syndrome)
Scleroderma-70	Diffuse scleroderma, rarely CREST syndrome
Anti-ribonuclear protein	SLE, mixed connective tissue disorder, undifferentiated connective tissue disease
C3 and C4	Reduced in SLE, autoimmune chronic active hepatitis Increased in biliary obstruction, nephrotic syndrome, acute phase response
ANCA	c-ANCA: Wegener's granulomatosis > Polyarteritis nodosa p-ANCA: Polyarteritis nodosa > Wegener's granulomatosis Can be increased with drugs (e.g. penicillins, sulfonamides, quinolones, phenytoin, thiazides)
Anti-glomerular basement membrane (antibody directed at type 4 collagen)	Goodpasture's disease

Continued

TABLE 6.23 Autoimmune markers—cont'd	
Anti-smooth muscle	Autoimmune chronic active hepatitis, EBV
Anti-mitochondrial	Primary biliary cirrhosis, chronic active hepatitis, Idiopathic cirrhosis
Anti-gliadin, anti-endomyseal, anti-transglutaminase	Coeliac disease
Anti-intrinsic factor and parietal cell antibody	Pernicious anaemia
Anti-TSH receptor	Autoimmune thyroid disease – Graves' and Hashimoto's thyroiditis
Anti-acetylcholine receptor MuSK antibody – muscle specific receptor tyrosine kinase antibody	Myasthenia gravis

Short Synacthen test

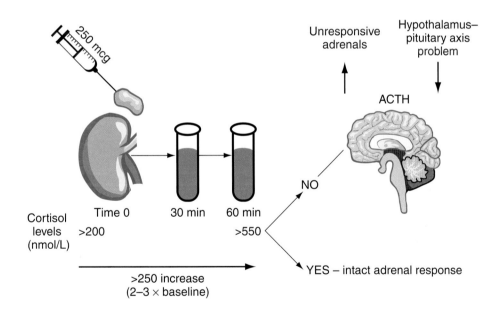

FIGURE 6.74 Short Synacthen test

In the traditional test, baseline ACTH and cortisol are measured with cortisol levels at 30 and 60 minutes after injection of 250 mcg intravenous bolus of synthetic ACTH ('Synacthen'). The cortisol level measured is the total (i.e. the free and albumin bound cortisol). The significance of the results remains highly controversial.

Thyroid function tests

A highly specific free T4 assay is now available, which, combined with TSH, provides fundamental information about this important endocrine axis.
- Euthyroid: normal T4, T3 and TSH
- Hyperthyroidism
  - increased T4 and T3
  - increased TSH if secondary to hypothalamic–pituitary disease
  - decreased TSH if primary thyroid disease
- Hypothyroidism
  - reduced T4 and T3
  - decreased TSH if secondary to hypothalamic–pituitary disease
  - increased TSH if primary thyroid disease
- Euthyroid sick syndrome
  - low total T3, normal/low T4 and TSH, increased reverse T3
  - present in severe non-thyroidal illness
  - TSH low for reduced T3 level, but increased T3 receptors maintains euthyroid state
  - TSH secretion decreased by starvation, stress, cytokines and drugs (e.g. dopamine, steroids, opioids)
- Euthyroid hyperthyroxinaemia
  - increased T4 with variable T3 and TSH
  - increased peripheral conversion T4 to T3
  - caused by drugs (e.g. amiodarone), hyperemesis, acute psychiatric illness, hyponatraemia.

Iron studies

- Iron deficiency: low serum iron and ferritin, high total iron-binding capacity
- Chronic infection and inflammation: low or normal serum iron, high ferritin, reduced total iron-binding capacity
- Haemochromatosis: high serum iron and ferritin with low total iron-binding capacity
- Sideroblastic anaemia: high serum iron with low total iron-binding capacity.

Tumour markers

More useful when used to assess response to therapy rather than as diagnostic tests. Basic understanding of these markers is relevant for the management of oncology patients.
- Alpha fetoprotein: increased in hepatocellular carcinoma, germ cell tumours, pregnancy
- CA-19.9: pancreatic, colorectal and cholangiocarcinoma
- CA-125 and CA-72–CA-74: ovarian tumours
- CA15-3: breast
- Carcinoembryonic antigen: colorectal, liver, lung, breast, cervix, pancreatic, thyroid, bladder
- Human chorionic gonadotrophin: testicular and trophoblastic tumours, pregnancy
- Prostate-specific antigen: prostate adenocarcinoma, prostatitis, benign prostatic hypertrophy
- Calcitonin: thyroid medullary carcinoma
- Neuron-specific enolase: neuroblastoma, small cell lung carcinoma
- Mast cell tryptase
- Increased in anaphylaxis.

Miscellaneous other tests

- HbA1C (glycosylated haemoglobin A1C)
  - surrogate marker for blood glucose reflecting the average level over the preceding 4 weeks to 3 months.

- Angiotensin converting enzyme; increased ACE may be seen with:
  - sarcoidosis
  - lymphoma
  - pulmonary TB
  - silicosis
  - asbestosis.
- Brain natriuretic peptide (BNP)
  - BNP is a neurohormone mainly secreted by the left ventricle in response to pressure and volume overload
  - produces natriuresis, a decrease in systemic vascular resistance and a reduction in cardiac filling pressure
  - elevation is proportional to severity of heart failure and correlates with mortality
  - false positives seen in asymptomatic left ventricular dysfunction, chronic pulmonary hypertension, unstable myocardial infarction, atrial fibrillation, pulmonary embolism, lung cancer.
- Beta 2 transferrin
  - marker for CSF leak
- C-reactive protein
  - an acute phase protein non-specifically elevated in acute and chronic inflammatory conditions, malignancies, infarction, autoimmune and connective tissue disorders, pregnancy and the oral contraceptive pill
  - other acute phase reactants that rise are complement and coagulation factors, fibrinogen, proteinase inhibitors, metal-binding proteins (haptoglobin, ceruloplasmin), superoxide dismutase
  - albumin, pre-albumin and transferrin fall as an acute phase response.
- Erythrocyte sedimentation rate
  - non-specific inflammatory marker
  - markedly elevated (>100 mm/hr) in multiple myeloma and other malignancies, temporal arteritis, polymyalgia rheumatica, severe infection
- Procalcitonin (PCT)
  - Under normal metabolic conditions, PCT is only present in the C cell of the thyroid gland
  - high levels of PCT are seen in blood with severe bacterial infections and sepsis
  - may help differentiate infectious from non-infectious causes of SIRS
  - false positives (with usually low levels of PCT) with burns, trauma, autoimmune and chronic inflammatory diseases, thyroid cancer, surgery
- C1 esterase inhibitor
  - deficient in hereditary angioneurotic oedema
- Plasma pseudocholinesterase
  - reduced in liver dysfunction, organophosphate poisoning, pregnancy, hereditary deficiency and with plasmapheresis.

Haematology

Blood counts and coagulation profiles are commonly requested on critically ill patients. Candidates must be familiar with common pathological patterns.

Blood counts
The differential diagnosis for common abnormalities of the complete blood count are provided in Table 6.24. Platelet disorders are summarised in Figure 6.75.

TABLE 6.24 Disorders of red and white blood cells

Abnormality	Differential diagnosis
Anaemia with low MCV	Iron deficiency, thalassaemia, sideroblastic anaemia
Anaemia with high MCV	Folate or vitamin B12 deficiency, alcohol abuse, chronic liver disease, hypothyroidism, reticulocytosis, myelodysplasia, drugs (anticonvulsants, antimetabolites)
Anaemia with normal MCV	Anaemia of chronic disease, chronic renal failure, pregnancy, haemolysis, bone marrow failure, mixed haematinic deficiency (e.g. iron and B12)
Haemolytic anaemia (low haptoglobin, high LDH, mildly increased bilirubin, reticulocytosis, haemoglobinaemia, haemoglobinuria, positive Coombs tests if immune mediated)	Intrinsic red cell defects: membrane (e.g. hereditary spherocytosis), enzyme (e.g. glucose-6-phosphate dehydrogenase deficiency, pyruvate kinase deficiency) or haemoglobin (e.g. thalassaemia) Extrinsic insults: immune (e.g. beta-lactam antibiotics, SLE, CLL, haemolytic disease of the newborn, blood transfusion reactions), microangiopathic haemolytic anaemias, infection (e.g. malaria), hypersplenism, paroxysmal nocturnal haemoglobinuria
Polycythaemia	Primary: polycythaemia rubra vera Secondary: chronic hypoxaemia, tumour production of erythropoietin (hepatoma, renal cell carcinoma, fibroids) Relative: haemoconcentration
Pancytopenia	Reduced marrow production: cytotoxic agents, idiosyncratic drug reactions (sulfonamides, phenytoin, carbamazepine, gold), severe B12 deficiency, autoantibodies (SLE), marrow infiltration (TB, malignancy), myelofibrosis, myelodysplasia Increased peripheral cellular destruction: SLE, HIV infection, hypersplenism, paroxysmal nocturnal haemoglobinuria
Neutropenia	Infection (bacterial, viral, TB), cytotoxic agents, idiosyncratic drug reactions (clozapine, carbimazole, sulfonamides, beta-lactam antibiotics), hypersplenism, or any other cause of pancytopaenia
Neutrophilia	Infection (bacterial), inflammation (trauma, surgery, infarction, haemorrhage, malignancy, vasculitis), corticosteroids, myeloproliferative disorders
Lymphopenia	Infection (viral and the atypical pneumonias), sarcoidosis, corticosteroids, uraemia, any cause of pancytopenia, common and often non-specific in critical illness
Lymphocytosis	Infection (viral, TB, toxoplasmosis, syphilis, brucellosis, whooping cough), thyrotoxicosis, leukaemia (especially CLL), lymphoma
Atypical lymphocytes	Viral infections (EBV, CMV, HIV), toxoplasmosis, leukaemia, lymphoma, lead poisoning, drug hypersensitivity
Monocytosis	TB, brucellosis, protozoa, leukaemia, lymphoma, myelodysplasia, inflammatory bowel disease, convalescence from any infection
Eosinophilia	Allergic disorders, Addison's disease, parasitic infections, sarcoidosis, polyarteritis nodosa, leukaemia, lymphoma, melanoma, irradiation, convalescence from any infection

Continued

TABLE 6.24 Disorders of red and white blood cells—cont'd

Abnormality	Differential diagnosis
Basophilia	Infection (TB, viral), hypothyroidism, inflammatory bowel disease, post-splenectomy, leukaemia (especially CML), systemic mastocytosis, haemolysis, polycythaemia rubra vera
Reticulocytosis	Acute blood loss or haemorrhage, any cause of premature red cell destruction
Leuckoerythroblastic picture (immature myeloid and erythroid elements)	Myelofibrosis
Leukaemoid reaction (marked granulocyte outpouring)	Severe sepsis, trauma, metastatic neoplasm, acute haemolysis
Acanthocytes (spiculated red cells or spur cells)	Alcoholic liver disease, hypothyroidism, anorexia nervosa, abetalipoproteinaemia
Howell-Jolly bodies (remnants of nuclear proteins)	Post-splenectomy, hyposplenism, megaloblastic anaemia, leukaemia
Auer rods (needle-like intracellular inclusions within blast cells)	Acute myeloid leukaemia
Heinz bodies (haemoglobin precipitates)	Glucose-6-phosphate dehydrogenase deficiency
Burr cells (irregular crenated cells)	Uraemia, pyruvate kinase deficiency, lymphosarcoma, peptic ulcer disease
Target cells (ring of pallor with central and a peripheral rim of staining)	Chronic liver disease, sickle cell disease, thalassaemia, post-splenectomy
Basophilic stippling	Lead poisoning, thalassaemia
Anisocytosis (variation in cell size)	Iron deficiency, thalassaemia, megaloblastic anaemia
Poikilocytosis (variation in cell shape)	Iron deficiency, thalassaemia, myelofibrosis
Left shift (immature white cells)	Infection
Right shift (hypersegmented polymorphs)	Uraemia, chronic liver disease, megaloblastic anaemia

Platelet Count

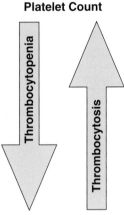

- Failure of platelet production: hereditary, drugs, alcohol, viral infection or part of a pancytopenia
- Increased platelet consumption: immune (ITP, drugs, viral infections, SLE, lymphoproliferative disorders); non-immune (DIC, TTP, cardiopulmonary bypass)
- Dilution: massive blood transfusion
- Splenic pooling

Thrombocytopenia

Thrombocytosis

- Primary: essential thrombocytopenia, myeloproliferative diseases
- Reactive: inflammatory disease (rheumatoid arthritis), bleeding, post-splenectomy

FIGURE 6.75 Disorders of platelets

Heparin-induced thrombocytopenia (HIT) is an acquired disorder of hypercoagulation and thrombocytopenia initiated by heparin. Traditionally it has been divided into two types:

- Type 1 (non-immune mediated) is relatively common, has an earlier onset, is not associated with thrombosis and is caused by direct heparin reaction with the platelet membrane leading to platelet aggregation and a small drop in platelets.
- Type 2 (immune mediated) occurs later after exposure to heparin and is clinically more important as it is associated with thrombosis. The key pathogenesis of HIT type 2 is the generation of IgG antibodies, which are triggered by complexes of platelet factor 4 and heparin on platelet surfaces leading to platelet aggregation and thrombin generation. The diagnosis requires a low threshold for suspicion. The rule of 4Ts is a simple and effective method of identifying those patients with suspected HIT (Table 6.25).

Two types of tests can be employed to confirm HIT: either functional washed platelet assays or antigen assays.

Coagulation studies

Candidates should be familiar with interpreting coagulation studies and special tests to clarify the cause of derangements. The following is a brief outline of some useful investigations, including the thromboelastograph, followed by some coagulation test findings in a range of pathologic conditions (Table 6.26):

- APTT
  ○ test of the traditional intrinsic pathway
- PT
  ○ test of the traditional extrinsic pathway
  ○ the INR (international normalised ratio) is the PT expressed as a ratio of the control used by the specific laboratory usually for monitoring of warfarin therapy
- TCT
  ○ test of the traditional final common pathway of the coagulation cascade that converts fibrinogen to fibrin
- Bleeding time
  ○ most often used to detect the presence of qualitative platelet dysfunction and capillary defects

TABLE 6.25 Pre-test probability of HIT – the 4Ts			
	2	**1**	**0**
Thrombocytopenia (Count per microlitre)	>50% drop or nadir <20–100,000	30–50% drop or nadir 10–19,000	<30% drop or nadir <10,000
Timing (days)	5–10	>10	Too early
Thrombosis	New thrombosis/ skin necrosis	Recurrent thrombosis/ erythematous skin lesions	None
Other causes of Thrombocytopenia	No other cause	Possible other cause	Definite other cause

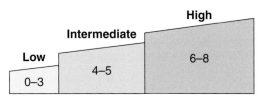

Source: Based on Lo G, Juhl D, Warkentin T, et al. Evaluation of pretest clinical score (4 Ts) for the diagnosis of HIT in two clinical settings. Journal of Thrombosis and Haemostasis, 2006; 4:760.

- ○ ristocetin-induced platelet aggregation is another useful test of qualitative platelet function
- ○ the Hess test is a clinical test where a tourniquet is applied to a patient's arm and petechiae are noted to arise under and distal to the cuff in conditions with prolonged bleeding time
- D-dimer
  - ○ specific for fibrin breakdown; increased in postoperative states, trauma, sepsis, venous thrombosis, malignancies
- Fibrin degradation products (FDPs)
  - ○ markers of fibrin and fibrinogen breakdown
- Protamine-corrected APTT
  - ○ the APTT after protamine (heparin antidote) is added to the patient's blood
- 50% normal plasma PT and APTT
  - ○ the PT or APTT after an equal volume of a control specimen (with normal coagulation factors) is added to the patient's blood
- Reptilase time
  - ○ assists with the differentiation of causes of an increased TCT
  - ○ reptilase is a thrombin-like molecule that converts fibrinogen to fibrin, but is not inhibited by antithrombin3 or FDPs
- Echis time
  - ○ differentiates liver dysfunction from vitamin K deficiency; *Echis carinatum* venom converts pre-prothrombin to prothrombin. In vitamin K deficiency the venom therefore corrects the PT, while in liver dysfunction the PT remains unchanged. An alternative is the vitamin K corrected PT.
- Euglobulin lysis time
  - ○ a shortened time indicates the presence of increased systemic fibrinolytic pathway activators

- Urea solubility test
  - factor 13 stabilises fibrin. If it is deficient then 5M urea will dissolve it
- Procoagulant screen
  - requested in circumstances of a suspected primary coagulation defect causing abnormal intravascular clotting episodes
  - may include:
    - antithrombin 3 assay
    - protein C and S assays
    - APC resistance – factor 5 (Leiden) mutation
    - lupus anticoagulant and anticardiolipin antibodies
    - prothrombin gene mutation (G20210A)
    - fasting homocysteine assay.

TABLE 6.26 Disorders of coagulation

Condition	Findings
Unfractionated heparin therapy (anti-9, 10, 11, 12, 2a effects via enhanced antithrombin 3 activity)	Increased APTT, mildly increased PT, increased TCT, normal protamine corrected APTT, normal reptilase time
Low-molecular-weight heparin (anti-10a activity)	Normal APTT, PT, TCT, increased anti10a activity
Warfarin therapy and vitamin K deficiency (reduced factors 2, 7, 9, 10, protein C and S production)	Increased PT, mildly increased APTT, normal TCT, normal echis time
Liver synthetic dysfunction	Same profile as warfarin but prolonged echis time, 50% normal plasma PT and APTT corrects
Qualitative platelet dysfunction (uraemia, postcardiopulmonary bypass, antiplatelet drugs, beta-lactam antibiotics, corticosteroids, vasculitis, vitamin C deficiency, paraproteinaemias	Increased bleeding time
von Willebrand disease	Mildly increased APTT, increased bleeding time, reduced vWB multimers and factor 8 levels
Disseminated intravascular coagulation	Increased APTT, PT, TCT, reduced fibrinogen (extremely low in snake envenomation), increased FDPs and D-dimer, reduced platelets, fragmented red cells, normal reptilase time if sufficient fibrinogen
Thrombolytic therapy	Increased PT, APTT, TCT, low fibrinogen, 50% normal plasma PT and APTT corrects (unless very early with lytic agent also in sample)
Hypofibrinogenaemia	Low fibrinogen, abnormal reptilase time if fibrinogen very low, abnormal functional (e.g. thrombin clottable fibrinogen) and immunological (e.g. fibrinogen antigen assay) tests

Continued

TABLE 6.26 Disorders of coagulation—cont'd	
Condition	Findings
Dysfibrinogenaemia (liver disease, congenital)	Variable fibrinogen, abnormal reptilase time, normal immunological fibrinogen assay, abnormal functional assay
Haemophilia A and B (factor 8 and 9 deficiency respectively)	Isolated increase in APTT, 50% normal plasma APTT corrects, low factor 8 or 9 assay level
Isolated factor 13 deficiency	Normal APTT, PT, TCT but abnormal urea solubility test
Lupus anticoagulant	Increased APTT, TCT; 50% normal plasma APTT abnormal, abnormal reptilase time, associated lupus anticoagulant and anticardiolipin antibodies
Inhibitors of factor 8 or 9	Same pattern as lupus anticoagulant without the lupus-associated antibodies, positive factor 8 or 9 inhibitor assay
Recombinant factor 7a therapy	Variable – usually some shortening of the PT and APTT
Activated protein C (drotrecogin alpha) therapy	Variable – increased APTT
Direct thrombin inhibitors (e.g. lepirudin)	Increased APTT

The thromboelastograph

Thromboelastography/ometry provides an assessment of global haemostatic function rather than the traditional measurements of PT and APTT. The normal thromboelastogram is illustrated in Figure 6.76 and has parameters such as r (reaction time), K (clot formation time), the α angle (slope from r to K value), the MA (maximum amplitude), CLI (clot lysis index) and A_{60} (amplitude 60 minutes after MA). Normal values appear in Table 6.27 and some abnormalities are shown in Figure 6.77.

Haematologic datasets

Thrombotic thrombocytopenic purpura

- A classical pentad of fever, thrombocytopenia, and microangiopathic haemolytic anaemia, renal and neurological defects. It is thought to be related to an abnormal metalloproteinase (ADAMTS13). The condition is seen with certain infections, drugs (e.g. calcineurin antagonists, clopidogrel), pregnancy, SLE, and with graft versus host disease. The laboratory findings are:
  - low platelets
  - reduced haemoglobin with polychromasia, schistocytes and spherocytes
  - increased reticulocytes
  - reduced haptoglobin and increased lactate dehydrogenase
  - unconjugated hyperbilirubinaemia with urinary urobilinogen
  - variable neutrophilia
  - increased urea and creatinine (greater in haemolytic uraemic syndrome)

Pre-eclampsia

- Characteristic biochemical and haematological features, include:
  - increased uric acid
  - increased urea and creatinine

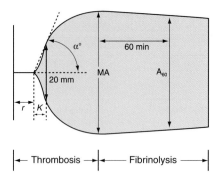

FIGURE 6.76 Normal thromboelastogram
Source: Based on Curry A, Pierce J. Conventional and near-patient tests of coagulation. Continuing Education in Anaesthesia, Critical Care and Pain 2007, 7:49.

TABLE 6.27 Normal values

	Value	Process	Blood component
r time	6–8 minutes	Initial fibrin formation rate	Plasma clotting factors and inhibitor activity
K time	3–6 minutes (curve amplitude 20 mm)	Fibrin build-up and cross-linkage	Fibrinogen, platelets and intrinsic clotting factors
α angle	50–60°	Speed of solid clot formation	Thrombocytopenia and hypofibrinogenaemia decrease angle
MA	50–60 mm	Absolute strength of fibrin clot	Platelet number, function and fibrin interaction
CLI	>85%	Loss of clot integrity due to lysis	
A_{60}	MA–5 mm	Clot retraction/lysis	

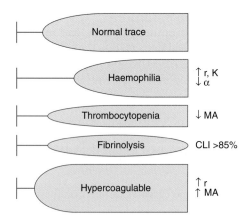

FIGURE 6.77 Abnormal thromboelastographic patterns
Source: Based on Curry A, Pierce J. Conventional and near-patient tests of coagulation. Continuing Education in Anaesthesia, Critical Care and Pain 2007; 7:50.

○ proteinuria
○ in HELLP syndrome, a variant of pre-eclampsia, there is microangiopathic haemolytic anaemia, elevated liver function tests (AST, ALT, LDH) and low platelets
○ PT, APTT and fibrinogen are normal.

'CAPPS' (catastrophic antiphospholipid syndrome)
• Noteworthy for being associated with a solitary abnormality in the coagulation profile – an isolated elevation in the APTT.

Haemophagocytic syndrome
• Characterised by the following laboratory findings:
    ○ cytopenias
    ○ features of haemolysis
    ○ increased triglycerides
    ○ massively increased ferritin
    ○ increased FDPs
    ○ low fibrinogen.
• Causes are varied and include malignancy (e.g. T-cell lymphoma, autoimmune diseases, infections such as EBV, influenza)
• Bone marrow shows activated macrophages with haemophagocystosis.

Analysis of body fluids

Sampling of urine, pleural, ascitic, cerebrospinal fluid and joint fluid may useful in the diagnosis of a range of conditions. The following series of tables are useful to facilitate interpretation of results (Tables 6.28–6.32).

TABLE 6.28 Urine	
Parameter	**Significance**
White cells	Seen in urinary tract infection, renal calculi, interstitial nephritis, glomerulonephritis, vasculitis, infarction Dipstick test for leucocyte esterase detects whole or lysed white cells
Red cells	Dysmorphic red cells: crenated cells that originated in the glomeruli in glomerulonephritis and have passed through the tubular osmotic gradients Dipstick test positive for haemoglobin (free or bound to red cells) or myoglobin. Differentiated on urine microscopy
Protein	Increased in glomerulonephritis, nephrotic syndrome, multiple myeloma, urinary tract malignancies, pyelonephritis
Casts	Hyaline: Tamm-Horsfall mucoproteins: clear and cylindrical, can be normal Red cell: anuclear cells with clear cylinder formations (mucoproteins), seen in glomerulonephritis, subacute bacterial endocarditis White cell: seen in pyelonephritis, interstitial nephritis, vasculitis, infarction Granular: degenerated casts, non-specific to many renal parenchymal diseases Fatty: oval fat bodies (cholesterol esters) in clear cylinders (mucoproteins), seen in diabetic nephropathy and nephrotic syndrome Epithelial: seen in the recovery phase of acute tubular necrosis Eosinophiluria: seen in interstitial nephritis and atheroembolism

Continued

TABLE 6.28 Urine—cont'd

Parameter	Significance
Crystals	Calculi: calcium pyrophosphate, calcium oxalate, magnesium–ammonium–phosphate, urate, cysteine Sulfonamides Methotrexate Acyclovir Oxalate with ethylene glycol Radiocontrast agents
pH (normally 4.5–8)	<6.0 with acidosis and pre-renal failure >7.0 with alkalosis and alkalinising agents, renal tubular acidosis, urease producing bacteria (e.g. *Proteus mirabilis*)
Glucose	Elevated blood glucose with diabetes mellitus and renal glycosuria
Ketones	Dipstick test detects acetone and acetoacetic acid but not beta-hydroxybutyrate Positive in starvation, alcoholic and diabetic ketoacidosis, carbohydrate-free and high fat and protein diet
Bilirubin and urobilinogen	Conjugated bilirubin increased if excess production or biliary obstruction A yellow foam forms when the sample is shaken Urobilinogen absent in biliary obstruction
Nitrite	Positive with most bacterial infections that convert nitrate to nitrite. Some organisms (e.g. *Streptococcus faecalis* and Gram-positive cocci) do not produce nitrite
Urinary cystatin C	Predictor of severity of acute tubular dysfunction in a range of renal pathologies including contrast nephropathy
Specific gravity (normally 1.005–1.030)	Increased in hyperglycaemia, proteinuria, SIADH, intravascular dehydration, radiocontrast agents Decreased in diabetes insipidus, glomerulonephritis, pyelonephritis, renal failure
Urinary electrolytes	Sodium: marker of hydration status and concentrating ability • Increased urinary losses in hypoadrenalism, salt losing nephropathy, acute tubular necrosis, excess salt loads, SIADH • Decreased excretion in hyperaldosteronism, Cushing's syndrome, intravascular dehydration, pre-renal failure, hepatorenal syndrome Osmolarity: like sodium is a marker of hydration status and concentrating ability but also reflects excreted osmotically active substances (e.g. mannitol, radiocontrast, glucose) Potassium: may help clarify source of potassium loss (e.g. renal versus extra-renal) • Increased renal losses in hypomagnesaemia, acute tubular necrosis, loop and thiazide diuretics, hyperaldosteronism, Cushing's syndrome, amphotericin B Chloride: may help clarify the mechanism of metabolic alkalosis • Cl⁻ responsive (urinary Cl⁻ <10 mmol/L) – intravascular volume depletion (e.g. diuretics, vomiting) • Cl⁻ resistant (urinary Cl⁻ >10 mmol/L) – intravascular volume expansion and hypokalaemia (e.g. hyperaldosteronism) Calcium: may clarify cause of deranged calcium homeostasis • Increased urinary losses with loop diuretics, idiopathic hypercalcuria, hypoparathyroidism, vitamin D intoxication, renal failure, renal tubular acidosis, sarcoidosis • Decreased excretion in hyperparathyroidism, malabsorption syndromes, vitamin D deficiency, thiazide diuretics

Continued

TABLE 6.28 Urine—cont'd

Parameter	Significance
Colour	Yellow: normal urochrome pigment Clear: low osmolality (diuretics), diabetes insipidus Milky: lipiduria, chyluria, urinary tract infection Pink: urate, haematuria Red: haematuria, beeturia Tea-coloured: haemoglobin, myoglobin, metronidazole, porphyria, povidone-iodine contamination Orange: rifampicin, conjugated bilirubin Blue-green: phenols (propofol metabolites, amitriptyline, Listerine™, triamterene), methylene blue, *Pseudomonas aeruginosa* urinary tract infection, chronic obstructive jaundice with biliverdin excretion Purple: Hartnup disease, Indican discolouration in chronically catheterised patients with bacterial overgrowth Grey-black: homogentisic acid in alkaptonuria, melanogens in disseminated melanoma, Addison's disease, alpha-methyldopa

TABLE 6.29 Pleural fluid

Parameter	Significance
Appearance	Normally pale yellow Haemorrhagic in trauma, malignancy, pulmonary infarction, post-pericardiotomy Turbid, purulent if parapneumonic or empyema Milky if chyle present
Protein	Pleural fluid: serum ratio <0.5 in a *transudate* (pleural fluid protein <30 g/L) e.g. heart failure, liver failure, nephrotic syndrome, protein-losing enteropathy, hypothyroidism, pulmonary embolism, fluid overload Pleural fluid: serum ratio >0.5 in an *exudate* (pleural fluid protein >30 g/L) e.g. parapneumonic, empyema, subphrenic abscess, oesophageal rupture, pancreatitis, malignancy, pulmonary embolism
Lactate dehydrogenase	Pleural fluid: serum ratio <0.6 in a *transudate* Pleural fluid: serum ratio >0.6 in an *exudate*
Glucose	Less than half serum glucose seen in bacterial infections, malignancy, rheumatoid arthritis, SLE
pH	<7.3 with empyema, often with raised lactate
White cells	Neutrophilia: parapneumonic effusion, empyema, PE Lymphocytosis: TB, rheumatoid arthritis, SLE, sarcoidosis, malignancy
Cytology	Malignant cells Mesothelial cells are normal or increased in mesothelioma Multinucleated giant cells in rheumatoid arthritis
Other findings	Acid-fast bacilli with TB Chylomicrons and triglyceride in chylothorax Amylase greater than serum in ruptured oesophagus, pancreatitis, malignancy, bacterial pneumonia Haematocrit >50% of blood with haemothorax

TABLE 6.30 Ascitic fluid

Parameter	Significance
Serum: ascitic albumin gradient	>1.1 g/dL (transudate): cirrhosis, cardiac failure, alcoholic hepatitis, portal vein thrombosis <1.1 g/dL (exudate): pancreatitis, malignancy, TB, nephrotic syndrome, bowel obstruction or infarction
Lactate dehydrogenase	Transudate <225 U/L Exudate >225 U/L
Glucose	Often normal in spontaneous bacterial peritonitis and low in secondary bacterial peritonitis
Amylase	Increased in pancreatic ascites
pH	<7.0 suggests bacterial infection
Triglyceride	Increased in chylous ascites
White cells	Bacterial peritonitis: WCC >250 x 10^6/L or >500/mm^3 Polymorphonuclear cells in bacterial infection Mononuclear cells in TB or fungal infection
Gram stain and culture	Spontaneous bacterial peritonitis usually monomicrobial Secondary bacterial peritonitis usually polymicrobial and a perforated viscus should be sought
Cytology	Malignant cells may be seen

TABLE 6.31 Cerebrospinal fluid

Parameter	Significance
Appearance	Normally clear Turbid with infection Blood-stained with subarachnoid haemorrhage and traumatic taps Yellow with xanthochromia (takes 6–12 hours to develop after blood has entered the CSF)
White cells	Normally scant monocytes In a traumatic tap expect 1 white cell per 500 red cells Polymorphonuclear leucocytosis with bacterial infection Lymphocytosis with viral, TB, cryptococcus and listeria infections Mixed lympho/monocytosis in Guillain-Barré syndrome and Status epilepticus
Red cells	Increased in traumatic tap and subarachnoid haemorrhage
Protein	Mildly increased in infection – TB > bacterial > viral Increased in Guillain-Barré syndrome, vasculitis, sarcoidosis and any CNS inflammation (including in situ CSF drains, blood in CSF) Oligoclonal band in multiple sclerosis
Glucose	Normally at least 75% of serum glucose Less than half serum glucose in bacterial, TB, and fungal infections, as well as vasculitis and sarcoidosis
Other findings	Xanthochromic index with spectrophotometry in subarachnoid haemorrhage after 6–12 hours Increased lactate in bacterial and fungal meningitis

TABLE 6.32 Joint fluid

Parameter	Significance
Appearance	Normally clear to light yellow
White cells	Infection, gout, pseudogout, inflammatory arthritides (e.g. rheumatoid arthritis, HLA-B27 associated arthritis)
Red cells	Traumatic tap, traumatic or spontaneous coagulopathy-related haemarthrosis
Protein	Levels greater than 30 g/L seen in infection and inflammatory arthritides
Lactate dehydrogenase	Levels greater than 300 IU/L seen in rheumatoid arthritis, gout or infection
Glucose	Less than half serum glucose seen in infection or severe inflammation
Crystals	Gout: monosodium urate, which are needle-shaped negatively birefringent under red polarised light Pseudogout: calcium pyrophosphate dihydrate, which are rhomboidal crystals positively birefringent under red polarised light

References

The following sources have been used as reference material in the preparation of this chapter.

Badr A, Nightingale P. An alternative approach to acid-base abnormalities in critically ill patients. Continuing Education in Anaesthesia, Critical Care and Pain. 2007; 7: 107–11.

Bersten AD, Soni N. (eds) Oh's Intensive Care Manual. Elsevier; 6th edn: 2009.

Collins J, Stern EJ. Chest Radiology: The Essentials. Lippincott Williams and Wilkins; 2nd edn: 2007.

Conti M, Moutereau S, Zater M, et al. Urinary cystatin as a specific marker of tubular dysfunction. Clinical Chemistry and Laboratory Medicine. 2006; 44: 288–91.

Curry, A, Pierce, J. Conventional and near-patient tests of coagulation. Continuing Education in Anaesthesia, Critical Care and Pain 2007; 7: 45–50.

Fauci AS, Braunwald E, Kasper DL, et al. Harrisons Principles of Internal Medicine. MGraw-Hill Professional; 17th edn: 2008.

Hall JB, Schmidt GA, Wood LDH. Principles of Critical Care. McGraw Hill; 3rd edn: 2005

Hampton JR. The ECG in Practice. Churchill Livingstone; 3rd edn: 2008.

Hampton JR. 150 ECG Problems. Churchill Livingstone; 3rd edn: 2008.

Hobbs G, Mahajan R. Imaging in Anaesthesia and Critical Care. Elsevier; 1st edn: 2000.

Hopkins R, Peden C, Gandhi S. Radiology for Anaesthesia and Intensive Care Medicine. Cambridge University; 2nd edn: 2009.

Irwin R, Rippe J. Irwin and Rippe's Intensive Care Medicine. Lipincott Williams and Wilkins; 6th edn: 2007

Joyce C, Saad N, Kruger P, Foot C, Blackwell N. Diagnostic Imaging in Critical Care: A Problem Based Approach. Elsevier: 2010.

Kaddoura S. Echo Made Easy. Churchill Livingstone; 7th edn: 2009.

Lo G, Juhl D, Warkentin T et al. Evaluation of pretest clinical score (4 Ts) for the diagnosis of heparin-induced thrombocytopenia in two clinical settings. Journal of Thrombosis and Haemostasis 2006; 4:759–65

McRae R and Esser M. Practical Fracture Treatment. Churchill Livingstone; 4th edn: 2008.

Miller RD. Miller's Anesthesia. Churchill Livingstone; 6th edn: 2009.

Nicholson DA, Driscoll PA. ABC of Emergency Radiology. BMJ Publishing Company; 1st edn: 1996.

Norwitz E, Schorge J. Obstetrics and Gynecology at a Glance. Wiley-Blackwell; 3rd edn: 2010.

Phelan D, Ruboletta F, Brown K. European Society of Intensive Care Medicine Patient-centred Acute Care Training On-line; 2nd edn.

Pierce L. Guide to Mechanical Ventilation and Intensive Respiratory Care. Saunders: 2005.

Pinsky M, Brochard L, Mancebo J, Hedenstierna G (eds). Applied Physiology in Intensive Care Medicine. Springer; 2nd edn: 2009

Venkatesh B, Morgan T, Joyce C, et al. Data Interpretation in Critical Care Medicine. Butterworth Heinemann; 1st edn: 2003.

Warrell DA, Cox TM, Firth JD, et al. Oxford Textbook of Medicine. Oxford University Press; 5th edn: 2010.

Watkinson P. The Stewart Hypothesis of Acid–Base Balance. Anaesthesia UK. www.frca.co.uk.

White H and Venkatesh B. Applications of transcranial Doppler in the ICU: a review. Intensive Care Medicine 2006; 32: 981–94.

Chapter 7

Vivas

Spoon feeding in the long run teaches us nothing but the shape of the spoon.
EM FORSTER

Generic advice

The vivas are a searching component of the examination; in several sequential, short interviews the examiners are trying to ascertain the depth and breadth of candidates' knowledge, and whether they meet the standard of an intensivist capable of safe, independent practice. The examiners are characteristically assessing clinical judgement, prioritisation, interpretation of complex situations, anticipation of clinical actions and their sequelae. They are trying to determine if you are able to apply your knowledge and clinical experience; whether you are aware of potential pitfalls and whether you have an ability to think on your feet.

The time allotted to each viva will pass surprisingly quickly. You will usually be addressed by one examiner who is seated directly opposite you with a marking sheet. There may be a second examiner, who often remains silent. As you reply you may notice them putting ticks in boxes or making comments on the marking grid. Do not let this distract you. Some examiners prefer to complete the marking sheet after the candidate leaves the room, so do not panic if there is minimal writing on the grid during your viva.

There may be an observer in the room, who will normally position themselves behind you, so that you are not distracted by their presence. This person may be a junior examiner observing a more senior colleague in action, or a senior examiner observing a new examiner (as a form of quality control). All examiners are subjected to peer review at regular intervals.

The tone you should adopt during the vivas is that of a respectful but competent colleague. If you are an authority on a particular topic this will be obvious from the answers you give to the questions posed. If you have never been exposed to the particular scenario in question, this will also generally be obvious to the examiners. It is not appropriate to refuse to answer a question based on the fact you have not previously been exposed to that situation. It is better to say: 'While I have never performed this technique/seen this condition/caused this complication personally, the most appropriate course of action I would consider in that circumstance would be ...'

It is wise not to second-guess the topics a viva will cover from the opening statement presented, as they often cover many areas that may be unrelated. You must be nimble of mind to rapidly adapt to changing circumstances. (A recent viva began with a history of a patient with refractory leukaemia and multi-organ failure, but rapidly progressed to a searching discussion on ethics and dealing with difficult or disagreeing colleagues.)

Management of crisis or urgent situations is likely to crop up in more than one scenario. The verbalisation of your actions will score you marks. Useful statements during these vivas, such as: 'This is an emergency'; 'This is a critical situation'; 'I would immediately hit the arrest alarm and call for help', can be used to display your appreciation of the urgency of a situation.

Similarly, brief prepared answers for introductory statements can also be helpful. For example, 'This is an emergency. I would call for help and simultaneously conduct an assessment of the patient while I commenced resuscitation and treatment, paying particular attention to the airway, ventilation and circulation parameters ...' and then go on to address aspects particular to that case.

The advantage of this approach is that it takes only 20 seconds to say and covers a wealth of important information, showing how safe you are. Without such a system candidates often fumble around all of the above points, making significant errors of omission and wasting a lot of time. However, you should make sure your statements are appropriate to the given situation. Be aware that the examiners may fast-forward you through this part of the viva as you have already gained the points available, and move you on to a more specific question with more opportunity to gain marks. Note that at any stage they may interrupt you and ask for more detail. Also note that such an opening approach may not answer the specific question posed. If the opening question asks for specific investigations for a certain medical condition, then answer that directly. You must be quick on your toes and flexible to the situation. The best way to achieve this is with practice.

Do not forget that you are not expected to be an island. There are several situations where points will be allocated for an appropriate referral to another specialty (e.g. an obstetrician for a woman with eclampsia or a paediatrician for a paediatric critical care patient in a rural or district hospital). Remember also, that safe practice for certain cases will involve timely transfer to a specialised centre (e.g. a burns unit for a patient with significant burns or a specialised paediatric ICU for a child). Viva marks are awarded accordingly.

You should also be aware that investigations or equipment may be presented to you in association with vivas, particularly as part of an unfolding case scenario.

The examiners realise that the examination is a very stressful situation for candidates. They are aware that under such circumstances some people may freeze up or not perform at their best. Poor performance in one viva may adversely affect your performance in the next viva, even if you have expert knowledge on the material under discussion. However, performance under pressure is also part of your daily work and some degree of cool-headedness in a stressful situation is to be expected. At all times listen carefully to what is asked. Answer what is asked, rather than what you know.

Should you say something inappropriate or embark on a plan that is not within mainstream current thinking, the examiner will try to give you a chance to retract a particular statement – a lifeline. If this is the case, do not take it as a challenge to stand by the courage of your convictions. Arguing the point will rarely get you anywhere. Politely ask the examiner to repeat the previous question, then think carefully about the answer you gave. If it was patently absurd (e.g. 'I would give the patient 100 milligrams of adrenaline'), then simply apologise and give a more appropriate answer. If you suddenly have an insight that you did not have before, you can say: 'On reflection, my preferred course of action would be ...'. The viva can then continue. If the examiner asks you for a list of possibilities, enumerate these as logically as you can. If they then ask, 'Is there anything else?' with their pen poised over a tick box, it is likely you have forgotten something important and they are giving you another lifeline and a chance to score more points.

Remember that the focus of the examination is for you to prove that you are knowledgeable and safe to work as a specialist intensivist. It is perfectly reasonable to say what you normally do in a particular situation, or to outline a course of action based on your experience. However, if that course of action is revolutionary, non-mainstream, experimental or simply dangerous, you are probably better to keep it to yourself.

Do not enter the viva examination with the expectation that all examiners will be reassuring, friendly, smiling and gentle, as this is unlikely to be the case. Some examiners will go out of their way to put you at ease, but others may take a more formal, professional interrogative approach, although none will be overtly hostile. Do not feel intimidated or discriminated against if you feel that you have not received positive feedback from the examiners. One of the reasons that you are examined by several different examiners is to counterbalance this possibility. The marking system is as fair as possible and under constant review, so there is actually very little room for the personality of the examiner to play a part in the marks you receive for your answers.

Viva technique is extremely important and can only be achieved through practice. Practise with as many different senior colleagues as possible, including those with whom you do not feel at ease. Ask for an appraisal of your technique, not just your knowledge.

Make a conscious effort to adopt a confident posture and avoid anxious hand gestures. Speak slowly and clearly. Many candidates, in the stress of the situation, rush their answers and talk incredibly quickly, omitting critical information in the process. When asked a question, force yourself to pause for a couple of seconds and consider the question carefully. Try not to um and ah. Sound confident, but not arrogant.

Tape yourself and, agonising though it can be, listen to yourself and work out what you need to stop doing, change or improve. If you drive to work you could take advantage of this time to rehearse out loud responses to viva questions. This otherwise lost time provides an excellent opportunity for you to improve the speed and fluency of your dialogue. In addition to audio-taping, some candidates find video-recordings of themselves performing viva practice can be very helpful. It is usually excruciating to witness yourself in this way, but may reveal all sorts of mannerisms and oddities of body language that you will not become aware of in any other way. Spending a group study session making these video-recordings and then reviewing them together can be a very valuable investment of time.

If English is not your first language, seek advice from a trusted colleague about how easy you are to understand under the stress of an examination situation. Fluent, easy-to-understand English can become almost impossible to follow when it is sped up, particularly if the cadences and timing of your native tongue make a reappearance. If this is a problem for you, taping as described above may be helpful, but may not be enough. If you are struggling, paying for one or two sessions with a professional voice (acting) coach may pay dividends. We know of several candidates for whom this has been a breakthrough step in passing the exam.

Format

For information about the specific format of the exam you are sitting see Chapter 1.

Viva topics for the EDIC, DICM and CICM Fellowship examinations

It is impossible to cover, in any great detail, all the topics that could reasonably be asked in the vivas. This section concludes with a list of the major topics relevant to all of the exit examinations, of which you should have comprehensive knowledge. Please note that this list is representative of the subjects often covered and is intended as a guide only. Topics are not presented in order of likelihood of being asked. If you can glance through this list confident of being able to hold a thorough discussion on each of the topics, then you are probably in very good shape for the viva examination.

Note that equipment, procedures and data interpretation may be asked about in the context of any viva. Questions about monitoring of physiologic parameters cross these domains and are commonly asked in some form (e.g. how to insert a device to measure cardiac output followed by questions probing understanding of haemodynamic indices). The pharmacology pertaining to drugs commonly encountered in the ICU are important examinable topics and are covered on the DVD. Paediatric issues are specifically addressed in Chapter 10. The examiners will want you to be aware of potential pitfalls of any course of action you advocate. As the date of the exam approaches, it may be helpful for your study group to devise other viva topics for each of you to practise. You can also work through the list below.

Those approaching the Fellowship examination of the CICM would be well advised to analyse recent examiners' reports carefully, as subjects that have been answered poorly in the past often recur in subsequent examinations. For example, a written question on the assessment of the airway and intubation that was answered very poorly one year, was followed by a clinical scenario station with intubation of a manikin in the subsequent exam. Similarly, a poorly answered written question on brain death criteria and testing was followed by a viva on the subject at the next sitting.

The questions and marking grid for each viva are determined in detail at the examiners' meeting beforehand in order to be as scrupulously fair as possible. Almost always the introductory information that you are given to read in the 2 minutes before the viva starts will lead into a broad, opening discussion, with subsequent questions leading down an increasingly specific route. For example, the scenario of a fitting pregnant woman at 36 weeks gestation will usually begin with description of appropriate resuscitation, investigations and calling for the obstetrician. This is not the time to launch into a dissertation on the molecular biology of eclampsia, however well you know the area. The examiner will then guide you in the direction they want you to go. For example, asking for a differential diagnosis (think and answer systematically – 'causes related to the pregnancy'; 'causes unrelated to the pregnancy'; 'intra-cerebral causes'; 'extra-cerebral causes') may lead swiftly to you being asked to interpret typical laboratory investigations for eclampsia, followed by the rest of the viva being spent on discussing the mechanisms of action and use of magnesium in critical care.

A particularity of the CICM vivas is the occurrence of a communication station and procedure station. These topics were dealt with in detail in Chapter 5.

Possible viva topics
Airway management
- Difficult airway algorithms
- Techniques of awake fibre-optic bronchoscopic intubation
- Ancillary equipment for management of the difficult airway.

Bariatric patients
- Specific management difficulties
- Bariatric surgical complications.

Burns
- Airway management
- Management of inhalation injury
- Fluid management
- Abdominal compartment syndrome

- Diagnosing infection in burns patients
- Antibiotic management.

Cardiovascular problems
- Myocardial ischaemia
- Complications of coronary artery revascularisation surgery – particularly bleeding and hypotension in the immediate postoperative period
- Post-cardiac-arrest care and prognostication
- Valvular heart disease
- Hypertrophic obstructive cardiomyopathy
- Care of the patient with endocarditis
- Aortic disease, including dissection and ruptured aneurysms
- Intra-aortic balloon pumps.

Collagen vascular diseases
- Systemic lupus erythematosus
- CREST
- Scleroderma
- Polymyositis
- CAPS
- Rheumatoid arthritis patients in the ICU
- Ankylosing spondylitis patients in the ICU
- Hereditary and acquired (e.g. von Willebrand disease, haemophilias, platelet disorders, disseminated intravascular coagulation, disorders of coagulation).

Endocrine disease
- Thyroid diseases, including myxoedema coma and thyroid storm
- Adrenal diseases, including hypoadrenalism
- Phaeochromocytoma
- Diabetes.

Fluid replacement and transfusion medicine
- Maintenance requirements for fluid and electrolytes
- Composition of replacement fluids
- Differences between colloid and crystalloid therapies
- Assessment of fluid status and fluid responsiveness
- Electrolyte disturbances
- Blood products and their administration
- Strategies to minimise necessity for blood transfusion
- Definition and risks of massive blood transfusion
- Recombinant factors (e.g. recombinant factor VIIa).

Gastrointestinal problems
- Acalculous cholecystitis
- Acute pancreatitis
- Upper and lower gastrointestinal bleeding, including stress ulceration
- Liver failure.

Infection control
- Universal precautions and isolation precautions
- Sepsis management, including the role of steroids
- Nosocomial infections
- Multi-drug-resistant organisms

- Common and classical ICU infections
- Infections in immunosuppressed hosts including HIV.

Medical crises
- Basic and advanced cardiac life support and resuscitation committee guidelines
- Medical emergencies (e.g. airway obstruction, hypoxia, anaphylaxis, status asthmaticus, severe hypertension, shock, hypo/hyperthermia, aspiration of gastric contents, pericardial tamponade, massive bleeding, near drowning, near hanging, status epilepticus)
- Complications of procedures (e.g. laryngospasm, tension pneumothorax, increased ventilator pressure, arterial puncture at central venous cannulation, intra-arterial drug injection)
- Thromboembolism management, including preventative strategies
- Electrical safety in the ICU
- Evacuation of an ICU
- Bioterrorism threats
- Triage and pandemic management.

Neurology
- Traumatic brain injury, including prognostication
- Cerebral protection strategies
- Strategies for detecting and reducing ICP
- Hypoxic-ischaemic brain injury
- Cerebrovascular disease
- Subarachnoid haemorrhage
- Muscular disorders (e.g. myasthenia gravis, myotonic and muscular dystrophy, familial periodic paralysis, Guillain-Barré syndrome, tetanus)
- Chronic diseases (e.g. multiple sclerosis, motor neurone disease, epilepsy, Parkinson's disease)
- ICU encephalopathy.

Nutrition
- Enteral and parenteral
- Micronutrients, vitamins and essential minerals
- Post-pyloric feeding
- Agents to increase gastric motility.

Obstetric patients
- Management of the pre-eclamptic or eclamptic patient
- Management of the patient with HELLP syndrome
- Management of the unconscious or fitting patient
- Amniotic fluid embolism
- Post-partum haemorrhage
- CPR in the pregnant patient
- Neonatal resuscitation
- Normal physiological changes in the pregnant woman.

Oncology
- Management of neutropenic sepsis
- Tumour lysis syndrome
- Common patterns of infection
- Post bone marrow transplant patient – graft versus host disease/hepatic veno-occlusive disease

- Management of respiratory failure
- Prognostication of the oncology/haematology patient in ICU.

Pain and sedation management in the ICU
- Acute postoperative pain management
- Safety considerations for patient-controlled and continuous infusion techniques
- Care of the drug-dependent patient in the ICU
- Characteristics, pathways and complications of chronic pain
- Approaches to sedation in the ICU.

Renal disease
- Preservation of renal function
- Acute renal failure in the ICU
- Chronic renal disease
- Renal replacement in the ICU.

Respiratory medicine
- Investigations (e.g. spirometry, flow-volume loops, DLCO)
- Effects of cigarette smoking
- Postoperative pulmonary complications
- ARDS
- Advanced management of refractory hypoxaemic respiratory failure
- Management of acute severe asthma
- Mechanical ventilation
- Pneumonia
- Principles, practice and evidence base for NIV
- VAP
- Obstructive sleep apnoea.

Scoring systems in ICU
- Strengths and weaknesses of common scoring systems (e.g. GCS, APACHE 2 and 3, SOFA).

Statistics and research
- Study design
- Types of data
- Statistical tests
- Systematic reviews and meta-analysis
- Evidence-based medicine.

The ICU patient outside the ICU
- Caring for the ICU patient transferred for CT/MRI scanning
- Intrahospital transport of the critically ill patient, including policy documents related to this
- Medical emergency teams, outreach and post-ICU follow-up services.

Toxicology
- Diagnosis and treatment of common toxidromes.

Transplantation medicine
- Types and complications of immunosuppressive therapy
- Management of the post-transplant patient

- Criteria for diagnosing brain death, and conduct of brain death test
- Discussing organ donation with families, including donation after cardiac death.

Trauma
- EMST/ATLS algorithms
- Assessment and management of specific injuries (e.g. head, spinal cord, torso, pelvic trauma)
- Burns
- Fat embolism syndrome.

Welfare issues
- Interpersonal conflict and communication problems in the ICU
- Resilience and fatigue
- Recommended working hours
- Rostering strategies to combat fatigue
- Substance abuse and dependence
- Professional liability
- Risk management and quality improvement.

Vivas for the Primary examination of the CICM

As with the two written papers, the CICM Primary orals test knowledge of the basic science that forms the foundation to intensive care practice. Many questions seek knowledge of the basic sciences as they occur in everyday clinical practice, for example, the physiology of massive blood loss, glucose control, anatomy relevant to central venous line insertion, drugs involved in the emergency management of hyperkalaemia and pharmacology of noradrenaline. Some consider this to be a particular strength of the CICM Primary examination, and something that differentiates it from other primary exams (which separate physiology and pharmacology). Note that there is some overlap with the final examination, but the emphasis is on the basic science of that subject. At the orals the topic to be discussed is posted outside the station and may include a diagram, photo or piece of equipment. The college have emphasised that accurate and clear diagrams can help efficiently answer questions and explain principles.

A detailed syllabus exists for the Primary examination and this forms the foundation of the knowledge base required. All questions are sourced directly from that syllabus. Candidates should have a sound understanding of those topics, and confidence to express their understanding of the subject material in both written and oral form. The examination is specifically constructed to test whether or not candidates are able to integrate and express basic physiological and pharmacological principles as they relate to various situations relevant to intensive care practice. Chapters 3 and 4 offer plentiful information for candidates approaching this obstacle.

Chapter 8

Clinical cases in the ICU

Knowledge is of no value unless you put it into practice.
ANTON CHEKHOV

Introduction

In this chapter we outline a generalised approach to tackling the clinical component of the FCICM, EDIC and DICM examinations. Areas that require specific attention will be highlighted and examples of common and important clinical cases will be outlined in the form of diagnostic problems or specific patient groups.

BOX 8.1 Clinical cases covered in this chapter

Diagnostic problems

1. Why does this patient have severe respiratory failure?
2. Why is this patient failing to wean from ventilation?
3. Can you extubate this patient?
4. Why is this patient shocked?
5. Why is this patient not passing urine?
6. Why is this patient jaundiced?
7. Why is this patient not waking up?
8. Why is this patient weak?
9. Is this patient brain dead?
10. Why is this patient febrile?
11. What injuries has this multiple trauma patient sustained?
12. How is this patient with multi-organ failure progressing?

Specific patient groups

1. The patient with chronic obstructive pulmonary disease
2. The cardiac arrest survivor
3. The post-cardiac surgical patient
4. The patient with a subarachnoid haemorrhage
5. The patient with a head injury
6. The patient with a spinal injury
7. The patient with an intra-abdominal catastrophe
8. The patient who has had an abdominal aortic aneurysm repair

Continued

BOX 8.1 Clinical cases covered in this chapter—cont'd

9. The obstetric patient
10. The transplant patient
11. The oncology patient
12. The patient with burns
13. The patient receiving extracorporeal life-support
14. The bariatric patient
15. The long-stay patient

A generic approach to the clinical case

When the examiners are preparing the cases to use in the exam they are able to choose from all of the patients currently receiving care in the unit that is hosting the exam. This can range from the routine cardiac surgical patient who is about to be discharged to the ward to the newly admitted and still being worked-up multi-trauma patient. Do not be lulled into a false sense of security because the venue for your exam does not usually manage burns, spinal injuries, transplant patients, or whatever you feel least comfortable with. It is our experience that specialised patient groups are sometimes managed outside the local major referral centre. For example, a burns patient occurred in our clinical exam, despite the fact that our exam venue *never* saw burns patients and the local major referral centre was nearby.

The purpose of the clinical case is to evaluate your ability to perform a systematic, appropriate assessment focusing on either a body part, a body system and/or the whole patient. You should be able to elicit the physical signs present, evaluate their importance, and, if required, demonstrate or explain your methods of doing so. Equally important is your ability to rapidly process the clinical information you have obtained and rationally present your thoughts in a meaningful and polished way. The essence of the clinical case is for you to demonstrate a specialist approach to the issue at hand.

For the clinical cases in the FCICM exam and the short cases in the EDIC the process will formally commence with the examiners presenting you with focused information about the patient you are going to see, typically followed by a question they would like you to address during your assessment. Do not forget the question! It is hopeless to give a beautiful rendition of the causes of shock in a post-cardiac surgical patient on an intra-aortic balloon pump and three inotropes, when you were actually asked why they are slow to wake up. We advise that you devote all of your attention to the examiners at this point and resist the urge to start looking around the room while this crucial information is being delivered. Listen carefully to the examiners, just as you would to a colleague handing over a patient.

There is only a short time available for you to make a thorough assessment. In order to do this well you must develop economy of movement. A routine that ensures that nothing is missed, but where every action is deliberate and purposeful, and nothing is repeated. We came to call this 'the dance' and it is described below. It must be appreciated that this description is only one possible approach. It aims to illustrate a helpful plan for those starting to approach clinical cases for the examinations. Feedback from the first edition of this book has verified that these are helpful recommendations, but care must be taken to ensure that the style is not mechanical and is varied appropriately for the specific patient presented. Some examiners have noted that overcompliance with a routine such as this is producing 'clones'. Individuality, flare and skilful physical examination technique are therefore likely to be highly rewarded.

We recommend that you move to the end of the bed and pause briefly to make a global assessment of the patient and the cubicle, while reviewing your game plan for the given scenario. For example, if shock is the focus of the viva, run through the differential diagnosis for causes of shock in your mind, and you can use this as the framework for your examination and presentation to the examiners.

If the patient appears conscious, now is the time to introduce yourself. If not, then you can wait until you commence your physical examination. For example, whether the patient is conscious or not say: 'Hello Mr Jones, my name is Fred Smith. I am a doctor and I am going to examine you'.

Move to your right as you look at the bed. If the monitor, infusions or ventilator are located on this side, now is the time to ask what medications and fluids are being given, notice any pertinent information displayed on the monitor (e.g. atrial fibrillation with a rapid ventricular response) and enquire about the ventilator settings. You are unlikely to be examined in your own unit and therefore may not be familiar with the ventilator, monitors and infusion pumps in use. The examiners will happily provide the details you need to know, but make an effort to appraise what is being instituted and avoid treating the examiners as your servants. Increasingly, large, easily visible labels are being used to make it easier to determine what is being infused (e.g. fentanyl).

Now turn and walk to the other side of the bed, looking carefully at floor and bedrail level so that you do not miss anything, such as wound drains or intercostal catheters. It is important to avoid spending excessive amounts of time on these things before progressing to examine the patient and significant practice is needed to do this efficiently without missing important information.

Environmental clues
The cubicle
Key observations to make include:
- infection control measures (e.g. signs, gowns, gloves at the entry to the cubicle)
- special waste disposal bins (e.g. for cytotoxic agents)
- signs that the patient may have been in the room for a long period of time (e.g. large quantities of photographs)
- weaning or activity plans fixed to the wall
- environmental observations (e.g. increased ambient temperature for burns patients, distinctive smells such as melaena stool)
- medications (e.g. vials of specific antibiotics).

Infusions
When you ask about the medications and fluids being infused, this may alert you to important possible diagnoses or pathophysiology.
Examples of this include:
- heparin infusions, suggesting venous thromboembolism or an acute coronary syndrome
- vasopressin infusion, suggesting distributive shock
- nimodipine, which almost always implies a subarachnoid haemorrhage
- the ratio and quantity of vasopressor versus inotropic drug, which may enable a grasp of the individual's haemodynamic disturbance
- activated protein C implies severe sepsis.

You must also seek the important negative observations. If the patient is not alert and not receiving sedation, ask what agents have previously been administered and when the last dose was. If the patient is unable to move spontaneously or in response to pain it is important to ask if they have received a neuromuscular blocking drug recently.

Do not miss total parenteral nutrition and blood products.

Ventilator

Review the ventilator settings:

- mode – often unit-specific preferences, therefore difficult to draw conclusions about the underlying pathophysiology
- fractional inspired oxygen – comment on the A–a gradient if possible
  - (e.g. it is reasonable to state that there is a significantly increased A–a gradient if the SpO_2 is less than 95%, with an FiO_2 greater than 0.3).
- ventilator strategy – tidal volume, rate, PEEP, I:E ratio
  - (e.g. protective lung ventilation with low tidal volumes, increased PEEP; airway obstruction strategy – low rate, low PEEP, increased inspiratory flow rates).
- where relevant, ask to assess auto PEEP with an expiratory pause manoeuvre and ascertain the plateau pressure with an inspiratory pause manoeuvre
- estimate dynamic lung compliance: tidal volume/driving pressure (peak pressure minus PEEP).

If non-invasively ventilated, ask for the settings and whether the patient has been invasively ventilated recently.

If not intubated, clarify oxygen requirement and delivery mode (nasal prongs, Hudson mask, Venturi mask, non-rebreather mask).

Monitor

A wealth of information may be available here. Ask yourself the question: Why are these variables being measured in this patient?

Ensure all vital signs are noted and if they are not displayed, ask for them. For example, heart rate, blood pressure, respiratory rate, SpO_2, ECG rhythm and temperature are basic vital signs in the critically ill. The end-tidal CO_2 trace can provide useful information.

Note other parameters commonly measured in specific patient groups. For example, in brain-injured patients, ICP, CPP and $EtCO_2$ are usual.

If a specific device, such as a pulmonary artery catheter or PiCCO, is present, then the last set of measured and calculated variables should be asked for. Be prepared to perform the measurements yourself, but in the interests of time you will usually be provided with this data.

Very occasionally, a rare device, such as a left atrial pressure line or portal venous pressure line, will be present. If there is any information displayed that you are unfamiliar with, ask what the numbers represent.

Equipment

The following is a list of common ICU equipment that you may encounter and should comment on:

- intravascular catheters – note all central venous lines, pulmonary artery catheters, PiCCO™, LiDCO™, FloTrac™, angiogram sheaths – all sites of skin penetration need to be assessed for infection
- CRRT machine – note the mode, settings, type of dialysate and buffer and the vascular access being used
- active cooling devices
- special bed types (e.g. Edgerton bed for spinal injury patients; bariatric beds for obese patients)
- intra-aortic balloon pump – settings, augmentation, timing
- pacing:
  - external, transvenous or epicardial with a pulse generator
  - mode, underlying rate and rhythm, pacing and sensing thresholds
- intercostal catheters – note the number and location, assess the site of entry and specifically note swinging, draining and bubbling

- surgical drains – note location, nature and volume of content
- urethral or suprapubic catheters – note the colour and volume of urine (e.g. haematuria, tea colouring with myoglobinuria)
- intracranial pressure monitors or external ventricular drains – note the colour and volume of cerebrospinal fluid being drained
- external fixators – spinal, pelvic and limb devices and assess the pin sites
- sequential compression limb devices
- physical therapy items – hand weights, wheelchairs, tilt trolley, Jordan frames.

Systematic clinical examination

Strict infection control procedures must be adhered to. Make sure you remove your jacket, watch and any other items of jewellery, except a plain wedding band. Ensure your arms are bare below the elbows. If you have long hair it should be tied back and off your face. You must wash your hands with soap and water or alcohol gel before examining each patient. If you decide to use your own stethoscope, ensure that you clean it before and after each patient use. Most units require that you wear gloves and a plastic apron before approaching the patient. Under certain circumstances you may be also required to wear a facemask, gown and/or a faceshield.

Begin by introducing yourself to the patient (if you have not already done so). Remember that you are a guest and should demonstrate respect for the ICU staff looking after the patient. All interactions with the patient should be performed with gentleness, and dignity should be maintained. The examiners should be consulted before inflicting painful stimuli, such as a sternal rub or application of nail bed pressure.

Take down the bed rail – ask for assistance if you need to. You must have good access to the patient.

While preserving modesty, uncover the patient. This is particularly important for conscious patients. One approach is to fold the bedclothes in towards the midline on both sides, ensuring that the genital area is covered but the groins visible. Important findings on the lower limbs and groins will therefore be noticed early. In female patients, ensure that the breasts are only exposed when necessary. If the patient is being actively warmed, note this and ask if you may briefly expose them more fully.

If the patient is in an awkward or inappropriate position, such as on their side facing away from you, or sitting up for an abdominal examination, then ask if you may reposition them. You will almost always be told no. However, this means the examiners have also examined them in this position and feel that all the relevant information can still be obtained. Look from top to toe for scars, rashes, devices, old line sites, wounds, pallor, bruising, bleeding, petechiae and other signs. Ask what lies beneath any dressings or bandages. Make sure that you have practised examining patients in chairs as well as in bed – remember that the exam is performed in a working ICU.

Economy of movement remains essential here as you have limited time and want to look slick and professional. You may already have a routine you feel comfortable with. If not, we suggest the following approaches.

Where you start will be determined by the specific question you have been asked to answer. For example, a request to assess for brain death must commence with neurological examination focused on the brainstem reflexes. For a question that requires a multisystem assessment, we always start with determining the GCS. We then examine the hands, upper limbs, head, neck, chest, abdomen, groins, lower limbs, then ask to examine the back, although you will often be told that this is not possible.

Often you will be asked to examine a particular system. For example, the examiner might ask you: 'Please examine Mr X's chest and present to me your findings.' In such cases it is useful to have a routine for examining each system, including the cardiovascular, respiratory, gastrointestinal, neurological and integumentary systems. We would strongly recommend practising examination of each individual system so that you appear well rehearsed and fluent at the time of the exam.

Look for or ask about pressure areas, including oral and corneal, enteral feeding tolerance, bowel motions and the nature of tracheal secretions.

Your physical examination will conclude either when you decide that you have completed all that you wish to do at the bedside or when the examiner states that your time is over. You may be told that time is almost over: 'What else do you want to do and what would you be specifically looking for?' If appropriate, conclude by asking for the results of relevant investigations. Be wary of parroting a pre-formulated shopping list of items (e.g. ABG, ECG, BSL, CXR, etc.). Always give a reason for wanting each piece of additional information and limit this to the most useful and relevant requests. For example: 'I would like to see the CT scan to confirm my diagnosis of a subarachnoid haemorrhage and the 4 vessel angiogram for localisation of the aneurysm, which I predict will involve the right posterior cerebral artery.'

You should remove your apron and gloves and wash your hands while formulating your presentation.

Presenting to the examiners

We have identified three distinct presentation styles. The examiners will allow you to use the one that you are most comfortable with:

- style 1 – say nothing until you commence the presentation at the end of the examination.
- style 2 – talk as you go about your findings and their interpretation (e.g. 'I note the blood-stained CSF in the EVD and I suspect a subarachnoid haemorrhage, but this could also be from a traumatic insertion of the drain').
- style 3 – comment on key findings as you go along (e.g. 'I note blood-stained CSF in the EVD'). A summation of all the major findings and their interpretation is given in the presentation at the end. This was our preferred technique. It shows the examiners that you are noticing all the findings; however, some of the less relevant observations can be omitted in the final presentation, as they have already been demonstrated. The focus of the presentation can concentrate on the answer to the clinical question posed. We suggest that you practise all three styles and choose the one that best suits you.

All of these styles have pros and cons that will become evident during practice sessions. The significance of any particular finding may only become evident as other signs are noted. Pointing out *every* finding may send signals to the examiner that the candidate cannot discriminate between the important and the irrelevant. Some candidates find that pointing out major findings as they proceed helps them to remember them during the presentation.

The potential to vary these styles is only limited by the individuality of the candidates and we strongly encourage this. For example, as variants of style 3, some candidates appear to effectively talk to the patient about their findings as a method of cementing in their minds and showing the examiners what they have found: 'I see you've got lots of spider naevi on your chest'. Others interact with both the patient and the examiner: 'Your central line looks quite red at the insertion site' (to the patient), then to the examiner: 'May I ask how old the line is?'

During the presentation ensure your back is to the patient so that you can maintain eye contact with the examiners and not have your gaze wander back to the patient or monitors. Choose a position for your hands that is not distracting. The tone to set here is of a junior consultant discussing a patient with senior colleagues. Never fabricate signs that you wish were present or ignore signs that you cannot explain.

Regardless of the style of presentation you choose you will be expected to answer the question posed by the examiners. This may require you to formulate a provisional or differential diagnosis (supported by your examination findings). You may also be asked to comment on relevant investigations and management issues.

Dealing with complex issues of medical ethics, decision-making capacity, living wills, end-of-life care and changing from active treatment to comfort care, is a key part of the everyday practice of an intensivist. Other challenging topics that may arise include managing the Jehovah's witness or consenting for HIV testing in the ICU. Do not be surprised therefore, if after discussing the medical management of a case with the examiners you are questioned about these aspects of the patient's care. You need to convey to the examiners that your approach is one of honesty, empathy and clarity.

A common question might be: 'What is the prognosis and what would you tell the family?' Useful responses might include:

- 'Based on the following observations I feel that the prognosis for a meaningful recovery are ...'
- 'I would arrange to meet the key family members in a private room and organise not to be interrupted. My usual practice is to invite the bedside nurse and, where appropriate, the unit social worker. I begin by discovering what the family understand about the patient's condition and then explain the situation to them simply, inviting them to ask questions throughout.'
- In a case where the prognosis is grim you might say: 'I would ask the family if Fred had ever discussed with them what he would wish for if he was in this situation'. 'I would ask the family what Fred's view would be were he here with us now in the room.'
- 'I would arrange to meet the family again soon. My usual practice is to offer a series of meetings, as in my experience it takes time for families to come to terms with situations such as ...'
- With a Jehovah's witnesses, you might say: 'First, it is necessary to clearly establish what derivatives of blood, if any, the patient would be willing to receive. Limiting the number of unnecessary blood tests for these patients is vital. Use of iron supplements and erythropoietin should be considered early. Consideration should be given to procedures such as cell salvage, cardiopulmonary bypass, dialysis and plasmapheresis ....'
- Regarding the issue of consent for HIV testing, you might say: 'Ideally, consent should always be obtained prior to testing for HIV, however, this may not be possible, for example in an unconscious patient. In such cases, HIV testing without consent should only be performed if it leads to a change the management of the patient ...'

The candidate should tailor a generic assessment to accommodate the focused approach demanded by a specific case. It is worth taking the time to consider and practise strategies for likely potential cases.

For FCICM candidates

Note that as for other parts of the exam, the examiners' reports over previous years provide a wealth of helpful information. In the clinical cases, candidates are repeatedly criticised for looking ill at ease at the bedside, being disorganised in their examination, failing to notice key pieces of equipment at the bedside, failing to prognosticate and incapable of correctly performing a neurological assessment. The key to avoiding these errors is sustained, repeated practice under the constructively critical eyes of senior colleagues.

For EDIC candidates

The clinical component of the exam consists of one long case and two to three short cases. For the long case in the EDIC you will be given a patient to review and allowed 30–40 minutes to familiarise yourself with them. During this time you will have access to the patient's notes, radiology and laboratory results and any other relevant information. You will also be expected to have completed a thorough examination of the patient. The nurse by the patient's bedside is an invaluable resource and will often provide you with a lot of useful information. Take a few minutes at the beginning to orientate yourself as it is unlikely you will be examined in your own unit and therefore you may be unfamiliar with the infusion pumps, ICU charts or the clinical information system.

Having a systematic approach to reviewing the notes, radiology, laboratory results and examination will save you time. Jot down key points on a piece of paper, so that you can refer back to them if necessary. At the end set aside 5–10 minutes to gather your thoughts, write out your opening sentence summarising the case and make notes on the potential management options. It is worth making notes as you will usually be taken away from the bedside to be examined. You can often predict the initial line of questioning that the examiners will pursue. Remember it is what we do every day in the ICU and the examiners want to reassure themselves that you are a competent intensivist who is safe and can be left in a clinical capacity to run the ICU.

We would strongly recommend practising long cases before the exam, being strict with the time you allocate yourself. Ask your senior colleagues or consultants to listen to you present cases. Previous long cases have included patients with polytrauma, post-surgical complications, sepsis with multi-organ failure, severe pancreatitis, acute liver failure, weaning difficulties, severe asthma, Guillain-Barré syndrome, post-transplant, critical illness polyneuropathy and post-cardiac arrest.

Short cases for the EDIC may focus on a clinical sign (e.g. drug rash, bronchial breathing, heart murmur, splinter haemorrhages), an item of equipment (e.g. chest drains, pulmonary artery catheters, intra-aortic balloon pump) or specific clinical examination (e.g. brainstem testing). Candidates are not expected to undertake practical procedures during the EDIC exam.

Candidates must have a systematic approach to examination of each organ system. Each short case will take around 10–15 minutes. Typical examples of short cases are show in Table 8.1.

TABLE 8.1 Typical EDIC short cases	
Critical illness polyneuropathy	The case might begin with a neurological examination of a patient who has been in the intensive care unit for several weeks and is difficult to wean. The discussion could then revolve around causes of failure to wean, different methods of weaning and the risk factors for critical illness polyneuropathy.
Non-invasive ventilation	The case may involve a patient with COPD receiving non-invasive ventilation via a facemask. The discussion could then include modes of non-invasive ventilation, the evidence for the use of non-invasive ventilation in different patient groups and the variety of methods available.

Continued

TABLE 8.1 Typical EDIC short cases—cont'd	
Renal replacement therapy	The case could begin at the bedside of a ventilated patient on haemofiltration. Topics discussed may be the definition of acute kidney injury, the differences between haemofiltration, haemodialysis and haemodiafiltration, anticoagulation, renal replacement fluids and filtration rates.
Ventilator-associated pneumonia	The case might start with a respiratory examination on a patient who is sedated and mechanically ventilated. The main finding is bronchial breathing in the right lung. The discussion may then revolve around ventilator-associated pneumonia and antimicrobial therapy.

For DICM candidates

The DICM does not have a traditional clinical component by the bedside. Instead, candidates are given a long case where they are asked to review a written case history and subsequently asked questions based on the case history. The short cases for the DICM do not involve patient examination by the bedside.

Diagnostic problems

1. Why does this patient have severe respiratory failure?

Possible cases

- Exacerbation of chronic obstructive pulmonary disease or asthma
- Severe pneumonia
- Chest trauma
- Cardiogenic pulmonary oedema
- Acute respiratory distress syndrome.

Appropriate thoughts

Consider the cause(s) of severe respiratory failure. An *anatomical* approach for systematically assessing for lung pathology includes consideration of:

- large airways, e.g. tracheal stenosis
- small airways, e.g. asthma, COPD
- lung interstitium, e.g. fibrosing lung disease
- alveoli, e.g. cardiogenic and non-cardiogenic pulmonary oedema
- pleural space, e.g. pleural effusion, pneumothorax
- chest wall, e.g. obesity, multiple rib fractures, neuromuscular diseases
- brain, e.g. metabolic encephalopathy, brainstem injury
- ventilator and circuit, e.g. asynchrony.

Evaluate whether this is part of a more global process, e.g. nosocomial pneumonia in a head-injured patient, ARDS with septic shock, Guillain-Barré syndrome with respiratory muscle failure and aspiration.

The examination

The cubicle

- Metered aerosol inhalers or nebuliser devices at the bedside imply reversible airway obstruction.

- Isolation procedures may suggest the patient has an infection with a multi-resistant organism.

The monitor

High-grade temperature may suggest an infective cause, e.g. nosocomial or community-acquired pneumonia.

High $ETCO_2$ readings may be seen when permissive hypercapnoea is part of a protective ventilatory strategy. Low or normal $ETCO_2$ readings do not necessarily reflect the arterial CO_2 ($PaCO_2$) in the setting of large ventilation–perfusion mismatches. The CO_2 trace can give valuable information about airway limitation. Remember the $ETCO_2$ value for later comparison with the $PaCO_2$ as a guide to V/Q mismatch and functional dead space.

Giant V waves on the tracing may indicate severe pulmonary hypertension with tricuspid regurgitation. The numerical CVP reading should be interpreted with caution as an index of right ventricular preload in the setting of severe respiratory failure.

Infusions

- Bronchodilator infusions (e.g. aminophylline, salbutamol, magnesium) may imply reversible airway obstruction.
- Note the choice of antibiotics, e.g. linezolid may imply VRE.
- Heavy sedation and drug paralysis, in the absence of a head injury, raise the possibility that ventilator asynchrony has been an issue.
- Immunoglobulin – this is seen in the management of vasculitic diseases, Guillain-Barré syndrome and myasthenia gravis.

Ventilation

If the patient is receiving non-invasive ventilation, but has severe respiratory failure, consider whether they might soon progress to needing invasive ventilation or if a decision has been made not to progress to endotracheal ventilation and, if so, why this may be.

- Assess the A–a gradient – if this is unremarkable consider neuromuscular disorders.
- Evaluate the ventilation strategy – you must mention protective ventilation settings or the zero PEEP, prolonged I:E ratio in severe airway obstruction.
- Determine dynamic lung compliance, intrinsic and total PEEP and plateau–peak airway pressure differences, as this may provide supportive evidence of your presumptive diagnosis.

Equipment

- Intercostal catheters – look for continuous bubbling, especially from multiple drains, which implies a bronchopleural fistula is present. Do not confuse the bubbling in chamber 3, due to continuous suction, with the important bubbling in chamber 2 in a multiple chamber drain set-up.
- Invasive haemodynamic monitoring – pulmonary artery catheters (e.g. PaOP and right heart pressures) or PiCCO data (e.g. ITBVI, EVLWI) may help differentiate primary respiratory from cardiogenic causes.
- Nitric oxide or inhaled prostacyclin – implies pulmonary hypertension or refractory ARDS.
- Intra-aortic balloon pump – may suggest that cardiogenic pulmonary oedema is a problem.

On examination

A detailed cardiorespiratory system examination, including peripheral signs (i.e. hands, skin, face), should be conducted. This includes assessment of the trachea, chest expansion, percussion and auscultation, and timing of heart sounds.

You must be able to elicit and differentiate between the clinical findings of pleural effusion, consolidation and bronchospasm.

Specifically assess:

- general appearance –, e.g. Cushingoid habitus from steroid dependency, morbid obesity, malnutrition in cystic fibrosis, hyperexpanded chest in COPD, prone positioning in refractory hypoxaemia
- hands, e.g. stigmata of infective endocarditis, finger clubbing, tar staining, interosseous muscle wasting
- skin, e.g. steroid purpura and thinning, vasculitic rashes, burns
- head, e.g. alopecia associated with chemotherapy, upper airway oedema, Horner's syndrome
- trachea – deviation from midline, previous tracheostomy scars, tracheal tug and reduced crico-sternal distance with hyperinflation
- praecordium – signs such as a deviated apical impulse, S3 and 4 gallops and left-sided murmurs favour a cardiogenic cause
- evidence of chest trauma e.g. bruising, rib fractures, flail segments and old ICC sites.

Useful questions
'What are the volume and character of the tracheal aspirates?'

Useful statements
'I suspect that this elderly man has severe respiratory failure because of an infective exacerbation of COPD. He has a hyperexpanded chest with a tracheal tug, scattered bilateral polyphonic wheezes with copious purulent sputum.'

'The severe respiratory failure in this patient appears to be due to several causes, which include painful chest wall trauma, bilateral haemopneumothoraces with ongoing air leak, and poor lung compliance, which may be related to pulmonary contusion, aspiration pneumonitis or ARDS. Furthermore, he has a fever with purulent sputum, raising the possibility of a nosocomial pneumonia.'

Topics for discussion
- Management of refractory ARDS, severe bronchospasm and bronchopleural fistula
- Risk factors, diagnosis and management of ventilator-associated pneumonia
- Timing of tracheostomy (early versus late)
- Non-invasive versus invasive ventilation in immunosuppressed patients
- End-of-life decision-making in exacerbations of COPD and neuromuscular disorders such as motor neurone disease.

2. Why is this patient failing to wean from ventilation?

Possible cases
- Patients with major chest trauma
- People with Guillain-Barré syndrome or other neuromuscular disorder, such as myasthenia gravis
- Any ICU patient who has had a protracted illness.

Appropriate thoughts
Consider the causes of failure to wean:
- Is there adequate cognitive function? What is the GCS?
- Is there adequate peripheral muscle strength and neurological function?

- Has the original problem that caused the patient to be ventilated been treated?
- Is there a new problem causing an ongoing systemic inflammatory response?
- Is there untreated cardiac disease, e.g. heart failure/mitral regurgitation/aortic stenosis?
- Is there a respiratory component? What are the tracheal aspirates like?
- Can the patient cough and clear secretions?
- Do they have a ventilator-associated pneumonia?
- What are the ventilator settings?
- Is there a mechanical chest wall component, e.g. flail chest/morbid obesity?
- Is the patient adequately nourished? Are they being overfed?

The examination
The cubicle
Many personal items suggest that the patient has been in ICU for some time.

The monitor
- What is the oxygen saturation (SpO_2)? What does it suggest about the A–a gradient?
- Is tachycardia evident, possibly suggesting ongoing inflammatory response?
- Is there a fever? Ongoing sepsis may be delaying the weaning process.

Infusions
- TPN, antibiotics or inotropes suggest that there is still an active medical problem requiring treatment.
- There may be few or no infusions, suggesting that weaning difficulty is the reason for the patient's continued ICU stay.

Ventilation
- What mode of ventilation is the patient receiving?
- What are the ventilator settings – FiO_2, PEEP, respiratory rate, pressure support, I:E ratio?
- What is the respiratory rate/unassisted tidal volume/rapid shallow breathing index?

Equipment
- Is there a bedside inhaler or nebuliser?
- Is there one or more intercostal catheters?
  - Are they bubbling or swinging?
  - How much drainage is present?

On examination
- What is the patient's level of consciousness? Can they interact with the physiotherapist and respond to instructions to cough? (Remember, the brain is the most important organ of respiration!)
- Purpura/striae/'tissue-paper' skin/Cushingoid appearance suggest chronic steroid use.
- Is there a tracheostomy? If so, it may suggest the patient has been in the ICU for some time.
- What does the chest wall look like? Is there a flail segment, or bruising suggestive of rib fractures and chest trauma? Is the patient obese?
- Is expansion equal? Is there anything focal to find on auscultation, e.g. crackles/wheeze/rubs? Can the patient cough and clear secretions?

- What is the patient's cardiovascular status? Are they well perfused? Is there a murmur, suggesting a valve lesion that is contributing to weaning difficulties?
- What is the patient's nutritional state? Are they cachectic? How are they being fed?
- How strong is the patient? Can they lift their head off the pillow? Can they lift their arms up off the bed? For how long? What is their grip like? Are reflexes present? (critical illness polyneuropathy/Guillain-Barré syndrome)
- Is there a source for sepsis? Has the condition that caused the need for mechanical ventilation been corrected?

Useful questions
'When did the patient last receive paralysis or sedation?'
'What do the tracheal aspirates look like?'
'Is the patient tolerating their feeds?'
'Does the patient have diarrhoea?'
'I would like to see the most recent chest X-ray and arterial blood gases.'
'Please, could you tell me the trend in temperature and fluid balance over the last 48 hours.'

Useful statements
'I believe that the reasons for this patient's difficulty weaning are multifactorial. The A–a gradient is high, with a normal CO_2 and minute volume of 12 litres per minute, suggesting there is ongoing respiratory impairment. The patient is cachectic with marked loss of muscle bulk. There is generalised weakness with areflexia, suggesting critical illness polyneuropathy. There is a sacral pressure sore, which may be infected.'

Topics for discussion
- Strategies used to wean from mechanical ventilation
- The use of objective criteria to predict successful weaning
- The role of non-invasive ventilation in the weaning process
- The role for early tracheostomy to facilitate weaning
- The use of automated weaning modes in weaning from mechanical ventilation.

3. Can you extubate this patient?

Possible cases
- Routine postoperative surgical patient
- Following the resolution of respiratory failure
- Head and neck surgical patients
- Patients with intra-oral sepsis, e.g. Ludwig's angina
- Patients with upper airway burns.

Appropriate thoughts
This is an extension of the weaning problem that progresses to the removal of the endotracheal tube and liberation of the patient from the ventilator.
- Why was this patient intubated in the first place and has this been resolved?
- Are there any additional focal, systemic or logistical barriers to extubation?

Consider specific airway issues that may make re-intubation difficult or impossible, in addition to practical issues, such as further surgery planned in the next 24 hours and availability of staff with good airway skills in the hours following the extubation (e.g. What time of day is it now? What is the current departmental workload?).

The examination

Establish that the patient meets the criteria for successful weaning from ventilation, as for Diagnostic problem 2, including that:
- the conscious state is appropriate and the patient is strong enough
- the cardiorespiratory function is satisfactory and the patient has an effective cough
- the original condition requiring mechanical ventilation has been corrected.

It is important to now establish whether there will be difficulties maintaining an airway:
- What size is the endotracheal tube?
- Seek to assess airway patency. Ask to perform a leak test, listening for air leaking around the deflated cuff. Follow this with an occlusion test, by covering the end of the endotracheal tube with your thumb (and the cuff deflated) and seeing if the patient is able to breathe around the tube. Remember to reinflate the cuff afterwards!
- Depending on the context, perform direct laryngoscopy to assess the laryngeal pathology.

Useful questions

'What was the airway like at the time of intubation?'
'What was the Cormack and Lehane grade and Mallampati score?'
'Are they still being fed? If not, for how long have they fasted?'

Considerations
- What is the time of day?
- What airway skills do the staff who will be present have?
- Is there a planned trip to theatre today?
- Have they already had a trial of extubation and failed? If so, why did they fail?

Useful statements

'I do not believe that this patient can be extubated because they do not have a leak present on deflation of the cuff on their endotracheal tube. They fail the occlusion test and on direct laryngoscopy there is marked mucosal oedema with grossly swollen vocal cords. I would consider percutaneous tracheostomy (if it seems that the problem will persist for some time) or repeat my assessment daily until the patient is ready to be safely extubated.'

Topics for discussion
- Assessing a patient for potential extubation and discussion of parameters that may be used to predict successful extubation, e.g. arterial blood gases near premorbid values, respiratory rate <25 breaths/min, maximal negative inspiratory airway pressure >−25 cmH_2O, airway occlusion pressure >6 cmH_2O, tidal volume >5 mL/kg, minute ventilation <10 L, vital capacity >10–15 mL/kg, FRC >50% predicted value, rapid shallow breathing index (ratio of breaths/min to tidal volume) <100
- Indications for percutaneous tracheostomy
- Management of post-extubation stridor
- Management of a difficult airway
- Awake fibre-optic intubation technique
- The management of upper airway burns.

4. Why is this patient shocked?

Possible cases
- Sepsis as a primary cause of admission or a sequela of nosocomial infection
- Hypovolaemic shock, e.g. trauma or post-surgical patient with ongoing blood loss, burns patient with ongoing fluid loss
- Cardiogenic shock in association with acute pulmonary oedema.

Appropriate thoughts
Consider the classification of shock and frame your examination to answer which one applies to your patient (often there is more than one):
- hypovolaemic (concealed or revealed): in an exam setting this will most probably have been detected and already treated, although treatment may be continuing during the examination
- obstructive: tamponade/tension pneumothorax/thromboembolism
- distributive: sepsis/anaphylaxis/neurogenic/adrenal insufficiency/liver failure/AV shunt
- cardiogenic: myocardial infarction/myocarditis/cardiomyopathy/cardiac valvular pathology.

The examination
The cubicle
- Blood or melaena on the sheets.

The monitor
- Heart rate and rhythm as a consequence or a cause of shock or the underlying process
- BP and MAP – are they supported (vasopressors, inotropes, IABP) or native? What has the trend been? Does the arterial waveform suggest a particular pathology?
- CVP – is the waveform suggestive of a specific pathology? What has the trend been? Be ready to elaborate on the uses and limitations of the CVP
- Invasive haemodynamic monitoring – PiCCO, pulmonary artery catheter or FloTrac. 'Can I examine the most recent data?'
- SpO_2 – is the trace adequate?
- $ETCO_2$ – compare the value to the blood gas $PaCO_2$ for a large V/Q mismatch due to severe bronchoconstriction or a large PE.

Infusions
- Fluids (crystalloid, colloid) and rates
- Blood products
- Inotropes and vasopressors. What dose?
- Activated protein C implies sepsis
- Heparin suggests an acute coronary syndrome, atrial fibrillation or thrombo-embolism.

Equipment
- 'Level One' rapid infuser.
- Intra-aortic balloon pump. Is it functioning appropriately?
- Is there pacing? Is it working properly?
- Intercostal drains? Are they swinging or bubbling? What and how much is draining?

- Surgical drains? What and how much is draining?
- What has the recent urinary output been like?
- Is there suggestion of spinal pathology, e.g. patient on an Edgerton bed, halo brace?

On examination
Systematically address each of the categories of shock:
Hypovolaemic shock
- What is the patient's fluid balance?
- Are they actively bleeding?
- Is there occult blood loss?
- Check for haemothorax and distending abdomen
- Check for evidence of pelvic, limb and scalp trauma
- Are there other major fluid losses (e.g. intra-abdominal in pancreatitis)?

Obstructive shock
- Does the patient have a tension pneumothorax? E.g. has one of the intercostal catheters become blocked?
- Is cardiac tamponade a possibility?
- Could this be a pulmonary embolus?

Distributive shock
- Does this patient have sepsis? Are they febrile, with warm vasodilated peripheries? Is a source of infection apparent?
- Is this neurological shock due to spinal cord injury? (Be very cautious about this diagnosis; it is easy to miss hypovolaemic shock in these patients.)
- Could this be anaphylaxis or Addisonian crisis?

Cardiogenic shock
- Rate
- Rhythm
- Pre-load
- Afterload
- Pump function (Is there an echocardiograph?)

Useful questions
'I would like to see the most recent CXR, ECG and the results of echocardiography.'
'I would like to review the arterial blood gases, renal function and troponin.' (Look for the trend in the lactate.)
'What is the trend in their haemoglobin/transfusion requirement?'

Useful statements
'I think the major cause of this patient's shocked state is sepsis; however, globally depressed cardiac function as part of the sepsis syndrome is likely to be present as well. Echocardiography would be useful to look for this.'

Topics for discussion
- The relative advantages and disadvantages of PiCCO, LiDCO™, FloTrac™, oesophageal Doppler, pulmonary artery catheters and echocardiography in the management of shock
- The concept of volume responsiveness and how it may be assessed
- The use of vasopressin in inotrope-refractory shock
- The role of corticosteroids in sepsis
- Surviving sepsis guidelines
- What is the role of acute revascularisation in cardiogenic shock due to acute myocardial infarction?

- The use of levosimendan in the management of acutely decompensated congestive cardiac failure
- The use of intra-aortic balloon pumps.

5. Why is this patient not passing urine?

Possible cases
- Dialysis-dependent chronic renal failure
- Post-renal transplant patients with an intercurrent problem
- Acute renal failure related to numerous causes, including shock, multi-organ failure, rhabdomyolysis, hepatorenal failure, nephrotoxic drugs, intravenous contrast agents or ruptured abdominal aortic aneurysm.

Appropriate thoughts
- Is this acute, acute on chronic or chronic renal failure?
- Is there a pre-renal cause? (This is the most frequent cause in the ICU – see Case 4, Why is the patient shocked?)
- Is there raised intra-abdominal pressure, causing an abdominal compartment syndrome?
- Is there a renal cause? (ATN, glomerulonephritis, interstitial nephritis.) Are there nephrotoxins present? Is there evidence of a vasculitis?
- Is there a post-renal cause? Is the catheter blocked? Are the ureters blocked? Has the patient had pelvic brim surgery?

The examination
The cubicle
- Machines for continuous renal replacement therapy or intermittent haemodialysis. What mode is in use (CVVHF, CVVHD, CVVHDF, SCUF, SLED)? What is the hourly volume removal rate? What filter lifespans have been achieved?
- Bags of dialysate fluid – lactate or bicarbonate buffer?

The monitor
- CVP may reflect volume status (be aware of limitations)
- Renal perfusion pressure (MAP – CVP)
- ECG may show signs of hyperkalaemia.

Infusions
- Inotrope or vasopressor agents to maintain organ perfusion
- N-acetylcysteine or sodium bicarbonate for imaging procedures with contrast
- Sodium bicarbonate for metabolic acidosis.

Ventilation
- High FiO_2/PEEP may be due to fluid overload with pulmonary oedema.

Equipment
- Dialysis access – dialysis catheter (and dressings from previous insertion sites), AV fistula, Tenckhoff catheter.
- IDC – note urine colour and volume in the tubing and drainage bag. If an hourly measure bag is not being used, it suggests that the problem is chronic. If there is no IDC, this suggests the patient is anuric. A manometer connected to the IDC indicates that bladder pressures are being measured. Ask for recent values.
- If an intra-aortic balloon pump is present, consider a low position as a cause for oliguria.

On examination
- Perfusion of other end-organs – skin, peripheries, brain (if not intubated assess GCS)
- Abdominal scars from major vascular/abdominal surgery, palpable polycystic kidneys
- Signs of chronic liver disease, suggesting cirrhosis and hepatorenal syndrome
- Sallow skin colour of chronic renal failure or pallor of anaemia
- Signs suggesting diabetes mellitus – scarred finger tips from recurrent BSL testing, abdominal fat atrophy or hypertrophy from insulin injections
- Compartment syndromes – tense limbs, buttocks, abdomen to palpation.

Useful questions
'What was the urine output over the previous 8 hours?'
'Has the IDC been flushed recently?'
'Is there a recent urine dipstick test and microscopy?' Look for leucocytes and nitrite indicating infection, blood-reflecting urinary tract trauma, haemoglobin or myoglobinuria, dysmorphic red cells and casts in glomerulonephritis.
'May I see the results of any paired serum and urinary electrolytes to help distinguish pre-renal from renal aetiologies?'
'May I see an ABG to assess the metabolic and electrolyte derangements present'?
If the patient is a young female: 'Has a pregnancy test been performed?' (Consider eclampsia.)
'May I see the CXR?' (To assess pulmonary oedema or ensure the balloon pump isn't too low.)
If tense abdomen or limb compartment: 'What are the compartment pressures?'

Useful statements
'The causes for the patient's acute renal failure are likely to be multifactorial with aetiologies that include …'
'There is evidence that this patient has end-stage chronic renal failure, with a Tenckhoff catheter/AV fistula indicating chronic dialysis has been required.'
'This patient has acute renal failure, which is only one component of multi-organ failure.'

Topics for discussion
- Indications for commencing dialysis in the intensive care unit
- Acute kidney injury – RIFLE criteria
- Prevention and management of acute renal failure in rhabdomyolysis
- Prevention of contrast nephropathy
- Diagnosis and management of hepatorenal failure
- Basic principles of common renal replacement modalities, including CVVH, CVVHDF and SLED
- Filters – composition and strategies to prevent clotting
- Dosing of dialysis
- Renal protective measures.

6 Why is this patient jaundiced?

Possible cases
- Chronic liver disease with a complication
- Acute liver failure
- Haemolysis
- Post-liver transplant.

Appropriate thoughts
- Is this pre-hepatic, hepatic or post-hepatic jaundice?
- Is this an acute decompensation of chronic liver disease? If so, what is the cause of the decompensation?
- Is this patient a candidate for a liver transplant?

The examination
The cubicle
- Dialysis machine – is there multi-organ failure or hepatorenal syndrome?
- 'Level 1' infuser – implies haemodynamically significant blood loss and possibly haemolysis as a source of the jaundice
- Smell of melaena – is there peptic ulcer disease or porto-systemic hypertension?

The monitor
- ICP (some centres use these in severe hepatic encephalopathy; others believe that the risks of bleeding and infection outweigh the benefits)
- High CO, low SVR.

Infusions
- Blood products
- Octreotide or terlipressin suggests a variceal bleed
- 10% dextrose suggests depleted liver reserves.

Ventilation
- The patient may be receiving a 'protective lung ventilation strategy' with high FiO_2 if multi-organ failure co-exists with a hepatic dysfunction.

Equipment
- Minnesota tube
- Blood in nasogastric drainage
- Possibly an ICP monitor.

On examination
- Signs of chronic liver disease and decompensation
- Look for IV track marks
- Determine liver size, texture and pulsatility. Is there splenomegaly or ascites present?
- Splenomegaly and lymphadenopathy – is there an underlying haematological malignancy with haemolysis?

Useful questions
'What did the liver ultrasound show?'
'What have the blood glucose measurements been?'
'What is the urine output?'
'What are the PR findings – blood/haemorrhoids?
'I would like to see the arterial blood gases, biochemistry and haematology for this patient.'
'What is the most recent prothromin time? (with or without FFP?)'

Useful statements
'I believe this patient has acute on chronic liver failure, in view of the widespread stigmata of chronic liver disease. This deterioration may have been precipitated by …'

Topics for discussion
- The management of variceal haemorrhage – resuscitation, octreotide, endoscopic banding, transhepatic intravenous portosystemic shunts, surgery (portosystemic shunts, oesophagectomy)
- Causes of renal failure in the patient with hepatic failure
- The diagnosis and management of hepatorenal syndrome and hepatopulmonary syndrome
- The management of ascites
- The features and causes of decompensation in chronic liver disease
- The causes and management of fulminant liver failure (including complementary and herbal therapies)
- The diagnosis and management of spontaneous bacterial peritonitis
- The Child–Pugh classification
- The criteria for liver transplantation
- The complications of liver transplantation.

7. Why is this patient not waking up?

Possible cases
- This is a common, 'everyday' ICU problem, which can affect any patient.

Appropriate thoughts
Broadly speaking, these patients can be divided into two groups:
- Does this patient have a primary focal neurological cause? (meningitis/encephalitis/thromboembolic CVA/cerebral haemorrhage/cerebral abscess)
- Is this due to a global encephalopathic process? (systemic infection/uraemia/liver failure/drugs or toxin effect/'ICU' encephalopathy).

The examination
The cubicle
- Dialysis machine.

The monitor
- Is there a fever?
- What is the ICP?

Infusions
- Sedative and analgesic infusions
- Nimodipine for subarachnoid haemorrhage
- Noradrenaline to maintain organ perfusion or cerebral perfusion pressure.

Ventilation
- If patient requires considerable ventilatory support, it suggests they are still acutely unwell.

Equipment
- External ventricular drain (with blood in it?) Could there be increasing hydrocephalus?
- ICP monitor?
- CRRT?

On examination
- It is important to establish whether the patient is awake, but unable to move (e.g. cervical spine pathology/locked-in syndrome).
- Assess the Glasgow Coma Score. Broadly speaking, this can be divided into awake GCS 13–15), profoundly comatose (3–8) or depressed level of consciousness (GCS 9–12). Assess the patient's pupillary responses, mental state, look for neck stiffness if appropriate.
- Is the patient agitated? If so, assess the cause – inadequate analgesia, hypoxic or hypotensive, septic, withdrawing from drugs or alcohol, full bladder with blocked catheter.
- If the patient is unconscious but not sedated, what are the brainstem reflexes doing? If they have received neuromuscular blocking drugs, what is the twitch response to the 'train of four' nerve stimulation?
- Is there marked muscle wasting?
- What is the tone, power and coordination? Are reflexes present? If not, is critical illness polyneuropathy a possible cause, especially if more marked in the lower limbs and in the proximal muscle groups?
- Check the skin for IV track marks.
- Look for craniotomy wounds.
- Look for sources of ongoing sepsis.
- Is the patient jaundiced? Are there signs of chronic liver disease?

Useful questions
'When did the patient last receive paralysis or sedation?'
'What other medications are they receiving?'
'Has the patient had a recent CT scan of the head? If so, may I please see it.'

Useful statements
'I believe that this patient has had a subarachnoid haemorrhage, as shown by the blood in the EVD …'

'I believe the reasons for this patient failing to wake up are multi-factorial – he has multi-organ failure as demonstrated by the fact that he is receiving dialysis, is jaundiced and requiring mechanical ventilation with a high A–a gradient. His sedative infusions have only been ceased for 24 hours and may take considerably longer to be metabolised. Additionally, he has ongoing sepsis from his intra-abdominal collections.'

Topics for discussion
- Sedation in the ICU
- Diagnosis of brain (stem) death
- The role of routinely ceasing all sedation every 24 hours in ICU patients
- Treatment of 'ICU psychosis'
- Assessment and management of delirium in the ICU.

8. Why is this patient weak?

Possible cases
- Primary neuromuscular conditions: Guillain-Barré syndrome, tetanus, botulism, myaesthenia gravis, old polio, CVA, acute myositis
- Associated with a systemic condition: connective tissue disorder, infection, critical illness polymyoneuropathy
  Generalised weakness may form part of 'failure to wean'.

Appropriate thoughts

- Is this primary weakness or weakness due to protracted illness/ICU stay?
- If it is primary weakness, then at what level? Consider muscle, neuromuscular junction, peripheral nerves, spinal cord, brain (upper versus lower motor neuron).

The examination
The cubicle

- Wheelchair, walking aids, handweights and limb splints from physiotherapist.

The monitor

- May show hyper- or hypotension and arrhythmias if autonomic dysfunction is a feature of the illness
- ICP monitor/EVD – subarachnoid haemorrhage, intracranial haemorrhage, traumatic brain injury.

Infusions

- Immunoglobulin is given for Guillain-Barré syndrome, myasthenia gravis and vasculitis
- Gentamicin can augment the effect of neuromuscular blockers.

Ventilation

- High levels of pressure support if breathing spontaneously
- How much PEEP? The patient is likely to be at risk of atelectasis, lobar collapse and pneumonia if generally weak.

Equipment

- Possibly plasmapheresis, although this is less common than it used to be
- Edgerton bed, suggesting spinal cord injury.

On examination

- Assess the GCS and level of consciousness.
- Examine the cranial nerves carefully; particularly evaluate the gag, cough and swallow reflexes.
- A tracheostomy would suggest prolonged need for mechanical ventilation due to respiratory muscle weakness or inability to cough and clear secretions.
- Check the patient's unassisted vital capacity.
- Look for purpura and 'tissue paper' skin, suggesting chronic corticosteroid use.
- Look for stigmata of connective tissue disorder/vasculitis.
- Assess muscle bulk. If wasting is present, is it symmetrical? Is it global or is the distribution predominantly proximal or distal?
- Are fasciculations present? (Suggests a lower motor neuron process, e.g. motor neuron disease).
- Assess tone, power and coordination. Is the weakness upper motor neuron or lower motor neurone in type? Is it symmetrical?
- Are reflexes present, exaggerated or absent?
- Is there sensory loss? Which pathways/columns are affected?
- Is this a myopathy or neuropathy? If it is a neuropathy, is it motor or sensorimotor?
- Try to locate the lesion: cerebral cortex, brainstem, anterior horn cells (motor neuron disease, polio), the peripheral nerves (Guillain-Barré syndrome, critical illness polyneuropathy), the neuromuscular junction (myasthenia gravis, botulism) or the muscle itself (acute myositis, periodic paralysis).
- Make an assessment of the patient's nutritional status.
- Look for evidence of any ongoing issues requiring treatment such as sepsis, thromboembolic disease.

Useful questions
'How long has this patient been in intensive care?'
'What was the initial reason for their admission?' Try to distinguish between a primary weakness (e.g. Guillain-Barré) or weakness secondary to prolonged ICU admission for another cause (e.g. abdominal sepsis).
'I would like to see the patient's head CT, the results of nerve conduction studies and muscle biopsy (if relevant) and the CK level and trend (if relevant).'

Useful statements
'I believe the causes of weakness in this patient are multi-factorial – he has evidence of chronic corticosteroid use causing myopathy; there has been a protracted intensive care stay with abdominal sepsis – the absent reflexes on the left suggest critical illness polyneuropathy; he is malnourished and in addition there is a longstanding right-sided hemiparesis with increased tone and brisk reflexes.'
'I would like to see the head CT; the results of nerve conduction studies; the results of nerve/muscle biopsy (where relevant); the patient's CK and the recent trend.'

Topics for discussion
- Immunoglobulin versus plasmapheresis for Guillain-Barré syndrome
- Corticosteroids in Guillain-Barré syndrome
- Risk factors for critical illness polyneuropathy
- Functional status at 1 year in ICU survivors
- Rehabilitation after critical care
- The treatment of tetanus.

9. Is this patient brain dead?

It should be realised that variations according to local legislation and standard of practice would be incorporated into examinations in different countries and this represents Australian guidance. Brainstem testing was covered in detail in Chapter 5.

Possible cases
- Patients with subarachnoid haemorrhage
- Patients with severe head injury
- Patients with severe hypoxic brain injury

Appropriate thoughts
In addition to absent brain stem reflexes, the diagnosis of brain death requires that an irreversible cause for the coma has been identified, that the patient is normothermic without metabolic or endocrine derangement and that their condition is not affected by sedative drugs or neuromuscular blockers.
Organise your thoughts in terms of:
- the underlying diagnosis
- the duration of the current neurological status
- exclusion of reversible causes
- the brain death examination
- neuroimaging.

The examination
The cubicle
- Often innocuous

The monitor
- Abnormally elevated ICP measurement
- Bradycardia with hypertension
- Exclude hypothermia.

Infusions
- Ensure there is no sedation
- When was the last dose of neuromuscular blocker given?
- Nimodipine suggests SAH as the underlying diagnosis.

Ventilation
- No spontaneous breaths on ventilator.

Equipment
- ICP monitor. Ask for its duration. (Calibration drift becomes a significant problem after 5–7 days.)
- EVD with blood-stained CSF draining.
- Evidence of recent cooling, such as a cooling blanket or cooling machine, might suggest an out-of-hospital cardiac arrest and hypoxic ischaemic encephalopathy.
- Copious urine drainage (development of diabetes insipidus).

On examination
Before you start to examine the patient, ask: 'Please may I have a torch, cotton bud, tongue depressor, otoscope, ice cold water and a 20 mL syringe, the peripheral nerve stimulator, end-tidal CO_2 monitor, Mapleson C circuit (for apnoea testing, to allow PEEP and to observe the bag for any effort at respiration) or oxygen catheter and a laryngoscope (to test gag with direct vision).'
- Ask whether a 'train of four' stimulus at 40 mv has been performed. If not, ask for a nerve stimulator to perform this yourself. (You will probably be told this is not necessary, but always be prepared to perform any bedside test for which you ask the result.)
- Perform a GCS. Check response to voice before you touch the patient.
- Response to pain (grimace CN VII) should be tested by pressing on the supra-orbital ridges (V), the temporomandibular joints (CN V) and a nail bed on each limb. (Beware of spinal reflexes, which do not preclude the diagnosis of brain death.)
- Test pupillary response to light (CN III).
- Test corneal reflexes (CN V).
- Look in both ears to check that the canals are not occluded and the tympanic membranes are intact. Ask an assistant to hold the eyelids open for you, then inject 20 mL of ice-cold water into each ear canal in turn. Movement of the eyes towards the side of the stimulus is an intact vestibulo-ocular response (CN III, VI and VIII). It is a good idea to put a towel on the pillow, and hold a kidney dish under the ear to avoid making everything wet.
- The oculo-cephalic (doll's eye) reflex is not part of the Australian brain death tests.
- Check for a gag under direct laryngoscopic vision. Check for a cough using a tracheal suction catheter (CN IX and X).
- Test for spontaneous ventilation – ventilate first with 100% O_2. Passively oxygenate during the test, using either a Mapleson C circuit attached to the ETT or an O_2 catheter in the ETT. If the starting CO_2 is normal, allow it to rise to 60 mmHg (8.0 kPa) with a pH <7.3, or 20 mmHg (2.6 kPa) higher than the baseline if the patient has COPD. The rate of rise of CO_2 during apnoea is approx 3 mmHg/min (0.4 kPa/min).

Useful questions

'Has an irreversible cause been established for the patient's coma?'
'What is the patient's temperature?'
'How long has the patient had this neurological state?'
'When did the patient last receive sedation or paralysing agents?'
'Is the patient's metabolic and endocrine status normal?'
'Is there a possibility that the patient could be poisoned/influenced by a toxin?'
'What has the urine output been in the last 24 hours?' (Diabetes insipidus?)
Ask to see the most recent CT scan of the head or whether any other form of neuroimaging has been performed, e.g. 4-vessel cerebral angiogram.

Useful statements

'This person is brain dead because an irreversible cause has been established for their coma; they are normothermic; their metabolic and endocrine status is normal, they have not received sedatives or muscle relaxants for 24 hours and a systematic examination of brain stem function revealed all brainstem reflexes to be absent. Finally, the patient remained apnoeic during an appropriately conducted test of respiratory function.'
'I am unable to say clinically that this person is brain dead because they do not meet the preconditions for testing. An irreversible cause has not been established for their coma/The patient is hypothermic/still under the influence of sedating drugs ...'
'Although this patient with hypoxic–ischaemic brain injury is not brain dead because ... I believe that the prognosis is likely to be very poor as this is the fourth day after the injury, they have only extensor motor responses, pupillary response is absent bilaterally and persistent myoclonus is present. My next step would be to meet with the family ...'

Topics for discussion

- What is the differential diagnosis of fixed dilated pupils?
- What are the requirements in your jurisdiction for certification of brain death?
- How would you diagnose brain death in the presence of a cervical spine fracture or severe facial injuries?
- When would you order a 4-vessel cerebral angiogram?
- What is the role of radio-isotope imaging in diagnosing brain death?
- What is the difference between post-coma unresponsiveness, locked-in syndrome and brain death?
- How would you talk to the family about organ donation?
- What are the management problems of the organ donor prior to donation?

10. Why is this patient febrile?

Possible cases

- Any ICU patient!

Appropriate thoughts

- Infectious cause? – upper and lower respiratory tract, urinary tract, endocarditis, meningitis, burns patients, patients with intra-abdominal sepsis/collections, acalculous cholecystitis
- Non-infectious cause? – pancreatitis, head injury/subarachnoid haemorrhage, drug or toxin effect, DVT, florid connective tissue disease
- hyperthermic emergency? – hyperthyroidism, neuroleptic malignant syndrome, malignant hyperpyrexia, heat stroke.

The examination

The cubicle

- Are there lots of cards, photos, personal items in the cubicle? If so, it suggests the fever may be a new problem rather than the reason for the ICU admission.
- Isolation procedures suggest a multi-resistant organism.

The monitor

- Temperature – could it be masked (age, steroids, immunosuppressants, dialysis, ECMO)?
- Is there a systemic inflammatory response? Look for a tachypnoea (or low $PaCO_2$), tachycardia and hypotension.

Infusions

- Antibiotic infusions
- Norepinephrine for septic shock
- Heparin (DVT/PE as cause of fever)
- Blood products.

Ventilation

- FiO_2?
- Protective ventilation strategy?
- If the patient has an FiO_2 of 30% with pressure support ventilation, primary chest pathology is less likely to be the cause of fever.

Equipment

- Intra-abdominal drains? Duration and contents?
- Are there intercostal drains? What is the appearance of fluid in the drains?
- Is there a external ventricular drain? Duration and latest CSF culture results?
- Is there a rectal tube? Is there severe diarrhoea, e.g. *Clostridium difficile,* chemotherapy induced mucositis?
- Is there active cooling in progress? This may mask a fever.
- Is there an epidural catheter? Examine for local infection.
- What colour is the urine? Myoglobin might suggest rhabdomyolysis from a compartment syndrome or pressure necrosis, or possibly a malignant hyperpyrexia.
  In surgical patients the focus of 80% of infections is the surgical site, the lines, the chest or the urine.

On examination

- Look at the skin for scars, old and new. Look at all wounds for erythema, discharge. Is there a pacemaker or other prosthetic device in situ, track marks of IV drug use? Ask to see under all bandages and dressings.
- Are there any skin sources of sepsis, e.g. bed sores, cellulitis? Ask to see the back of the patient. Look at all line sites. Is there a vasculitic rash present?
- Check for neck stiffness. Feel all over the scalp for wounds and pressure areas. Palpate over the sinuses, parotids and mastoids. Look in the mouth and at the teeth. Ask to look in the patient's ears and eyes (Roth's spots, choroidoretinitis, endophthalmitis, bullae on the tympanic membrane, acute otititis media, blood or CSF).
- Check carefully for vasculitic and embolic phenomena and murmurs suggestive of endocarditis.
- Check for increased tone in the limbs, suggesting neuroleptic malignant syndrome.
- Palpate for organomegaly and lymphadenopathy, suggesting a haematological malignancy.
- Palpate for tenderness and fullness in the RUQ (acalculous cholecystitis).

- Palpate the thighs and calves for swelling, suggestive of DVT. Include the upper limbs, especially if there is a long-term vascular catheter or reason to suspect a procoagulant pathology.

Useful questions

'What do the tracheal aspirates look like?'

'Is the patient tolerating their feeds? Have they had their bowels open?'

'Does the patient have diarrhoea?'

If the patient is a woman of appropriate age, in the appropriate context: 'Has the patient had a PV examination to ensure there is no retained tampon or other intrauterine device?'

'How long have the lines been in situ?'

'What medications is the patient on?' Specifically: 'Has the person had an anaesthetic recently (malignant hyperpyrexia)?' 'Are there any neuroleptic medications (neuroleptic malignant syndrome)?' 'Is the patient receiving antibiotics (the penicillins in particular cause drug fevers)?'

'I would like to see the most recent CXR, the trend in the white cell count and microbiology results.'

Useful statements

'I believe there are several potential causes for fever in this patient – x, y, z. This is how I would proceed from here to establish the diagnosis …'

'In this (burns) patient I would like to inspect all the burn and donor sites when the dressings are next changed. I would perform burn biopsies (not skin swabs) to diagnose burn/graft/graft site infection.'

Topics for discussion

- The role of activated protein C in the management of sepsis
- The role of vasopressin in inotrope refractory septic shock
- The role of corticosteroids in the management of septic shock
- The role of double Gram-negative antimicrobial cover in Gram-negative sepsis
- Multi-resistant organisms on the ICU
- Surviving sepsis guidelines
- Catheter-related blood stream infections
- Ventilator-associated pneumonia
- The management of venous thromboembolism in the critically ill patient
- Care bundles
- Special issues related to neutropaenic sepsis (see diagnostic problem no. 11. 'The oncology patient' on p. 258).

11. What injuries has this multiple trauma patient sustained?

Possible cases

- The majority of these patients have sustained blunt trauma due to vehicle collisions, but falls are also common.

Appropriate thoughts

- At what stage of the illness is this patient?
- Is the resuscitation phase still ongoing?

- Is the patient now stable, although still in the acute phase? Has a tertiary survey been performed? Are there any peripheral injuries that were initially overlooked?
- Will the patient require ongoing surgical management?
- Has the patient been ill long enough to be experiencing complications, such as nosocomial pneumonia?
- Is the patient in the rehabilitation phase?

The examination
Infusions
- Look for crystalloids, blood and blood products. At what rate? What volume has been given to date?
- Noradrenaline suggests that the patient may still be hypovolaemic, has a new problem such as sepsis or that cerebral perfusion pressure is being targeted in traumatic brain injury. It might also be targeting a low SVR due to neurogenic shock from high spinal trauma.
- Hypertonic saline or mannitol suggest active ICP manipulation.
- Higher dose sedation and neuromuscular blocking agents suggest management for severe brain injury.

The monitor
- Is the ICP elevated?
- Tachycardia
- Hypotension, despite resuscitation efforts; consider ongoing bleeding, neurogenic shock and SIRS reaction
- $ETCO_2$ monitoring in TBI – is the level appropriate?

Ventilation
- High inflation pressures and poor gas exchange may suggest pulmonary contusions or pulmonary oedema (e.g. aggressive volume resuscitation, cardiac injury, aspiration pneumonitis, neurogenic pulmonary oedema).

Equipment
- Is there a cervical collar in place?
- An Edgerton bed suggests spinal injury.
- Look for intercostal catheters. Are they swinging or bubbling? How much blood is in them and over what period?
- Look for intra-abdominal drains and assess their contents.
- What is the urine output rate? Is it dark, smoky coloured urine, suggesting myoglobinuria?
- Look for orthopaedic devices, e.g. external fixators, traction, plaster of Paris (risk of DVT and fat embolism).
- An ICP monitor suggests TBI.
- A cooling blanket suggests management of refractory raised ICP.

On examination
Expanding the ATLS recommendations for trauma assessment is often the most practical approach to examination. Essentially, you should perform a rapid primary survey followed by a full tertiary survey:
- Is there a secure and patent airway?
- Is adequate ventilation being achieved? Is a flail segment visible? Are multiple rib fractures palpable?
- Ensure there is adequate IV access and that there is no obvious ongoing bleeding.

- Check the GCS and patient's ability to feel and move their limbs. Assess the pupillary response. If the patient has a severe brain injury, assess whether adequate cerebral perfusion pressure is being achieved.
- Examine the patient from top to toe:
  - Look for scalp wounds/Battle's sign/mastoid bruising/blood behind the haemotympanum/CSF from the nose or ears/facial bone fractures.
  - Is there subcutaneous emphysema across the anterior neck and chest wall? Auscultate for carotid bruits due to dissection in blunt neck trauma.
  - Is there chest wall bruising?
  - Is there a laparotomy wound? Is the abdomen soft or distended? Are intra-abdominal pressures being measured?
  - Palpate the pelvis for stability, but avoid 'springing' the pelvis. Check for perineal or scrotal bruising, suggesting urethral injury.
  - Examine the long bones by careful palpation. Look for evidence of a fasciotomy, suggesting a compartment syndrome. If there has been a severe chest injury, examine the clavicles and shoulders/scapulae carefully for associated injury.
  - Ask to roll the patient to examine their back and perform a PR.
  - If you suspect a spinal cord injury ask if you can look for a bulbo-cavernosus reflex and whether the patient is aware of the presence of enemas (rectal sensation).

Useful questions
For penetrating injury: 'What was the penetrating implement?'
For blunt injury: 'What was the mechanism and speed of injury?'
'Was the patient restrained?'/'What was the damage to the vehicle?'
'What was the GCS on the scene – before/after resuscitation?'
'Has the spine been cleared (including thoraco-lumbar views)?'
'What are the tracheal secretions like?' 'Are they blood-stained?'
'What have been the losses in the intercostal drains?'
'I would like to check the position of the endotracheal tube and intercostal catheters on the most recent CXR.'
'What are the nasogastric aspirates like?'
'Is the patient's tetanus status up to date?'
'Have compound orthopaedic injuries been appropriately scrubbed?'
'Is further surgery planned? When?'

Useful statements
'I would like to review all of the radiological investigations in this patient, in particular, cervico-thoraco-lumbar spine imaging, CT head/chest/abdomen and pelvis, chest X-ray, pelvis (and long bones as appropriate).'
  'I would like to liaise with the treating teams (neurosurgery, general surgery, orthopaedics) to plan this patient's ongoing management.'

Topics for discussion
- Management of major haemorrhage from severe pelvic fracture
- Management of traumatic brain injury, injury including indications for ICP monitoring and decompressive craniectomy
- The role of anti-seizure prophylaxis following head injury
- The management of refractory raised IP
- Thromboprophylaxis in the patient with spinal cord injury
- The role of methylprednisolone in spinal cord injury
- Management of abdominal compartment syndrome
- Trauma scoring systems
- The use of factor VIIa
- Assessment and clearing cervical spine injuries in an unconscious patient.

12. How is this patient with multi-organ failure progressing?

Possible cases
- Any ICU patient!

These patients require an exhaustive evaluation, as described at the start of this chapter.

Appropriate thoughts
Key issues to focus on are:
- which organs have failed?
- is the initial illness responding to treatment?
- is the diagnosis correct?
- is there an occult acute process (such as sepsis or ischaemic bowel) driving the organ failure?
- is it possible to provide more support to failed organ function than is currently being received? Is this appropriate?

Useful questions
'What was the initiating cause of the organ failure and is it responding to treatment?' (If the diagnosis is not known, or the condition is refractory to treatment the prognosis is usually poor. It is hard to treat someone if you don't know what is wrong with them.)
'What are the trends? Has renal recovery begun? Has the prothrombin time begun to decrease? Has ventilatory support escalated or diminished? How much inotrope/vasopressor is required? Is it escalating?'

Useful statements
'I believe that this patient with multi-organ failure due to ..., is slowly improving, as demonstrated by ...'
'I believe that this patient with multi-organ failure is very unlikely to survive because ...'
'The prognosis is very poor in this patient who continues to deteriorate on maximum medical therapy. I would like to meet with the family to discuss changing the goals of therapy to comfort care.'

Topics for discussion
- Pathophysiology of multi-organ failure
- Critical care illness scoring systems
- Withdrawal of therapy in the ICU
- Function at 1 year in ICU survivors generally and for specific illnesses, e.g. ARDS, TBI.

Specific patient groups

1. The patient with chronic obstructive pulmonary disease

Possible cases
- A patient with an acute exacerbation receiving either non-invasive ventilation or intubated and ventilated

- A patient with chronic severe COPD who is in the ICU for another reason, e.g. after cardiac surgery or post-thoracotomy for lung cancer
- Following lung reduction surgery.

Appropriate thoughts
- What stage is the patient at in their ICU course? Are they improving and ready to be weaned? Are they likely to need protracted ventilation and a tracheostomy?
- If the patient is receiving non-invasive ventilation, what management would you recommend if they continue to deteriorate?
- What is the patient's nutritional status?
- Has the person had previous ICU admissions?

The examination
As for clinical case Diagnostic problem 1: 'Why does this patient have severe respiratory failure?'
In addition:
- look for the scar of a previous tracheostomy.
- pay particular attention to other systems as relevant, e.g. the abdomen in patients with severe COPD who are in ICU post-laparotomy; look carefully for evidence of cardiac failure in the post-CABG patient.
- assess the patient's work of breathing and evidence of systemic inflammatory response to estimate their nutritional requirements.
- does the sternal wound/thoracotomy wound/laparotomy wound significantly worsen respiratory excursion? Is analgesia adequate? Can the patient cough effectively?
- is there evidence of aggressive physiotherapy, e.g. incentive spirometry devices at the bedside?

Useful questions
'What is the quantity and appearance of the tracheal secretions/aspirates?'
'Please may I review this patient's preoperative lung function tests and arterial blood gases on room air?'
'I would like to know the patient's functional status prior to admission to the intensive care unit/this episode.'
'How often is this patient receiving physiotherapy?'

Useful statements
'I believe that this patient with an infective exacerbation of COPD is currently improving on non-invasive ventilation as shown by ... However, in view of their previous good functional status, should they deteriorate I would consider intubation and ventilation ...'
'I believe that this frail patient with severe COPD post-CABG will require a tracheostomy. Despite aggressive physiotherapy his course has been complicated by postoperative pneumonia and, in addition, he appears to have a phrenic nerve palsy on the right post-cardiac surgery. He is now on his sixth postoperative day and it will be several days before weaning can be commenced – as shown by ... In addition, I would maximise the therapy of his COPD by adding...'

Topics for discussion
- The role of lung volume reduction surgery in the management of severe COPD
- The role of early versus later tracheostomy
- The role of non-invasive ventilation in the weaning process

- The role of and methods for optimising respiratory function using different options for analgesia and endotracheal tube tolerance
- The management of intercostal catheters in patients post-thoracotomy
- Perioperative risk assessment in the patient with severe COPD
- Advanced healthcare directives and severe COPD.

2. The cardiac arrest survivor

Possible cases
- Prognostication after hypoxic–ischaemic brain injury
- Assessment of general progress after cardiac arrest
- The post-cardiac arrest patient who is not waking up.

Potential variants include the patient after a massive myocardial infarction complicated by cardiac arrest who is being treated with inotropes/intra-aortic balloon pump/urgent revascularisation.

Appropriate thoughts
- Complications of the arrest/resuscitation attempts, e.g. burns from the defibrillator pads, sternal or rib fractures, aspiration pneumonia
- Cardiac consequences of the event, e.g. evidence of cardiogenic shock, needing inotropic support, IABP in situ, evidence of angiography/revascularisation
- Cerebral consequences of the event, especially the severity of hypoxic–ischaemic insult
- Causes of cardiac arrest other than myocardial infarction.

The examination
The cubicle
- Cooling device at the end of the bed if within the first 24 hours.

The monitor
- ECG leads – ischaemic changes (ST segment elevation or depression, Q waves or T wave inversion, territories), arrhythmia or features of heart block
- core temperature – expect 33.5–34.5°C if moderate therapeutic hypothermia during the first 24 hours
- MAP, CVP or other haemodynamic parameters (e.g. SVRI, CI) from a pulmonary artery catheter or PiCCO.

Infusions
- Vasoactive drugs – any combination possible, tailored to specific haemodynamic disturbance, with the most common scenario a mixture of cardiogenic and distributive shock (from a systemic inflammatory response).
- Sedative infusions – if none and an abnormal GCS, ask about the amount and type of medications that were administered, and when this was stopped.
- Neuromuscular blockade (e.g. vecuronium infusion) may be required if therapeutic cooling is in place to prevent shivering.
- If nimodipine is being delivered, consider SAH as the cause of the cardiac arrest.

Ventilation
- A high FiO_2/PEEP may reflect left ventricular failure with pulmonary oedema or aspiration.

Equipment
- Cooling blanket if early therapeutic hypothermia
- Pulmonary artery catheter or PiCCO
- EEG monitor if paralysed with neuromuscular blocker (e.g. to prevent shivering to facilitate cooling)
- If an EVD or parenchymal ICP monitor is present, consider a primary CNS cause for the arrest.

On examination
- If the patient is still receiving neuromuscular blockade, then a meaningful neurological examination cannot be performed.
- If the patient is hypothermic, comment that this may influence an accurate neurological assessment.
- Neurological examination – assessment for prognostication at 72 hours, unclouded by sedative drugs:
  - GCS – motor response of flexion to pain or better associated with better prognosis
  - pupil reactions to light – reactive pupils associated with better prognosis
  - generalised myoclonus is a poor prognostic sign
  - presence of spontaneous breathing – if absent and pupils are unreactive, need to determine if brain death has occurred
  - if localising signs (e.g. hemiparesis), consider a primary CNS cause for the arrest (e.g. SAH or intracranial haemorrhage).
- Defibrillation burns on chest wall or bruising from CPR.
- Other trauma from CPR, such as fractured sternum/ribs/liver laceration.
- Signs of secondary trauma incurred at the time of collapse (e.g. signs of head trauma).
- Evidence of a femoral artery puncture or vascular sheath consistent with access for coronary angiography.

Useful questions
- 'Could I please examine serial ECGs and see the results of coronary angiography and echocardiography if performed?'
- 'Could you please clarify the patient's history to aid prognostication, including time to basic and advanced life support, time to return of spontaneous circulation, resuscitation required, including the arrest rhythm, number of shocks, adrenaline boluses and other drugs required?'
- Has a formal EEG been performed and what are the results of this study (if the diagnosis of myoclonic jerks is uncertain)?

Useful statements
'This 70-year-old man has suffered a cardiac arrest requiring recurrent defibrillation for return of spontaneous circulation, as shown by the burns over his chest conforming to the shape of defibrillation pads.'

'The predicted prognosis for this 65-year-old cardiac arrest survivor, now 3 days post arrest and off sedation for 24 hours, is poor. He is experiencing generalised myoclonic jerks with stimulation, has fixed, dilated pupils and his limbs are extending in response to a painful stimulus.'

Topics for discussion
- Prognostication after hypoxic–ischaemic brain injury
- Evidence for vasopressin in cardiac arrest
- Benefits of therapeutic hypothermia in the cardiac arrest patient

- Strategies demonstrated to improve the survival of patients after acute myocardial infarction
- Risks and benefits of thrombolysis versus percutaneous intervention with angioplasty/stenting for acute myocardial infarction in patients generally, and specifically in the post-cardiac arrest patient, with and without cardiogenic shock
- The approach to discussing organ donation with relatives.

3. The post-cardiac surgical patient

Possible cases
- Routine patient progressing through ICU uneventfully after elective cardiac surgery (most often coronary artery bypass grafts and/or aortic/mitral valve replacement)
- Complications of elective surgical patients requiring more prolonged ICU management (e.g. take-back for bleeding, tamponade, graft occlusion with acute myocardial infarction, CVA)
- Patients requiring pre- and postoperative management of non-elective conditions (e.g. aortic dissection, acute endocarditis with conduction system dysfunction, shock from sepsis or acute valvular dysfunction, complicated myocardial infarction with VSD or acute valvular dysfunction).

Appropriate thoughts
- Try to ascertain if surgery has been elective or urgent.
- Determine if the course has been routine or complicated – look for complications.
- If shock is the main issue refer to Diagnostic problem 4.
- In all young people consider non-ischaemic causes of heart disease (e.g. infective endocarditis, congenital heart disease) or predisposing factors for premature ischaemia (e.g. type 1 diabetes, congenital hyperlipidaemia).
- In patients with structural heart disease and a fever, always consider endocarditis.

The examination
Infusions
- Vasoactive drugs – inotrope and vasopressor/dilator combination may suggest the nature of the haemodynamic disturbance.
- Haemostatic agents – if high drain losses, look for management strategies for coagulopathy (e.g. DDAVP, antifibrinolytics, aprotinin, recombinant factor 7a).
- Blood products – packed cells, fresh frozen plasma, cryoprecipitate or platelets for management of persistent postoperative bleeding.
- Fluid loads – colloid most often used.

The monitor
- ECG – HR, rhythm, pacing spikes, obvious conduction defects
- Arterial line trace – BP, slope of the upstroke (reduced if poor CO state), height of the dicrotic notch (low with reduced SVR state)
- CVP trace – note value and character (e.g. giant C and V waves with tricuspid regurgitation)
- Temperature – fever from sepsis or systemic inflammatory response.

Ventilation
- Increased FiO_2/PEEP – consider cardiogenic pulmonary oedema, atelectasis, ARDS, nosocomial pneumonia
- Increased A–a gradient with normal lung compliance from a PE.

Equipment
- Intra-aortic balloon pump – note amount and ratio of augmentation (e.g. 1:1–1:3).
- Pulmonary artery catheter (less often a PiCCO) – perform or ask for an up-to-date set of measured and calculated haemodynamic parameters.
- Pacing wires and pulse generator:
  - number and position of epicardial wires relative to the sternum (atrial usually on the patient's right and ventricular to the left)
  - pacing mode, rate, output (mV) and sensitivity (mA).
- Surgical drains – check patency and note the nature and amount of losses and presence of an air leak.
- Intercostal catheter or 'pleurocath' if a pneumothorax has been problematic (usually after removal of the surgical drains). Note swinging, drainage and bubbling with the respiratory cycle.
- Rapid infusion lines – commonly inserted in theatre.
- Dialysis catheter if CRRT has been required for management of acute (or chronic) renal failure.

On examination
- Look for peripheral stigmata of infective endocarditis – digital clubbing, Janeway lesions, Osler's nodes; also look for features consistent with IV drug abuse (e.g. needle track marks on the limbs).
- Look for marfanoid habitus – tall, long limbs, arachnodactyly, high arched palate, kyphoscoliosis.
- Look for eyelid xanthelasma, tendon xanthomata, corneal arcus.
- Check the pulse character (brachial or carotid arteries) – plateau or collapsing pulse.
- Check JVP character at 45 degrees of head up – if appropriate to sit up and is not obscured by a central line (e.g. prominent C–V waves of tricuspid regurgitation).
- Chest – palpate sternotomy wounds for stability and check for signs of infection.
- Look for surgical or traumatic scars.
- Undertake a structured cardiovascular examination.
- Palpate position and nature of apex beat, presence of thrills, heaves or a P2.
- Auscultate in the mitral, tricuspid, pulmonary and aortic areas (you will need to ask to put the IABP on hold or on a reduced ratio, if one is present).
- Time the heart sounds and any murmurs with simultaneous palpation of the carotid artery.
- Note radiation to the axilla or carotids and try to differentiate carotid bruits (balloon pump noise will make this difficult unless the augmentation rate is reduced).
- Look particularly for crackles in the chest and signs of a pleural effusion. A dull percussion note at the right base may reflect a phrenic nerve palsy, which may complicate cardiac surgery.
- Abdomen – distended from an ileus (e.g. 'pump pancreatitis', ischaemia from dissection or mesenteric embolism).
- Assess perfusion of the peripheries – classically warm and vasodilated in distributive shock and cold with prolonged capillary refill time (>3 s) in a low cardiac output state.
- Graft harvest sites – saphenous veins (open or endoscopic methods) or radial artery.
- Signs of a lower limb DVT – unilateral swelling and tenderness.
- Peripheral oedema – chronic congestive cardiac failure.
- If an IABP, check the femoral artery puncture site for bleeding and signs of infection and assess distal limb perfusion with a comparison with the opposite

side (skin temperature, pulses). Is it sheathed or not? (There will be a bigger hole in the artery.)
- Femoral artery puncture sites – recent coronary angiography, balloon pump or femoral bypass catheter access; note swellings from a haematoma or false aneurysm.
- Neurological status – reduced GCS (disproportionate to the amount of sedation that is being/has been administered) and signs of a hemiparesis suggest a CVA has complicated treatment.
- Check urine output.
- Oliguria (e.g. low cardiac output state, compromised renal perfusion from a low-lying balloon pump or dissection).
- Polyuria (e.g. 'cold' diuresis in hypothermia, mannitol given in theatre, frusemide therapy).
- Ventricular assist devices.

Useful questions
'Could you please provide surgical details?', e.g. the type of surgery (including number, type and location of grafts, type of valvular prosthesis, duration of cardiac bypass and cross-clamp time, need for filtering or mannitol on bypass, problems related to going on and coming off bypass).

'What have the drain losses been since the patient's return from theatre (especially in the first 24 hours)? If bleeding is problematic, 'What has been the preoperative exposure to anticoagulants, antiplatelet agents and could you please give me a history of a pro-coagulant disorder (including uraemia)?

'Could you please clarify the position of the surgical drains (e.g. mediastinal, pleural, pericardial)?

'Could I please review a recent 12-lead ECG? (Ask for serial ECG as appropriate)'

'What are the echocardiogram findings?' – recent transthoracic or transoesophageal study, if progress has not been straightforward.

If an IABP is present: 'Can I please check timing with augmentation ratio of 1:2 and check position of tip on a recent supine CXR? (Should be just above the left main bronchus). 'Could I please check for pulses with a Doppler ultrasound probe?' – if pulses were impalpable in the limb on the side of insertion.

'May I check the positions of the pulmonary artery catheter (tip in a pulmonary artery and not more lateral than the junction of the medial and middle thirds of the lung field diameter) and CVL (tip just above right atrium) on a recent CXR?'

If paced: 'When were the sensitivity and pacing thresholds last checked?' If fully paced: 'What has the underlying rhythm and rate been?'

Useful statements
'Twenty-four hours after coronary artery bypass grafting, with saphenous vein conduits, this 70-year-old man appears to have progressed well. He is extubated, has good pain control and is not requiring any vasoactive medications. He has well-perfused peripheries and an adequate urine output. The praecordial murmur, present on auscultation, is a pericardial rub of no clinical significance.'

'This patient, who is receiving infusions of adrenaline and GTN, has the following signs of a low cardiac output state ...'

'I suspect that this young woman is suffering from acute infective endocarditis involving the tricuspid valve because ...'

Topics for discussion
- Approach to post-cardiac surgical bleeding
- Causes of shock after cardiac surgery
- Management of atrial arrhythmias after cardiac surgery

- Indications for surgery for endocarditis and aortic dissection
- Comparison of different methods for the assessment of cardiac output
- Outcomes following off-pump versus on-pump coronary artery bypass surgery.

4. The patient with a subarachnoid haemorrhage

Possible cases
Spontaneous SAH caused by a ruptured berry aneurysm or arteriovenous malformation with:
- complications causing a reduced conscious state, necessitating intubation for airway protection (e.g. hydrocephalus, vasospasm, status epilepticus, intracerebral bleeding with mass effect or cerebral oedema)
- complications requiring ventilation (e.g. massive aspiration, neurogenic pulmonary oedema)
- requirement for high-dependency unit monitoring for tight control of blood pressure or management of electrolyte disorders (e.g. cerebral salt wasting, SIADH, diabetes insipidus).

Appropriate thoughts
- Where is the lesion? Which hemisphere? What territory?
- Is this patient following a straightforward course or have there been complications?
- Has the patient received definitive treatment yet? If not, what is the most appropriate treatment?

The examination
The monitor
- Note the MAP in conjunction with the infusions for BP control
- ICP monitoring, e.g. to detect rebleeding.

Infusions
- Nimodipine as prophylaxis against vasospasm
- Antihypertensives to control MAP in the setting of unclipped aneurysms
- Vasopressors to augment MAP in the setting of vasopasm (part of 'triple H' therapy)
- Sedatives.

Ventilation
- High FiO_2/PEEP may be due to aspiration or neurogenic pulmonary oedema.

Equipment
- EVD for management of hydrocephalus
- Femoral artery sheath if recent cerebral angiogram or endovascular coiling.

On examination
- Note GCS and pupil responses to light.
- Craniotomy scar if recent neurosurgery.
- Meningism (e.g. neck stiffness, Kernig's sign).
- Signs of conditions associated with berry aneurysms (e.g. polycystic kidney disease).
- Fundoscopy may show subhyaloid haemorrhages.
- Focal neurological signs

  ○ cranial nerves (e.g. CN III if a posterior communicating artery aneurysm)
  ○ long tracts (e.g. hemiplegia of leg more than arm if anterior cerebral artery haemorrhage)
  ○ brainstem signs (e.g. posterior circulation aneurysmal haemorrhage or brain death from raised ICP)
- Chest signs – purulent or frothy sputum if aspiration pneumonia or neurogenic pulmonary oedema.
- Urine output – looking for polyuria (e.g. suggesting diabetes insipidus or cerebral salt wasting).

Useful questions
Ensure there is no drug paralysis before commenting on neurological signs. 'Is the patient currently under the influence of paralysing drugs?'
If no sedative infusions and a reduced GCS: 'When did the patient last receive sedation? What drug(s) were used? For how long? What dose?'
'Could I please see the CT head scan and the results of the cerebral angiography?'
'Could you please tell me a recent serum sodium (if polyuria present)?'
'Has CSF from the EVD has been sent for culture?'

Useful statements
'This patient has most likely experienced a spontaneous subarachnoid haemorrhage complicated by hydrocephalus, on the basis of the EVD and nimodipine infusion.'

Topics for discussion
- Complications of spontaneous subarachnoid haemorrhages
- Aetiologies of subarachnoid haemorrhage – including berry aneurysms, non-aneurysmal perimesencephalic haemorrhages, arteriovenous malformations, trauma
- Severity grading – Hunt and Hess; World Federation of Neurosurgeons
- Definitive management of aneurysms – role and timing of clipping and coiling
- Prevention and management of vasospasm
- The role of 'triple H' therapy
- The conflict between protective lung ventilation strategies and the need for normocarbia in this group of patients
- Role of transcranial Doppler studies
- Cardiac complications of subarachnoid haemorrhage.

5. The patient with a head injury

Possible cases
- Isolated severe traumatic brain injury
- Head injury in a multiple trauma patient
- Not waking up after a experiencing trauma to other body regions (e.g. from fat embolism syndrome or secondary brain insults).

Appropriate thoughts
- Is this an isolated head injury or not?
- At what phase in the course of the illness is this patient? – first 48 hours? Day 4 or 5 with continued raised ICP despite maximal therapy?
- Are there other factors that will influence the management of the patient's head injury, e.g. multiple orthopaedic procedures required in the forthcoming days…?

The examination
The cubicle
- Cooling device at end of bed.

The monitor
- MAP, ICP, CPP usually displayed if an acute severe injury – should have a CPP
- 60–65 mmHg based on recent guidelines
- Note ICP waveform character:
  - normally three phases: P1 (percussion wave from arterial pulsations); P2 (rebound wave reflecting intracranial compliance); P3 (dicrotic wave from venous pulsations)
  - 'A' waves or plateau waves – high amplitude waves of 50–100 mmHg sustained for up to 15 minutes, associated with raised ICP with compromised cerebral blood flow
  - 'B' waves – sawtooth appearance with small changes in pressure every 0.5–2 minutes associated with poor intracranial compliance
  - 'C' waves – low amplitude oscillations up to 20 mmHg for approximately 1 minute with a frequency of approximately 5/min – can be normal and associated with variations in vasomotor tone
  - flat ICP trace – damped trace from blockage, compression or kinking of the measurement device.
- ETCO$_2$ monitoring:
  - 30–40 mmHg (4–5 kPa) satisfactory (if higher, may be inappropriate if ICP elevated)
  - chronic hypoventilation to CO$_2$ less than 30 mmHg (<4 kPa) also problematic – should be correlated with PaCO$_2$ from a recent blood gas analysis.
- Core temperature
  - no evidence for routine therapeutic hypothermia
  - can assist ICP control if refractory raised pressures
  - cooling to normothermia if febrile to >38.5°C is commonly performed.

Infusions
- Sedation – commonly narcotic and sedative (e.g. morphine and midazolam) or propofol infusions
- Neuromuscular blocker infusion, such as vecuronium (e.g. for management of shivering during cooling)
- Intravenous phenytoin for seizure prophylaxis or management
- Vasoactive drugs (most often norepinephrine infusion) for augmentation of MAP to maintain a CPP
- Cerebral osmotherapy –3% saline or mannitol infusions
- Thiopentone infusion if refractory raised ICP.

Ventilation
- High FiO$_2$/PEEP may reflect associated chest injuries, aspiration or nosocomial pneumonia.

Equipment
- EVD or parenchymal ICP monitor. If there is an EVD, note CSF pressure before drainage can occur, colour of CSF, frequency and volume of drainage from EVD. If the ICP waveform is flat, ask to close the EVD drain tap in order to assess it.
- EEG may show burst suppression if thiopentone required for refractory raised ICP or to detect seizures in a drug-paralysed patient.
- Tracheostomy is frequently required.

- Urinary catheter – note the colour and ask about the volume of urine in the previous 8 hours.
- If polyuria, consider diabetes insipidus, cerebral salt wasting or effects of osmotherapy agents.
- If the urine has a green colour and there is a propofol infusion, consider alternative sedatives as there is an increased risk of the propofol infusion syndrome (phenol metabolite accumulating).
- Jugular venous bulb monitoring performed in some units.

On examination
- Note patient's head position – midline, 30–45 degrees head up, no compression on the neck veins if raised ICP.
- Look for head wounds – traumatic or surgical, including from previous ICP monitors/EVDs or craniotomy.
- Check for stigmata of base of skull fracture – auroscope examination for haemotympanum, CSF otorrhoea or rhinorrhoea, Battle's sign (bruising over the mastoid region), racoon eyes (bilateral periorbital bruising).
- GCS – it is essential to apply a painful stimuli to each limb and both supraorbital ridges if not responding to voice to correctly assess motor response (ask first before causing pain). First clarify that the patient is not drug paralysed and whether they speak English.
- Check pupil size, shape, symmetry, direct and consensual light responses, afferent pupil defects (consider traumatic mydriasis if unilaterally dilated pupil, as well as raised ICP)
- Fundoscopy (e.g. retinal haemorrhages, papilloedema).
- Other cranial nerves as conscious state permits.
- In the unconscious patient check oculocephalic reflex (ensure cervical spine is stable first), corneal reflexes, jaw jerk, facial wincing in response to pain, gag and cough reflexes.
- Motor examination – tone, power if cooperative, reflex symmetry and briskness, plantar responses.
- Sensory testing is rarely rewarding unless the patient is co-operative and alert.

Useful questions
- 'Could I please see the CT head scan and review the full injury history to clarify the nature of relevant primary and secondary insults?'
- If the patient is polyuric: 'Could I please see recent paired urine and serum sodium and osmolality?'
- To assess the role of residual medication effects in the patient who is not waking up: 'When was sedation ceased? What type and duration of drugs were administered? What is the renal and hepatic function?

Useful statements
'This young man, with signs of trauma to his head, is experiencing refractory raised intracranial pressure despite multiple therapies, including heavy sedation, tight CO_2 control, osmotherapy, CSF drainage via an EVD and induced hypothermia with paralysis. I suspect he has a severe traumatic brain injury.'

Topics for discussion
- Indications for monitoring of ICP in traumatic brain injury
- Methods of monitoring ICP – advantages and disadvantages of each
- Conventional and experimental strategies for managing raised ICP in patients with severe traumatic brain injury, including the Lund approach and decompressive craniectomy

- Theoretical phases of traumatic brain injury (ischaemic, hyperaemic, vasospastic) and the influence of these phases on management
- Pros and cons of mannitol versus hypertonic saline as agents for osmotherapy
- Prognostication – what should the family be told?

6. The patient with a spinal injury

Possible cases
- Cervical cord injury with ventilatory dependency
- Multiple trauma patient with a spinal injury
- Patient with a spinal injury and intercurrent problem (e.g. severe sepsis).

Appropriate thoughts
- Has the spine been stabilised yet?
- At what phase of the injury is this patient?
  - acute: cardiovascular problems, ileus
  - sub-acute: recurrent atelectasis and segmental collapse
  - chronic: pain, psychological issues, urosepsis.
- Will this patient need a tracheostomy? Consider the timing with regards to the surgical plan (e.g. the tracheostomy may need to be delayed for several days after an anterior cervical stabilisation wound is created, to reduce the risks of infection).
- Are there other injuries?

The examination
The cubicle
- Edgerton spinal bed until spine is stabilised
- Pressure area prevention bed (e.g. nimbus mattress) after spine stabilised
- Equipment for moving patient (e.g. Jordan frame, poles with canvas).

The monitor
- Mild hypotension and bradycardia are common during the acute phase of spinal shock
- Patients with chronic spinal injuries above mid-thoracic level may experience hypertension from autonomic dysreflexia.

Infusions
- Methylprednisolone may be present if an acute blunt traumatic injury
- Low-dose inotrope/vasopressor infusions for management of bradycardia/hypotension.

Ventilation
- Expect mandatory breathing mode early after injury and a weaning mode with progress (e.g. PSV, CPAP)
- High FiO_2/PEEP may reflect aspiration, nosocomial pneumonia or from associated thoracic injuries
- Tracheostomy common for cervical injuries
- Devices to assist speech (e.g. Passy-Muir valves) in the subacute/chronic patient. You should be familiar with the various types of tracheostomies available.

Equipment
- Spinal immobilisation devices – skull tongs with traction, cervical collars (e.g. hard collar or Philadelphia collar), halo brace with thoracic jacket, sandbags
- Splints – hands, wrists, ankles to prevent contractures

- DVT prophylaxis with sequential calf compressors or anti-thromboembolic stockings
- Signs of spinal fixation surgery – scars, surgical wounds, drains
- Pacing wires – rarely for management of early bradycardia/asystole in high cervical cord injuries
- Nasojejunal feeding tubes – feeding intolerance is a common early problem.

On examination
- Determine neurological level of injury or define cord syndrome from motor and sensory examination.

Motor
- Myotomes
- Spinal reflexes
- Limbs and abdominal:
  ○ flaccid weakness initially, replaced by hyperreflexia and clonus with time
  ○ it is a rule of thumb that as limb reflexes return so does chest wall tone associated with progress in ventilatory weaning and involuntary, often distressing, muscle spasms commence
- Anal tone and bulbocavernosus reflex
- PR examination with gloved finger, then test for reflex anal contraction by pulling on urinary catheter to stimulate glans or clitoris
- A positive bulbocavernosus reflex signifies spinal shock is over. A persistent lack of sensorimotor function following return of the bulbocavernosus reflex suggests an established complete spinal cord injury
- Ask whether the patient senses rectal fullness following an enema.

Sensory
- Dermatomes
- Specific sensory tracts – dorsal columns, spinothalamic tracts
- The 'level' of the injury is described as the last spinal segment that is intact on either side of the body and may be separately described for motor and sensory function if there is a discrepancy (e.g. 'C5 sensory level' means sensation over the C5 – upper outer arm – dermatome has intact sensation but the C6 dermatome does not)
- Paradoxical, diaphragmatic breathing if spontaneous breathing and high cervical cord injury
- Priapism during spinal shock
- Pressure sores – early from spinal immobilisation devices and over time from chronic immobilisation
- Signs of other injuries in the multiple trauma patient.

Useful questions
- During examination: 'Can/how can I move the patient (especially their neck)?'
- 'Could I please look at the patient's back?' (Look for signs of localised trauma, surgery or pressure areas.)
- If the injury has been localised anatomically from examination: 'Could I please see imaging of this region (e.g. plain films, CT, MR studies)?'

Useful statements
'This patient has evidence of a cervical cord injury with complete C5 neurology with associated ventilator dependency.'
'The signs demonstrated on neurological examination are consistent with a central cord syndrome, with weakness affecting the upper limbs and relative sparing of the lower limbs.'

Topics for discussion
- Approach to weaning from ventilation
- Management of haemodynamic instability in the patient with spinal shock

- Evidence supporting high-dose corticosteroids for blunt spinal cord injury
- Supportive care for patient with a spinal injury – physical and psychosocial.

7. The patient with an intra-abdominal catastrophe

Possible cases
- Persistent sepsis; acute necrotising pancreatitis; abdominal trauma or peritonitis (e.g. perforated viscus – duodenal ulcer, appendix, diverticulum, appendix, bowel neoplasm, obstructed bowel, breakdown of a surgical bowel anastomosis)
- Massive blood loss from uncontrolled upper or lower gastrointestinal bleeding (e.g. oesophageal varices, angiodysplasia, tumour)
- Abdominal trauma.

Appropriate thoughts
- What is the cause of the problem?
- Has the problem been treated or is treatment still ongoing? (e.g. open abdomen with packs still present?)
- Is the patient being fed? Are they tolerating feeds? What is their nutritional status?
- What is required for this patient to continue to make progress?
- Could fungal sepsis be an issue?
- Could abdominal compartment syndrome be complicating this patient's situation?

The examination
The cubicle
- Note infection control warnings (e.g. isolation measures for multi-resistant organisms, such as MRSA, VRE or multiresistant *Acinetobacter*).

The monitor
- Note core temperature and HR and determine if the readings are consistent with SIRS
- JVP, MAP or other invasive parameters (e.g. PiCCO data) will help clarify volume status and any haemodynamic disturbance.

Infusions
- Vasoactive drug infusions – the vasopressor and inotrope strategy will reflect the haemodynamic disturbance(s); most commonly distributive and hypovolaemic shock
- Antibiotics – institution-specific, but may suggest the underlying problem (e.g. vancomycin for MRSA infection)
- TPN for failed enteral feeding or select abdominal problems (e.g. intestinal fistulae)
- Transpyloric feeding – for failed gastric feeding and often first-line in acute pancreatitis
- Blood products and/or fluid loads for hypovolaemia
- Octreotide infusion for variceal bleeding
- Omeprazole infusion for peptic ulceration
- Terlipressin infusion for hepatorenal syndrome.

Ventilation
- Increased FiO_2/PEEP may reflect basal atelectasis from reduced diaphragmatic excursion, ARDS, nosocomial pneumonia or associated chest injuries in a trauma patient.

Equipment
- Surgical drains and VAC dressings – number, location, nature of drainage material (fluid, bile, pus, blood, faeculent material), presence of suction or irrigation of tubes
- Stomas – location, mucosal integrity, nature of losses; feeding jejunostomy in necrotising pancreatitis
- Bladder pressure transducer if abdominal compartment syndrome has been suspected (>25 cmH$_2$0 is significant)
- Rectal tubes – diarrhoea, melaena, fresh blood, mucus
- Vascath for CRRT if renal failure has been a complication
- Minnesota tube if uncontrolled variceal bleeding
- Right internal jugular vein catheter or puncture site from a TIPPS procedure
- Large-bore peripheral cannulae/rapid infusion catheters if recent massive volume replacement.

On examination
- Check for jaundice – resorption of massive haematoma, biliary obstruction with ascending cholangitis, acute of chronic liver disease.
- Look for stigmata of chronic liver disease (e.g. leuconychia, spider naevi, gynaecomastia, caput medusae).
- Look for stigmata suggestive of alcoholism (e.g. Dupuytren's contracture, parotidomegaly).
- Examine abdominal wounds – surgical or traumatic, closed or open with mesh covering if tension, or increased intra-abdominal pressures prevented primary closure. Note if wounds appear recent or granulating, clean or infected.
- Percutaneous jejunostomy for feeding – pancreatitis.
- Look for Cullen's sign (periumbilical bruising) or Grey-Turner's sign (flank bruising) suggestive of haemorrhagic pancreatitis.

Useful questions
'Could I please see the results of recent abdominal imaging investigations or findings at laparotomy?'
'What was the recent serum amylase and lipase?' – if pancreatitis should be considered.
'What has the urine output been over the last 8 hours?'
'Could I please see the results of drain fluid cultures, surgical swabs or tissue biopsies, blood and urine cultures?' (Include cultures for bacteria and fungi if febrile.)

Useful statements
'This patient has evidence of multi-organ dysfunction. The most likely cause is persistent intra-abdominal sepsis. I would liaise closely with the surgical team managing the operative care of the patient. It is possible that they require repeat abdominal imaging +/– a further laparotomy.'
'The clinical findings of spider naevi, scleral jaundice and gynaecomastia are indicative of chronic liver disease. The Minnesota tube and rectal tube that is draining liquid melaena stool are consistent with recent uncontrolled variceal bleeding.'

Topics for discussion
- Management of acute pancreatitis – nutrition, antibiotics, determining the aetiology
- Diagnosis and management of abdominal compartment syndrome
- TPN versus enteral feeding for various abdominal pathologies
- Risk factors for fungal infection and the role of empirical fluconazole therapy in intra-abdominal sepsis
- Management of variceal bleeding.

8. The patient who has had an abdominal aortic aneurysm repair

Possible cases
- Postoperative monitoring after an uneventful elective AAA repair – open or endoluminal
- Management of complications after emergency or elective AAA.

Appropriate thoughts
- Was this intervention elective or urgent?
- Was there supra-renal extension?
- What was the supra-renal clamp time?
- If urgent, is there evidence of end-organ damage from prolonged hypotension/ hypovolaemic shock?
- Is there evidence of complications relating to the surgery? (e.g. hypoxic–ischaemic brain injury, spinal cord ischaemia, intestinal ileus or ischaemia, lower limb ischaemia, compartment syndromes of the limbs or abdomen, bleeding or sepsis, acute renal impairment)

The examination
The cubicle
- A dialysis machine may be present.

The monitor
- Note the BP – avoidance of hypertension in the early postoperative course (e.g. systolic BP <150 mmHg) is desirable.

Infusions
- Sedation and analgesia if ongoing ventilation is required.
- Transpyloric feeding or TPN may reflect intestinal ileus or ischaemia.
- Frusemide infusion – may facilitate removal of excess third space fluid as SIRS resolves.

Ventilation
- Increased peak airway pressures may reflect increased intra-abdominal pressure.
- An increase in FiO_2/PEEP may result from basal atelectasis caused by reduced diaphragmatic excursion or ARDS (which may also be suspected by a protective lung strategy with tidal volumes 6 mL/kg).

Equipment
- IDC – oliguria or anuria from acute renal failure (multifactorial aetiology including pre-renal and renal causes such as prolonged supra-renal clamping, hypotension, hypovolaemia or the abdominal compartment syndrome)
- Vascath for continuous or intermittent haemodialysis and/or haemofiltration
- Intra-abdominal pressure measurement – bladder pressure monitoring via a transducer.

On examination
- Look for transverse or midline laparotomy wound.
- Look for arterial catheters or puncture sites if an endoluminal repair.
- Look for lower limb perfusion; sensation, power and compartment tenseness should be noted.

- Jaundice may reflect unconjugated hyperbilirubinaemia from resorption of massive intra-abdominal haematoma.
- GCS, pupil reactions to light, evidence of myoclonus and a motor examination of limb tone, power and reflexes may demonstrate upper motor neuron pathology caused by a diffuse hypoxic–ischaemic brain injury.

Useful questions
'Could you please clarify for me the circumstances and nature of the surgery?' (i.e. emergency versus elective, open versus endoluminal technique, supra- versus infra-renal clamping, duration of shock before aortic cross-clamping and restoration of organ perfusion.)
'What has the urine output been over the past 8 hours?' If recently returned from the operating theatre, ask: 'Was mannitol and/or frusemide given intra-operatively?'
'Has enteral feeding been commenced and tolerated?'
'Have lower limb pulses been detected with Doppler (if they are not palpable)?'

Useful statements
'This patient, who has had an emergency repair of a ruptured abdominal aortic aneurysm, is suffering from a number of complications including enteral feeding intolerance because of an ileus, renal failure requiring CRRT and respiratory failure, likely to be caused by nosocomial pneumonia.'

Topics for discussion
- Outcomes of endoluminal versus open surgical techniques
- Management of common complications
- Indications for elective aortic repair
- The role of perioperative beta-blockers in elective aneurysm repair.

9. The obstetric patient

Possible cases
- Complications specific to pregnancy:
  - pre-delivery – ruptured ectopic pregnancy with hypovolaemic shock, DIC (e.g. septic abortion or intrauterine fetal death), pre-eclampsia with HELLP syndrome or acute fatty liver of pregnancy
  - post-delivery – amniotic fluid embolism, massive postpartum haemorrhage (e.g. placenta accreta/increta/percreta)
- Critical illnesses not specific to pregnancy – severe sepsis, multiple trauma, massive pulmonary embolism, subarachnoid haemorrhage, aortic dissection, decompensated valvular heart disease
- Complications of assisted fertility (e.g. ovarian hyperstimulation syndrome).

Appropriate thoughts
- Is this pregnant patient in ICU because of a problem related to the pregnancy or is the illness unrelated to her pregnancy?
- Has the fetus been delivered? If not, should it be and when?

The examination
The cubicle
- Cardiotocography machine near the bed.

The monitor
- Blood pressure: in pre-eclampsia, expect systolic BP >140 and/or diastolic BP >90 mmHg
- Very high CVP in massive PE with acute right heart strain or low in hypovolaemia
- High core temperature – sepsis including intrauterine source from prolonged rupture of membranes pre-delivery or endometritis postpartum.

Infusions
- Therapies for pre-eclampsia – $MgSO_4$, phenytoin, antihypertensives (e.g. hydralazine, GTN)
- Tocolytics, e.g. salbutamol (nifedipine more often used via NGT)
- Heparin – thromboembolism
- Blood products, fluid loads, haemostatic drugs (e.g. antifibrinolytics) for massive blood loss
- Oxytocin, to promote uterine contraction (e.g. following significant post-partum haemorrhage)
- Steroids for fetal lung maturation (e.g. betamethasone or dexamethasone)

Ventilation
- If spontaneous breathing, expect an increased RR, TV and MV with reduced $ETCO_2$ as a normal finding in pregnancy.
- Increased FiO_2/PEEP may reflect pulmonary oedema complicating severe pre-eclampsia or decompensated valvular heart disease.
- An increased FiO_2 and A–a gradient with normal lung compliance in PE.
- Remember that at term the normal pCO_2 is 27–32 and normal pH is approximately 7.47.

Equipment
- Large bore IV cannula/rapid infusion catheter for fluid resuscitation
- Arterial line and CVP for tight BP and volume management in pre-eclampsia
- CTG monitor for assessment of fetal well-being
- Angiocatheter sheath in femoral artery if a uterine embolisation procedure has been performed (e.g. for placenta increta).

On examination
- Check for generalised oedema – pre-eclampsia, ovarian hyperstimulation syndrome (also with pleural effusions and ascites).
- Look for bruising/ecchymoses/petechiae – liver dysfunction, DIC, low platelets in HELLP syndrome.
- Check for jaundice – fatty liver of pregnancy.
- Perform a fundal examination – height and correlation with gestational age, presenting part, lie, liquor volume.
- Is there a caesarean section scar? Occasionally with surgical drains.
- Check for lower limb DVT.
- Check clonus and reflexes if on magnesium infusion (they disappear as an early sign of magnesium toxicity).

Useful questions
If you suspect eclampsia/severe pre-eclampsia: 'Did the patient have a seizure? What, if any, neurological symptoms has she had?'
'What is the gestational age of the fetus and progress of the pregnancy to date?'
'Can I please see the results of the per vaginal examination?' If pre-delivery, note if membranes are intact or ruptured, if postpartum note the colour and volume of lochia.

'Can I check the fetal heartrate with Doppler?'
'What is the mother's blood group?'
'Could I please inspect a recent CTG trace?'
'Could I please see the results of a recent fetal ultrasound scan?'
If pre-delivery: 'Have steroids been given?'
If the mother has already delivered: 'What is the health status of the neonate?'

Useful statements

'This young woman has had an urgent caesarean section delivery for eclampsia. She is being treated with a magnesium infusion and phenytoin for seizures. I suspect she may have the HELLP syndrome as she is jaundiced with multiple petechiae visible on her trunk and limbs.'

'(Name) is a 25-year-old female in the third trimester of pregnancy. She appears to have been the victim of a motor vehicle accident. There is seatbelt bruising on abdominal examination and her right forearm is immobilised in a plaster cast. The fetus appears to be intact with a fetal HR of 130/min.'

Topics for discussion

- Minimal gestational age for viability and the timing of delivery in various common critical illnesses complicating pregnancy
- Complications of magnesium treatment and how to detect them
- Indication for and method of performing an ICU caesarean section when the mother has had a cardiac arrest
- Drugs contraindicated in pregnancy
- Management of common critical illnesses complicating pregnancy
- Management of ovarian hyperstimulation syndrome.

10. The transplant patient

Possible cases

- Liver, heart, lung and heart–lung transplant recipients most commonly for perioperative management, less often a late complication (e.g. sepsis, severe rejection episode)
- Renal or pancreatic transplant patients with a complication requiring ICU (e.g. need for CRRT in a haemodynamically unstable patient or infection with septic shock)
- Bone marrow transplantation – usually ICU admission for a septic complication in a patient with a haematological malignancy (e.g. respiratory failure requiring non-invasive ventilation or intubation and/or shock requiring inotropes).

Appropriate thoughts

Issues facing all transplant recipients can be considered as perioperative, early and late onset problems, related to:

- surgery
  - consider the specific anatomy and anastomoses formed to predict specific problems (e.g. early anastomotic leaks or thrombosis and late stenosis)
  - preservation injury with early poor graft function common to all transplants.
- infection
  - early bacterial and delayed opportunistic infections (fungal, viral, mycobacterial).
- immunosuppression
  - rejection – hyperacute (<12 hours – alloantibody related), acute (usually <1 month but remains a risk – T-cell related), chronic (vasculitis presenting as

vanishing bile duct syndrome, accelerated ischaemic heart disease, obliterative bronchiolitis 'OB' or nephrosclerosis)
- graft versus host disease – most relevant to bone marrow transplantation – acute (<100 days) or chronic with a triad of skin rashes, liver dysfunction and gastrointestinal symptoms and signs
- drug side effects (e.g. cyclosporin – renal toxicity, hypertension, hirsutism, rarely haemolytic uraemic syndrome)
- transplant-related malignancies (e.g. skin).

The examination
The cubicle
- Special waste disposal equipment for cytotoxic agents
- Infection control precautions if multi-resistant organisms or neutropenic sepsis.

The monitor
- Fever – sepsis, SIRS, rejection, drug fever
- CVP – high in right ventricular dysfunction (common after heart and lung transplants); prominent V wave on the waveform if associated tricuspid regurgitation
- ECG – note paced rhythm and conduction disturbances (common after heart transplants)
- Haemodynamic measured and calculated variables (arterial BP, pulmonary artery catheter or PiCCO data) – consideration of these, in association with the vasoactive drugs being administered, should enable the major disturbance(s) to be elucidated.

Infusions
- Immunosuppressant drugs (e.g. calcineurin antagonists, corticosteroids, anti-nucleotides, monoclonal antibodies)
- Antibiotics – may reveal the likely infective agent(s)
- Vasoactive drugs
- Distributive shock requiring norepinephrine or rarely vasopressin; often seen after liver transplantation
- Isoprenaline for chronotropy after cardiac transplant or additional agents if low cardiac output state (e.g. dobutamine and dopamine).

Ventilation
- Increased PEEP/FiO$_2$/reduced lung compliance – important causes to consider are cardiogenic pulmonary oedema, atelectasis, ARDS, ventilator-induced lung injury, nosocomial pneumonia (including opportunistic infective agents), aspiration, rejection of a lung transplant, idiopathic pneumonia in a bone marrow transplant recipient.

Equipment
- Examine location and drainage from drains – blood loss
- Intercostal catheters after lung transplant
- Mediastinal, pleural, pericardial drains after heart transplants
- Abdominal drains after liver transplants, as well as a biliary drain if a T-tube inserted (may be no drain if a Roux-en-Y anastomosis)
- IDC and wound drain most relevant for renal transplants
- Epidural for analgesia common for early management after lung transplants
- Pulmonary artery catheter occasionally used in liver transplant surgery
- Epicardial pacing common after cardiac transplants
- Right internal jugular vein spared from lines with cardiac transplants (to permit subsequent endocardial biopsies).

On examination
- Examine surgical wounds – sternotomy for heart, clamshell or sternotomy for lung, 'Mercedes Benz' for liver and 'lazy S' flank to iliac fossa incision for kidney transplants.
- Perform a focused examination of the organ system involved.
- Look for rashes – drug reactions or graft versus host disease.
- Look for signs of the underlying disease necessitating transplantation.
- IDC – check urine output (oliguria from hypovolaemia with bleeding, nephrotoxicity from calcineurin antagonists, abdominal compartment syndrome after liver transplantation complicated by bleeding, graft dysfunction after renal transplant).

Useful questions
In the early postoperative period determine results of key investigations to determine graft viability:
- liver – ultrasound (portal vein and hepatic artery patency, new haematomas); serial liver function tests, stability of blood glucose and coagulation profiles)
- lung – bronchoscopy
- heart – echocardiography
- kidney – ultrasound (renal flow)

'Have any graft tissue biopsies been performed and what did they show?'
'Could I please see the results of drain fluid biochemistry (e.g. creatinine in drain fluid suggests a ureteric leak after renal transplant) and culture?'

Useful statements
'This patient, who is day 1 post cardiac-transplant, is making good progress. This is demonstrated by the fact that he is warm and well perfused; he requires minimal inotropic support; he is alert with good gas exchange an adequate urine output and his pain is well controlled. I believe that he is ready to be extubated.'

'This patient, who is day 2 post lung-transplant, appears to have had some unexpected problems postoperatively. This is shown by the poor lung compliance, the high A–a gradient and the requirement for nitric oxide. Possible causes for this can be separated into recipient factors and donor factors …'

Topics for discussion
- Indications for organ transplant
- Approach to the investigation and management of new lung infiltrates in the transplant patient
- Complications of immunosuppression
- Management of acute rejection
- Prognosis after individual organ transplantation
- Issues regarding organ donation

11. The oncology patient

Possible cases
- Chemotherapy-related neutropenic sepsis
- Post stem cell transplantation – acute versus chronic graft versus host disease and their complications
- Complications of chemotherapy (including the acute abdomen) or radiotherapy
- Post major cancer surgery.

Appropriate thoughts
- This could be a complication of the malignancy, a side effect of the treatment or an infective complication of the immunosuppression.
- What treatments has this patient received to date (e.g. chemotherapy, radiotherapy, surgery)?
- What complications of the condition or its treatment have led to the need to be in the ICU?
- If sepsis is the problem, what are the possible sources and is this neutropenic sepsis?
- Are there end-of-life care/prognostication issues associated with the management of this case?

The examination
The cubicle
- Are infection control measures, such as contact precautions, in place? (Suggests infection with a multi-resistant or transmissable organism.)
- Special disposal bins for cytotoxic drugs.

The monitor
- Fever? tachycardia? hypotension? (Suggests sepsis, an inflammatory response due to drugs or rejection and/or intravascular fluid depletion from bleeding from coagulopathy, mucositis and/or diarrhoea.)

Ventilation
- Evidence of non-compliant lungs and protective ventilation strategy in patients with lung infiltrates (broad differential diagnosis)
- Low FiO_2 with low oxygen saturation on the monitor, suggesting chemotherapy with bleomycin and attempts to avoid oxygen toxicity.

Infusions
- Blood products, suggesting marrow suppression or active bleeding
- Chemotherapy agents
- Mesna, suggests haemorrhagic cystitis, particularly secondary to cyclophosphamide
- Palifermin (human recombinant keratocyte growth factor), suggests severe mucositis
- Rasburicase and/or bicarbonate, suggests tumour lysis syndrome
- G-CSF, suggests neutropenia
- Antibiotics may suggest a pathogen or given for prophylaxis against common serious pathogens (e.g. antifungals, antivirals)
- Inotropes and/or vasopressors.

Equipment
- Cardiac output monitoring equipment to aid management of complex shock states
- CRRT (e.g. tumour lysis syndrome with acute renal failure)
- An apheresis machine may be present.

On examination
- Chemotherapy-related issues – alopecia, long-term intravenous catheters (e.g. Hickman catheters, PICC lines), mucositis, Cushingoid fascies and myopathy from steroid therapy. Look for sources of sepsis with a head-to-toe approach outlined in the febrile patient case.
- Radiotherapy-related issues – ink/tattoo markings outlining the field; skin irritation if recent treatment, underling complications (e.g. thoracic region – early oesophagitis, risk of late fibrosing changes).

- Surgical issues – what operation has been performed? Is there evidence of previous surgery, suggesting this is for resection of metastases rather than curative resection or debulking of a primary lesion? Don't miss scars in less exposed areas (e.g. thoracotomy scars, breast surgery and reconstructions, partially shaved head after craniotomy). Look for effects of past surgery (e.g. lymphoedema of a limb).
- Nutritional issues – look for signs of malnutrition and cachexia (e.g. estimate BMI, examine muscle bulk and sites of classical wasting, such as the muscles of mastication and periorbital region; signs of hypoalbuminaemia, including peripheral oedema, ascites and pleural effusions).
- Signs suggesting specific problems:
  - Superior vena cava obstruction – facial plethora, swelling, Pemberton's sign
  - Stem cell transplant – look for cutaneous stigmata of acute or chronic graft versus host disease (allogeneic transplants).

Useful questions
- What treatments have been given?
- If stem cell transplantation has occurred, was it autologous or allogeneic? How long has it been since transplantation?
- What are the cell counts and coagulation indices?
- If the patient is in a single room or a cubicle, is it positive pressure isolation, suggesting immunosuppression, or negative pressure, suggesting a communicable respiratory pathogen is present (e.g. pulmonary TB)?

Useful statements
- 'You asked me to assess Lisa, a 23-year-old patient with sepsis, with regards to how she is progressing. I suspect that Lisa has had a recent allogeneic stem cell transplant, as evidenced by what appears to be cutaneous graft versus host disease. She appears to be improving with treatment as the noradrenaline that is still attached to her central line has been weaned off and …'
- 'John is a 78-year-old cachectic man, whom I suspect has had a previous thoracotomy and radiotherapy, and looks like he will die. He is on 100% oxygen, is requiring very high doses of adrenaline and noradrenaline and is anuric on CRRT.'

Topics for discussion
- Treatment of neutropenic sepsis, including the complexities of antibiotic management and the role of invasive versus non-invasive ventilation
- Expect discussions about prognosis and factors determining appropriateness of ICU management in oncology patients; discussing ethical issues associated with withdrawing and withholding therapies is common
- Problems associated with managing patients with a history of specific chemotherapy exposure and specialised therapy in the ICU (e.g. bleomycin lung injury with high-flow oxygen, anthracyclines and cardiomyopathy; diagnosis and management of graft versus host disease and other problems after stem cell transplantation)
- The differential diagnosis and management of specific clinical syndromes in the haematology-oncology patient:
  - Respiratory failure with pulmonary infiltrates – don't forget all-trans-retinoic acid (ATRA) syndrome and toxicity, such as bleomycin and amiodarone
  - Acute abdomen – neutropenic enterocolitis ('typhlitis'), infective diarrhoea, including clostridium difficile, CMV colitis, mucositis from chemotherapy, intestinal graft versus host disease, malignant obstruction and ileus
  - Haemorrhagic cystitis – cyclophosphamide, coagulopathy, viruses including CMV, adenovirus, HHV6.

12. The patient with burns

Possible scenarios
- Major burns (usually >25% body surface area) frequently with associated inhalational injury and trauma.

Appropriate thoughts
Problems and priorities may be considered in terms of three phases:

Resuscitation phase (0–36 hours)
- Airway burns, toxic gas injury – respiratory injury or systemic toxicity (carbon monoxide and cyanide)
- Burn shock and fluid resuscitation, consumptive coagulopathy
- Compartment syndromes requiring escharotomies or more extensive decompressions (limbs, including buttocks, chest wall, neck, abdomen)
- Definitive management of traumatic injuries and delineation of significant co-morbidities.

Post-resuscitation phase (day 2–6)
- Operative phase – debridement and grafting with recurrent trips to theatre
- Fluid therapy to address ongoing evaporative losses, anaemia from surgical blood loss and high nutritional requirements.

Inflammatory/infective phase (day 7 – complete closure of wounds)
- Clinical problem of differentiating sepsis from burns-related SIRS
- Extubation or tracheostomy.

The examination
The cubicle
- Increased ambient temperature to reduce heat loss
- Isolation room with strict infection control strategies
- Fibreoptic bronchoscope may be in the room – assessment of airway burns and for bronchial toileting.

The monitor
- Fever and tachycardia – sepsis or burns-related SIRS – a pulse rate 110–120 can be normal for up to 6/12 post burn.

Infusions
- Analgesia a priority (continuous narcotic infusions and ketamine for dressing changes commonly used) – combined with sedation to tolerate ventilation
- Feeding – enteral route preferred; continuous including while in theatre
- Fluids
  - Parkland formula-driven crystalloid resuscitation fluid (Hartmann's or normal saline) in first 24 hours – 1.5–2 times the calculated volume if an inhalation injury
  - colloid (4% normal serum albumin) – added after the first 12 hours and 20% albumin used by some to maintain a minimal serum albumin (e.g. >20 g/dL)
  - hypertonic saline – used in some units to minimise the volume of resuscitation fluid required (to reduce microcirculatory hypoperfusion related to tissue oedema)
  - later evaporative fluid losses met with extra crystalloid infusions (e.g. 5% dextrose) or more often extra free water added to enteral feeds

○ the free water loss in mL/hr = (25 + %TBSA burn) × BSA (as rule of thumb use 2 m^2). You will need to use this quick calculation with respect to the fluid balance, e.g. 50% burn = expect 150 mL/hour free water loss = 3600 mL/day in addition to other fluid requirements to maintain a neutral fluid
- Blood products – management of anaemia and consumptive coagulopathy related to surgery (packed cells, fresh frozen plasma, platelets)
- Insulin infusion – commonly required for glucose intolerance
- Antibiotics – prophylactic for theatre or for management of complicating infections
- Treatments for cyanide poisoning – rarely required (e.g. dicobalt edetate, hydroxocobalamin, sodium thiosulfate)

Ventilation
- Increased FiO$_2$/PEEP/reduced lung compliance/high peak inspiratory pressures – processes include ARDS, chest wall burn, pain or shivering restricting chest expansion, inhalational injury, nosocomial pneumonia, fluid overload, associated chest trauma
- Protective lung strategy (TV 6–8 mL/kg) and/or inhaled nitric oxide may reflect ARDS management
- A metabolic cart may be attached to the ventilator – nutrition in burns patients often tailored to calculated resting energy expenditure and adequacy assessment incorporates measured respiratory quotients
- Nebulised heparin or N-acetylcysteine sometimes used for inhalational injury.

Equipment
- Bladder transducer for measurement of intra-abdominal pressures
- Vascath and CRRT – compartment syndrome with myoglobinuria and acute renal failure
- CoolLine™ and CoolGard™ endovascular cooling device used for active cooling
- Temperature – skin temperature probe.

On examination
- Acknowledge that limited examination is possible – with care and appropriate questions the examiner will provide almost all the information that you need.
- Review all body surfaces and burn wounds at times of dressing changes.
- Look for signs of burn wound infection. Multiple cannulae or catheters emerging from various points in the dressings, especially if there is an odour of vinegar, suggest a pseudomonal burns infection.
- Clarify the extent of the wound that has been treated and the amount that still requires surgery.
- Make a head-to-toe examination for signs of associated traumatic injuries.
- Examine the eye for corneal injury – when oedema permits.
- Examine the mouth – torch and tongue depressor.
- Look for signs of inhalational injury (e.g. carbonaceous sputum on suctioning, burns to the face, singed eyelashes, eyebrows and nasal hair – signs of upper airway obstruction or hoarse voice in the non-intubated patient).
- Examine the neck for suitability for placement of tracheostomy – this site is often grafted early. If tracheostomy has been performed examine for infection.
- Abdominal examination includes asking if the urine output has been poor and whether bladder pressures have been performed.
- Assess for compartment syndromes – limb assessment should include each digit.
- Examine the febrile patient for other sources of sepsis (e.g. signs of nosocomial pneumonia, sinusitis with purulent nasal discharge).

- Identify all invasive lines for signs of infection and to ensure they are secure – look for potential sites for replacement – groins often spared and central line sites in the neck grafted as a priority.
- Urine output – >0.5–1 mL/kg/hr if adequate resuscitation; dark urine of myoglobinuria.

Useful questions
'Could I please see the results of the bronchoscopy examination?'
'What are the results of the urine test for myoglobinuria?'
'What has been the trend in the haematocrit?'
'May I review a recent arterial blood gas with lactate?'
'Has the patient had recent burn biopsies? What were the culture results?' (Wound swabs are not helpful in assessing burns infection.)
'What is the current surgical plan?'

Useful statements
'This patient is being treated for a major burn with at least 70% of the body currently dressed. They are intubated and I suspect a significant inhalational injury has occurred with carbonaceous sputum being suctioned, reduced lung compliance and a large A–a gradient.'

Topics for discussion
- Determination of the extent of burns – including depth and body surface area assessment using the 'Rule of nines' and Lund and Browder charts
- Nutritional therapy of the burns patient, including the role of immunonutrition
- Fluid therapy during different phases of post-burn management
- Diagnosis and management of inhalational injury
- Prognosis for severe burns
- Burns dressings (nanocrystalline silver, skin substitutes).

13. The patient receiving extracorporeal life support

Possible cases
- Patients with refractory potentially reversible respiratory failure (community-acquired pneumonia; H1N1 or other viral pneumonitis; pulmonary vasculitides) on VV ECMO
- Patients with the above problem compounded by severe haemodynamic disturbance on VA ECMO
- Patients with refractory heart failure on VA ECMO as a bridge to possible recovery (e.g. myocarditis) or as a bridge to decision about further therapy for irrecoverable myocardial function, e.g. VAD as destination therapy or VAD as a bridge to transplant
- Patients on a VAD (LVAD only or BiVAD, if significant co-existent right ventricular dysfunction), awaiting transplant. Usually in ICU because in the immediate post-insertion period or because of a complication such as bleeding, thrombosis or infection.

Appropriate thoughts
- Why does this patient need extra-corporeal life support?
- Is this V-A or V-V ECMO?
- Is there any evidence of the common complications of these therapies? Look for bleeding (including intracerebral), thrombosis (particularly intracerebral or within the circuit/oxygenator), sepsis (systemic, at the skin insertion site).

- For patients on ECMO – does this patient have a single (usually femoral) access cannula or two (femoral plus internal jugular)? Be able to give the pros and cons for both.

The examination
The cubicle
- Look for special personnel at the bed-side (e.g. perfusionists, a second ICU nurse).
- Look for signs of blood or blood products indicating recent haemorrhagic problems.

The monitor
- For patients receiving V-A ECMO or on a VAD, look at the arterial pressure trace for an indication of pulsatility (ECMO) and electromechanical dissociation (LVAD).

Infusions
- Intravenous heparin would be usual; if this is not present it may indicate a recent problem with bleeding
- Antibiotics, antivirals or immunosuppressive medication for treatment of underlying respiratory failure
- Antibiotics, antifungals for treatment of circuit or line-site related sepsis
- Unusually high dose sedative and analgesic infusions (drug absorption by the circuit and the membrane oxygenator)
- Inotropes – likely to be absent or in low dose in the presence of artificial cardiac support.

Ventilation
- Patients on ECMO will usually be on 'rest' ventilation – i.e. low frequency, very low volume (2–3 mL/kg) and sufficient PEEP to prevent atelectasis. The amount of FiO_2 delivered by the ventilator may give an indicator of how well the ECMO circuit is meeting the oxygen requirements – i.e. if the patient is receiving FiO_2 1.0 from the ventilator, the ECMO circuit is not matching their needs.
- Patients on a VAD may be on a protective ventilation strategy if they have associated multi-organ failure or severe ventilator-associated pneumonia.

Equipment
- For patients on ECMO, look at the amount of sweep gas and the concentration of oxygen being delivered by the membrane oxygenator device; if you are not familiar with ECMO devices ask for this information.
- Look at the cardiac output being delivered for patients on V-A ECMO and VADs; if you are not familiar with these devices, ask for this information.
- Check to see if a machine for regular measurement of ACT is present at the bedside.

On examination
- Check very carefully for signs of infection at the skin entry sites of the extra-corporeal circuit tubing.
- Check carefully for skin sepsis at all other sites of invasive lines or tubes – clinicians are often reluctant to change these in fully anticoagulated patients.
- Look of 'tube chatter' (a shuddering of the access catheter due to partial obstruction such as hypovolaemia, kinking or thrombus).
- Look for signs of vasodilatory septic shock, even if the patient is not febrile (fever may be masked by the cooling effect of the extracorporeal circuit).

- Look for clots in the membrane oxygenator device for patients on ECMO, which may be reflected in a widening of the transmembrane pressure on the ECMO monitor.
- Look for clots in the VAD device.

Useful questions
- 'How long has this patient been receiving ECMO/VAD support?'
- For all patients on extracorporeal life support: 'Please may I review the recent plasma free haemoglobin level and sequential coagulation results?'
- For patients on V-A ECMO or a VAD: 'Please may I review this patient's ECGs and echocardiograms?'
- For patients with predominant respiratory pathology: 'May I please review the sequential CXRs?' 'I wonder if a CT chest is available, although I realise that obtaining CT imaging in patients on ECMO is complex.'
- For all ECMO patients: 'Please may I review the blood gases from the arterial line and pre and post the membrane oxygenator?'
- For patients on ECMO: 'What has been the trend in the FiO_2 delivered by ECMO and the sweep gas in the last few days?'
- For all patients receiving extracorporeal support for several days (except for those patients where the examiners' question has revealed that the patient has irreversible pathology): 'Has this patient recently had an assessment of their function independent of support?' Be ready to demonstrate or explain how this is done.

Useful statements
- 'This patient is gravely ill. Their chances of survival will depend on the reversibility of their underlying pathology, and avoiding the common complications of systemic sepsis, bleeding or thrombosis.'
- 'This patient is gravely ill. Their chances of survival until a heart transplant becomes available depends on them recovering from this current problem of … and subsequently surviving the common complications of systemic sepsis, bleeding and thrombosis, which they will remain at risk of until the extracorporeal circuit is removed.'

Topics for discussion
- The role and evidence base for the use of ECMO in the management of refractory hypoxaemic respiratory failure
- How to wean a patient from extracorporeal life-support
- Difficulties in managing anticoagulation in these patients.

14. The bariatric patient

Possible cases
- Complications after laparoscopic banding or other bariatric surgery
- Any other ICU case complicated by morbid obesity.

Appropriate thoughts
- What is the underlying condition that has caused this patient to be critically ill?
- How does their obesity complicate the management of that condition?
- Is there any evidence of complications specifically related to this patient's morbid obesity?

The examination
Infusions
- Anything is possible depending on the underlying condition
- Diabetes is often a co-morbidity and an insulin infusion is likely.

The monitor
- Non-invasive BP monitoring may not be possible, or inaccurate (giving falsely high readings) due to the difficulties in finding cuffs large enough.

Ventilation
- Tidal volumes should be set on a mL/kg ideal body weight.
- PEEP may at 10 cmH$_2$O to increase FRC, decrease atelectasis and therefore improve lung compliance.

Equipment
- Bariatric devices such as special beds, chairs and hoists to reduce risks to the patient and to staff involved in patient care
- Sequential compression devices on the legs
- The patient's own home CPAP device.

On examination
You may need (and the examiners may expect you) to examine the patient from both sides of the bed, as to accurately visualise the left side of an extremely large person from the right side of the bed is not possible.
- Check the jaw, mouth opening and neck particularly with reference to airway problems.
- Look for evidence of heart failure.
- Look for signs of DVT.
- Look for signs of repeated attempts at invasive line access.
- Examine carefully under the skinfolds for signs of intertrigo.
- Ask particularly about skin care problems.

Useful questions
- 'Does this patient have home CPAP for obstructive sleep apnoea?'

Useful statements
'The severity of this patient's asthma/intra-abdominal sepsis/pneumonia is greatly increased by their morbid obesity. They are at increased risk of pressure area problems, venous thromboembolism and sepsis.'

'I would anticipate weaning difficulties in this patient due to the reduced FRC and expiratory reserve volume in obese patients compounded by the decreased static pulmonary compliance due to the heavy chest wall, with subsequent increased work of breathing. Emergency re-intubation may be difficult due to the problems associated with the airway in morbidly obese people and I would consider a tracheostomy. This may need to be performed in theatre due to difficulty in ascertaining the clinical landmarks in the neck.'

Topics for discussion
- The difficulty of obesity bias and maintaining the patient's dignity
- Problems associated with intubation and invasive lines in the morbidly obese patients
- Problems associated with appropriate drug-dosing in patients with morbid obesity
- The reasons for impairment of both left and right ventricular function in the bariatric patient

- Difficulties in diagnosing intra-abdominal pathology in the morbidly obese – difficulties with physical examination and performing investigations (many radiological investigations have weight limits for the electronic tables).

15. The long-stay patient

Possible cases
Admission for more than 2 weeks may be due to a number of problems – ventilator dependency with failure to wean (e.g. weakness from critical illness polyneuropathy or myopathy, Guillain-Barré syndrome, cervical spinal injury, severe chest injury), unresolving or recurrent sepsis (e.g. intra-abdominal collections from a perforated viscus), multi-organ failure from any cause (e.g. acute necrotising pancreatitis).

Appropriate thoughts
- Why was this patient admitted to ICU?
- Why are they still here? What needs to happen before they can be discharged?

The examination
The cubicle
- Personal items are common (e.g. photographs of the patient, their family and friends, get well cards, entertainment including television, reading material or music)
- A weaning plan or rehabilitation plan (e.g. for daily physiotherapy, occupational or speech therapy) may be displayed on the wall.

The monitor
- Observations of vital signs may be minimised if an isolated weaning problem or comprehensive as required for ongoing major pathologies.

Infusions
- Minimal IV therapy if an isolated, improving ventilation weaning problem
- Treatments required for slowly resolving problems (e.g. ongoing parenteral antibiotics for endocarditis).

Ventilation
- A weaning mode may be present (e.g. pressure support, assist-control). Note the amount of support needed by the patient (full ventilation at 2 weeks suggests there are other major unresolved problems).

Equipment
- Note the type of bed – should be suited to the prevention of pressure areas.
- With prolonged immobilisation DVT prophylaxis is important – note lower limb sequential compression devices, anti-thromboembolic stockings and bruises on the abdomen consistent with subcutaneous heparin injections.
- Limb splints to prevent joint contractures – must be well fitted to avoid causing pressure areas.

On examination
- Look for signs of a slowly improving patient (e.g. with an isolated weaning problem such as a cervical spinal injury), including being dressed in items of their own clothing, intact dentures, wearing of spectacles and interest in entertainment for stimulation.

- The patient's flat effect and poor eye contact may reflect depression.
- Pressure areas must be sought, with examination focusing on pressure areas, importantly inspecting the patient's back and buttocks, endotracheal tube or feeding tube resting sites on the nose and mouth.
- Examine for DVT in the lower limbs.
- Look for scars/wounds from multiple vascular access devices or traumatic injuries.
- Note eye integrity, personal hygiene, including mouth care, general grooming (e.g. shaving of facial hair).
- General examination as for diagnostic problem no. 2: 'Why is this patient failing to wean from ventilation?' helps define the relevant obstacles to success.

Useful questions
'What is the frequency and adequacy of bowel motions?' Constipation is a common problem.
If no signs of tube feeding or TPN: 'What has the patient's oral intake been over the past 24 hours?'.
'Have any psychoactive medications been prescribed?' These include antidepressants, anxiolytics, hypnotics or antipsychotics.

Useful statements
'This patient has been in ICU for several weeks, most likely because of ongoing intra-abdominal sepsis and multi-organ dysfunction. There is an open-meshed abdomen with multiple surgical drains, antibiotics and TPN are being delivered via a central line.'
'On examination there is a generalised flaccid paralysis, consistent with Guillain-Barré syndrome. This lady remains in ICU because of a failure to wean from ventilation. She has a pressure area on the sacrum and a unilaterally swollen calf that raises the possibility of a DVT.'

Topics for discussion
- Strategies for weaning patients from ventilation
- Supportive care of the immobile patient – physical, psychological, social, spiritual, practical (including financial) issues
- Communication issues with the patient's family/support network and ICU staff
- Physical and psychological rehabilitation after critical care.

Chapter 9

Critical care literature

Let every man judge according to his own standards, by what he has himself read, not by what others tell him.
ALBERT EINSTEIN

Introduction to the reference library

This section is intended as a reference guide to some of the most important papers in the literature. They have been selected on the basis of being practice-changing, highly contentious and/or widely debated among clinicians. A complete reference for each article is provided, followed by a succinct outline of the paper and comments about its significance. Highly select, high-yield resources that may be used to obtain essential theoretical information are also included and appraised.

The commentaries are a reflection of the authors' opinions about these articles and exam candidates are strongly encouraged to form their own opinions. Familiarity with the body of evidence supporting critical care practices is essential in order to become a well-informed specialist. One cannot claim to be an intensivist until one has formed an opinion about issues, such as the role of steroids in sepsis, how to titrate PEEP in ARDS, when to insert a pulmonary artery catheter or how to manage blood glucose, to name but a few of the most important issues. Knowledge of the evidence basis for conventional practices, as well as the inherent controversies in clinical practice, is essential before presenting for any critical care exit examination. Familiarity with this body of work also provides a contextual foundation that the reader can build upon as new developments arise.

This is not intended to be a complete list. Readers are encouraged to stay up-to-date with new developments and debates. Participation in evidence-based journal clubs (at work or online) will assist you to develop the skills needed to critically evaluate new articles.

It is not feasible to include papers that cover *all* of the subspecialty issues and the purpose of this chapter is not to replace a textbook that covers the full depth and breadth of intensive care medicine. It is important, however, to have an in-depth grasp of key literature from other specialties. Not only must intensivists stay abreast of new developments, they must be able to extrapolate the results to their critically ill patients and be able to comment on why specific recommendations may or may not be able to be followed. Such discussions also make for excellent viva dialogue. For example, the cardiology literature pertaining to acute coronary syndromes, particularly recommendations about anticoagulation, is not directly transferable to patients who have just had major surgical procedures.

It is essential to be familiar with the tools to specifically appraise articles about therapies, diagnostic methods and systematic reviews, and important to have a knowledge of basic statistical methods. The majority of these topics were covered in Chapter 3; statistics is covered in this chapter.

The topics have been arranged alphabetically and do not reflect the importance of one area over another. Articles within each subject have been carefully arranged in an order that reflects their relevance to issues, such as historic and significant developments in a particular field, and topics that are related to each other.

The following index is provided as a tool to assist the reader. All of the papers are presented with a more comprehensive indexing system on the DVD, which may further assist the usability of this material. The literature pertaining to paediatric intensive care medicine, addressed in Chapter 10, is also of relevance to the adult intensivist.

BOX 9.1 Index of topics covered

Airway management
Anaesthesia
Cardiovascular medicine
　Acute coronary syndromes
　Heart failure
　Surgery
Ethics
Fluids and electrolytes
　Glucose control
　Fluid therapy for resuscitation
Gastroenterology
　Feeding
　Gastrointestinal bleeding
　Pancreatitis
Haematology
Monitoring devices
Neurology
　Guillain-Barré syndrome
　Hypoxic–ischaemic brain injury
　Stroke
　Subarachnoid haemorrhage
Obstetrics and gynaecology
Pain medicine
Perioperative medicine
Quality
Renal medicine
　Dialytic therapies
　Prevention of radiocontrast nephropathy
Respiratory medicine
　ARDS
　Non-invasive ventilation
　Nosocomial pneumonia
　Thromboembolism
　Weaning
　Other issues
Resuscitation
Sedation
Sepsis
　Steroids

Continued

BOX 9.1 Index of topics covered—cont'd

Other interventions
Nosocomial infections
Antibiotic issues
Toxicology
Trauma
    Fluid management
    Burns
    Spinal injury
    Traumatic brain injury
    Other issues

Statistics

The assessment of statistics has evolved over the years from simple requests of definitions (e.g. mode, median and mean) to being provided with raw data that candidates are requested to describe before applying a relevant statistical test to analyse it. Knowledge of forest plots, box and whisker plots and specific types of analysis (e.g. meta-analysis) have also been required.

SAMPLE QUESTION

Make notes on meta-analysis.

Answer
Meta-analysis
- A statistical process that combines independent studies to allow an objective appraisal of the evidence.
- It may explain variability of effects seen in different trials.
- It aims to provide a more precise treatment effect of an intervention.
- It is subject to various errors when trials are included or excluded in error.
- Involves the same process of setting up a trial: formulation of hypothesis, data collection and analysis, reporting of results.
- Criteria for trial inclusion (e.g. published and unpublished trials) must be stated.
- Data collection forms should be standardised, allowing recording of the same information from different studies.
- Use of odds ratio or relative risk to standardise outcome measures.
- Use of 'fixed', 'random' effects model or Bayesian theory to combine data from various (e.g. sized) trials.
- There should be scrutiny of data if significant heterogeneity exists between trials (identified from the I^2 results).
- Graphical display on a forest plot (see text) illustrates results.
- A sensitivity analysis should be performed to assess the robustness of statistical tests used in the meta-analysis and the methodological quality assessing randomisation, publication bias and interim analyses (causing studies to stop).
- Make conclusions that are relevant to patient care, make clinical sense and reflect an accuracy of the meta-analysis performed (correct assumptions made on studies and appropriate combining of studies).
- Follow the Quorom (Quality of Reporting of Meta Analyses) statement.

Data

The value of having some statistical knowledge for the non-researcher is that it allows a better understanding of the literature. The main aim of research is to obtain meaningful information for the population based on a sample of it. To do this, data is collected; it is then described and information is inferred from it.

Data can be classified in different ways and analysed data can be quantitative or qualitative.

- Qualitative, or categorical, data refers to a quality (e.g. poor, below average, above average, good on a ratings scale), which can then be assigned a number when ranked (ordinal) or grouped (nominal).
- Quantitative data is numerical, which may be continuous or discrete. Continuous can be further considered if there is a zero point applicable (ratio) or not (interval).

Discrete refers to whole number variables or observations (also seen in qualitative data, e.g. number of ASA 4 patients in a group).

It is difficult to analyse raw data without presenting it in a more readable form, hence different methods exist for displaying and summarising data (descriptive statistics). This involves the use of such tools as histograms, tables and scatter plots. The data can be summarised using the median and range (quantitative and qualitative) or mean and standard deviation (quantitative). The more accurate the numbers assigned for qualitative data, the more precise the analysis.

Categorical data is often tabulated, which allows analysis with tests such as the Fisher exact test or chi-squared if larger than a 2×2 table.

Quantitative interval data is best displayed with tables and histograms. These are not simple bar charts, as the area of the histogram is important. They give an idea of central tendency, and distribution and scatter plots can be used when two sets of interval data are plotted together on X and Y axes. Correlation of the relationship and how it is defined can be performed.

Correlation is used for looking at independent variables and the Bland-Altman plot is used to look at different ways of measuring the same variable.

Summarising data

- Mode (most frequent observation): ideal for nominal data, ordinal data.
- Median (central observation): ideal for non-normally distributed interval data.
- Mean (sum of observations/number of observations): ideal for normally distributed interval data.
- Range: highest to lowest observation.
- Percentiles: division of observations usually into quartiles, which can be represented by box and whisker plots (Fig 9.1). These show outliers, range of results (whiskers), usually 25th and 75th centiles (box), and the measure of central tendency.
- Normal distribution curves (Fig 9.2) are described by their mean and standard deviation around the mean. The mode, median and mean coincide in a normal distribution. When data follows a normal distribution it is often termed parametric. A z-score is useful for comparing normal distributions.
- Non-normally distributed data should be analysed with non-parametric tests.

Inferential statistics – which test to use and when

- A one-sample t-test is useful to test a sample mean against a known population mean for parametric, normally distributed data (degrees of freedom [n–1] determine the t-distribution used).
- A Wilcoxon rank sum test is useful to test a sample median against a population mean for non-parametric data.

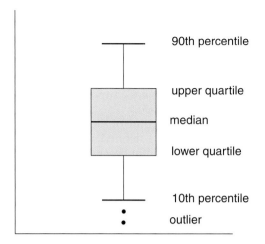

FIGURE 9.1 Box and whisker plot
Source: Myles P, Gin T. Statistical Methods for Anaesthesia and Intensive Care. Butterworth-Heinemann; 2000, Fig 2.4, p. 17.

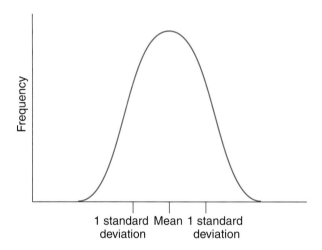

FIGURE 9.2 Normal distribution curve
Source: Myles P, Gin T. Statistical Methods for Anaesthesia and Intensive Care. Butterworth-Heinemann; 2000, Fig 2.3, p.13.

- A student's unpaired two sample t-test is used when two sample means are tested against each other to look for a difference. An equation and tables are then required to determine if a confidence interval exists, such that there is a significant difference between the means of the two groups. If the comparison is done for multiple groups the Bonferroni correction should be made, accounting for the number to prevent a chance result ($p < 0.05/n$).
- The Mann-Whitney U-test is used for non-parametric data when two sample medians are tested against each other.
- A student's paired two sample t-test is used when one sample acts as its own control and two interventions are assessed for significance on the one sample.
- A Wilcoxon matched pairs test is the equivalent for non-parametric data.

- ANOVA (analysis of variance) is similar to the paired t-test but can be used for two or more groups.
- Kruskall-Wallis is the test for non-normally distributed data with more than two groups.
- Fisher exact test and chi-squared tests are used for qualitative categorical data that is grouped. These compare two samples' proportions if the data is unpaired. If the data is paired a McNemar's test is used.
- Risk ratio is used to quantify the degree of significance of an association that has been found. In a clinical sense it is defined as the proportion of people with a known outcome exposed to a risk factor compared to the proportion of people not exposed to that factor. Accordingly, if the result is <1 there is less risk, >1 more risk of the outcome and if = 1 there is no association of risk.
- The odds ratio is appropriate with a retrospective study where the outcome is rare and the occurrence of the event is not known. It is an estimate of the risk ratio. Risk is overestimated with the odds ratio if the outcome is common, hence it is used when looking into uncommon events.
  The odds ratio and risk ratio can be used for prospective studies.
  Their calculation can be placed in a contingency table:

	Outcome 1	Outcome 2
Group 1	A	B
Group 2	C	D

$$\text{Relative risk ratio} = [A/\{A+B\}]/[C/\{C+D\}]$$
$$\text{Odds ratio} = \{A \times D\}/\{B \times C\}$$
$$\text{Odds ratio} \approx \text{Risk ratio if A and C are low}$$

The ratios are often described in context with their (CI) confidence intervals, such as 0.75 (95% CI, 0.65–0.90) at $p < 0.05$. This suggests the risk factor is statistically significant (CI < 1) and there is a $(1-0.75) \times 100\%$ reduction of risk.

If a significant risk is calculated for an intervention this should be put into the overall context of risk according to how frequently the event occurs. Absolute risk is the difference between the groups' outcome and is calculated using the relative risk (25%) in the example of the difference in the groups (e.g. 16% incidence is reduced to 12%). This gives the number needed to treat (NNT) of 25 (the reciprocal of 4% 1/0.04). This is the number of people who would need to receive the given therapy to see the desired treatment effect in one patient.

Trials

Results of trials are published with information such as the 'p value' (the exact value should be quoted), the power of the study (which should be determined when designing the study) and the errors (Type I and Type II).

The result of statistical significance must be related to clinical significance (clinical significance should be pre-determined).

Confidence intervals will reveal four conclusions:
- statistical and clinical significance
- clinical but not statistical difference
- inconclusive (more data required)
- no clinically or statistically significant difference.

With small numbers of data or non-normally distributed data, a non-parametric test should be used. Larger number of subjects should increase the power of the study. This also reduces the effect of different variables (which may influence outcome on their own such as age) in the study.

The null hypothesis is the assumption that there is no real difference in the population between control and intervention and the trial sets out to disprove this.

Type I error (α) occurs when the null hypothesis is incorrectly rejected (a difference is detected in the sample but is not true of the population). The lower the p value, the less likely this will occur.

Type II error (β) occurs when the null hypothesis is accepted in the sample but a real difference exists in the population. The cause of this event is usually due to small sample numbers, hence power (which is denoted by $(1-\beta) \times 100\%$).

Factors involved in study design

The following factors need to be considered in developing a study design:
- Select and study a subject (including a review of the literature for previous related investigations).
- Generate a hypothesis and hence a null hypothesis.
- Obtain ethics approval.
- Prospective versus retrospective study design.
- Randomisation (if prospective).
- Adequate power – sample size and avoidance of statistical errors.
- Selection or participation bias.
- Blinding (single, double and investigator).
- Single versus multi-centre.

Meta-analysis

Use of multiple studies can be displayed on a forest plot (Fig 9.3) where log odds ratio (or relative risk) is on the X-axis and the Y-axis is a line where no effect on outcome occurs. If the confidence intervals (denoted by horizontal lines) cross the

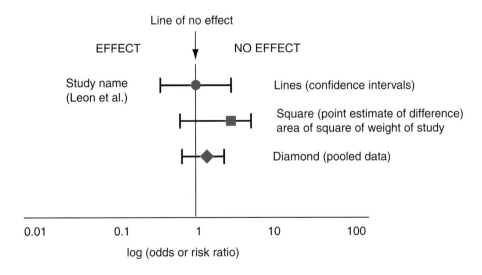

FIGURE 9.3 Forest plot
Source: Myles P, Gin T. Statistical Methods for Anaesthesia and Intensive Care. Butterworth-Heinemann; 2000, Fig 10.1, p. 115.

Y-axis there is no effect. Sizes of boxes on the lines reflect weighting given to that study (by sample size). A diamond reflects data that is pooled together.

I^2 is an important measure of heterogeneity between the results of included studies. If I^2 is more than 50%, and particularly if more than 75%, this suggests that the studies have significant inconsistency. It can also be used to determine heterogeneity in subgroup analyses between studies.

Diagnostic tests

There are various ways of analysing the data and displaying the results. Figure 9.4 shows a 2 × 2 table.

The following definitions are essential and often tested in the exams:
- sensitivity: the ability of a test to predict those with a condition having that condition. True positives/true positives + false negatives
- specificity: the ability of a test to predict those without a condition who do not have the condition. True negatives/true negatives + false positives
- negative predictive value (NPV): the likelihood of no condition with a negative test. True negatives/true negatives + false negatives
- positive predictive value (PPV): the likelihood of having the condition with a positive test. True positives/true positives + false positives.

NPV and PPV are dependent on how common the condition is in the population.

Receiver operator characteristic (ROC) curves are graphs of sensitivity on the Y-axis versus (1-specificity) on the X-axis (Fig 9.5). These provide a graphical representation of the balance between sensitivity and specificity of the test and account for the arbitrary cut-off levels made for the test. A gradient of 1 gives an ROC area under the curve of 0.5, which suggests the test has no predictive ability. A left-shifted line increases the ROC area and PPV of the test.

Gold standard test

		Positive	Negative	
Test outcome	Positive	True positive	False positive (Type 1 error)	**Positive predictive value**
	Negative	False negative (Type 2 error)	True negative	**Negative predictive value**
		Sensitivity	**Specificity**	

FIGURE 9.4 2 × 2 table for diagnostic test results
Source: Myles P, Gin T. Statistical Methods for Anaesthesia and Intensive Care. Butterworth-Heinemann; 2000, Fig 8.1, p. 95.

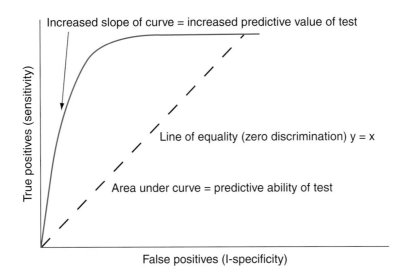

FIGURE 9.5 **A receiver operator characteristic (ROC) curve**
Source: Myles P, Gin T. Statistical Methods for Anaesthesia and Intensive Care.
Butterworth-Heinemann; 2000, Fig 8.4, p. 98.

Looking at papers

Most medical papers report initial research and have an order of importance related
to their findings:

- Randomised controlled trials look at the effect of an intervention on two equivalent
  groups (e.g. protective lung strategy versus traditional ventilation). These studies
  attempt to eliminate all possible sources of bias (selection, performance, exclusion
  and detection).
- Cohort studies involve the follow-up of two or more groups to determine if an
  event (drug, exposure to an agent) leads to differences in the subjects (e.g. smokers
  versus non-smokers). Eliminating differences between the two groups is the
  challenge with these studies when selecting participants.
- Case–control studies take a retrospective look at previous possible events (e.g.
  a drug, exposure to an agent) leading to an effect. The timing of the event
  determines which group the participant falls into (case versus control) and can
  change results.
- Surveys answer specific questions at a point in time (e.g. Does simulation improve
  crisis management?).
- Case reports involve single or small groups of patients with a condition (which
  may reveal an unusual effect of drug).

It is important that candidates are aware of the distinction between superiority
(historically, drug versus placebo trials) – where there is no known effective agent for
a condition – and non-inferiority trials, where a new drug is trialled against a known
effective agent (active control).

References

Continuing Education in Anaesthesia Critical Care and Pain Statistics I–V. British Journal of Anaesthesia 2007–08.

Greenhaigh T. How to read a paper. Papers that summarise other papers (systematic reviews and meta-analyses). BMJ 1997; 315: 672.

Guyatt G, et al. Basic statistics for clinicians I–IV. Canadian Medical Association Journal 1995; 152(4): 487–504.

Higgins J, Thompson S, Deeks J. Measuring inconsistency in meta-analyses. BMJ 2003; 327(7414): 557–60.

Myles P, Gin T. Statistical Methods for Anaesthesia and Intensive Care. Butterworth Heinemann; 2000.

Chapter 10

Paediatric intensive care

Children seldom misquote. In fact, they usually repeat exactly what you shouldn't have said.

AUTHOR UNKNOWN

Introduction

As a critical care physician working in a general ICU, you will require an adequate level of knowledge and skills to manage critically ill children who may need to be resuscitated and managed for a limited period of time before being transferred to a paediatric or neonatal unit. In addition to specific paediatric problems, familiarity with the paediatric management of conditions common to children and adults (e.g. acute severe asthma, acute kidney injury and trauma) is mandatory.

In both the EDIC and UK DICM paediatrics is not examined formally, but some knowledge is required and many intensivists working in smaller institutions may be called upon to help with the initial resuscitation and stabilisation of children.

In the FCICM exam candidates should be prepared to demonstrate that they can recognise acute problems and be able to resuscitate paediatric patients with life-threatening conditions, institute appropriate intensive care management, and, when required, prepare for transport to a paediatric or neonatal intensive care unit.

Box 10.1 sets out the contents of this chapter and, although the chapter focuses on Australian exam requirements, it provides an invaluable resource for all adult intensivists who may be involved in the management of sick children during their careers. Table 10.1, key paediatric facts, has combined all the useful equations and summarises important differences in children.

BOX 10.1 Contents of Chapter 10

Key paediatric facts
The paediatric component of the FCICM
Training in paediatric intensive care medicine in Australasia
    Training requirements
    Strategies for success
    Blueprint for the Paediatric Intensive Care Fellowship examination
The clinical component of the FCICM

Continued

BOX 10.1 Contents of Chapter 10—cont'd

Clinical cases
  1. Is this child suitable for extubation?
  2. The post-cardiac surgical paediatric case
  3. The child on extracorporeal life support (ECLS)
  4. The child post-transplant
  5. The child with a head injury
  6. The child with an acute kidney injury
Paediatric critical care literature
  Brain death and organ donation
  Burns
  Cardiovascular medicine
  Endocrine
  Fluids and electrolytes
  Haematology
  Neurology
  Nutrition
  Renal medicine
  Respiratory medicine
  Resuscitation
  Sedation and analgesia
  Sepsis

Key paediatric facts

TABLE 10.1 Key paediatric facts

Topic	Key fact
Weight	(Age + 4) × 2
	(2× age in yrs) + 8
	(formulas apply from 1 to 10 yrs)
	e.g. term neonate = 3.5–4 kg; 6 months = 6 kg; 1 yr = 10 kg
Airway differences	Narrowest part of airway is at cricoid cartilage
	Relatively large tongue and floppy epiglottis
	Anterior larynx at a higher level
	Large head
	Short trachea
	Obligate nose breathers
Endotracheal tubes	Size: Age (in yrs)/4 + 4
	Note term neonate = 3.5
	Type: Uncuffed generally previously used until >8 yrs (cuffed now acceptable at all ages)
	Insertion depth: oral = (age/2) + 12 cm
	nasal = (age/2) + 15 cm
	(applies from 1 to 10 yrs)

Continued

TABLE 10.1 Key paediatric facts—cont'd

Topic	Key fact
Intubation	Head in neutral position
	Prepare atropine (20 mcg/kg)
	Straight blade laryngoscope <2 yrs
	FRC smaller, so ventilate in 100% FiO_2 longer than in adult
	Consider orogastric tube, as easy to overinflate stomach
	Two-person technique to bag and use a Guedal airway
	Suction catheters 8 Fr <1 yr, 10 Fr >1 yr
Circulation	Blood volume is 80 mL/kg
	Cardiac output is HR-dependent in neonates
	Stroke volume is fixed due to less compliant left ventricle
	Assessment includes central capillary refill time (<2 sec) or core-peripheral temperature difference (<2°)
	Palpation of anterior fontanel (up to 1 yr) can aid assessment of fluid status
	Systolic BP: 80 + (age in yrs × 2)
Fluids	If intravenous access cannot be established quickly an intraosseous needle should be inserted.
	Resuscitation: 20 mL/kg 0.9% saline as rapid bolus (can be repeated twice) before considering packed cells at 10–20 mL/kg
	Deficit: % dehydration × wt × 10. This is then given over 24 hrs guided by serum sodium (48 hrs in DKA)
	Maintenance: based on 4, 2, 1 rule
	4 mL/kg/hr for first 10 kg of child's wt
	2 mL/kg/hr for next 10 kg of child's wt
	1 mL/kg/hr for every kg of child's wt up to 60 kg (100 mL/hr)
	Or daily rule of:
	0–10 kg 100 mL/kg/24 hrs
	10–20 kg 1000 mL + (50 mL/kg for each kg >10 kg)/24 hrs
	20 kg + 1500 mL + (20 mL/kg for each kg >20 kg)/24 hrs
	Safest fluid is 0.9% saline with 5% glucose, and 20 mmol/L potassium chloride (to avoid iatrogenic hyponatraemia)
	Urine output 1–2 mL/kg

Continued

TABLE 10.1 Key paediatric facts—cont'd	
Topic	**Key fact**
Resuscitation	Over 50% of arrests are respiratory
	Asystole most common rhythm usually due to hypoxia
	VF seen in poisoning and congenital heart disease
	Compressions in centre of sternum
	• <1 yr use hand encircling technique or 2 fingers
	• >1 yr use heel of 1 hand
	100 bpm with compression to ventilation ratio of 30:2 (one rescuer) or 15:2 (two rescuers)
	For VF/pulseless VT 4 J/kg for all shocks
	Adrenaline 10 mcg/kg as per ARC algorithms
Drugs	Weight-based until 40 kg
	Common drugs:
	• Amiodarone 5 mg/kg IV
	• Cefotaxime/ceftriaxone 30–50 mg/kg IV
	• Diazepam 0.2 mg/kg IV bolus
	• Fentanyl 1–5 mcg/kg IV bolus
	• Hydrocortisone 4 mg/kg IV bolus
	• Magnesium sulfate 0.2 mmol/kg IV
	• Midazolam 0.1 mg/kg IV bolus
	• Morphine 0.1 mg/kg IV bolus
	• Phenytoin 18 mg/kg IV loading dose
	• Propofol 2–5 mg/kg IV bolus
	• Sodium bicarbonate 1 mg/kg of 8.4%
	• Suxamethonium 1–2 mg/kg IV bolus
	• Thiopentone 2–5 mg/kg IV bolus
Approach to the sick child A: Airway & C spine B: Breathing C: Circulation D: Disability (AVPU) E: Exposure	Look, listen and feel
	Respiratory rate, effort and air entry
	Heart rate, pallor, capillary refill, BP
	Alert/responds to voice/pain/unresponsive
	Don't forget the glucose and temperature (heater)
Never forget	The glucose (children should be 'wet, pink and sweet'), give
	5 mL/kg 10% dextrose (for suspected or measured hypoglycaemia)
	Non-accidental injury
	Parental history and concerns

The paediatric component of the FCICM

There are usually one or two questions in the written section of the Fellowship examination with a paediatric focus. In addition, it is possible to encounter a paediatric-based scenario or procedure in the viva component of the examination, e.g. a procedure station requiring knowledge of the paediatric cardiac arrest algorithms. This can equate to 6–7% of the total marks of the whole examination. Examiners usually select cases and problems with relevance to the adult intensivist working in a mixed or rural ICU.

It is essential to have knowledge of the relevant anatomical, physiological, pharmacological and psychological differences between neonates, infants, small children and adults (Table 10.1). Some basic knowledge is also required of major neonatal conditions, such as congenital heart disease, persistent pulmonary hypertension, acute and chronic neonatal lung disease, tracheo-oesophageal fistula, diaphragmatic hernia, gastroschisis/exomphalos and necrotising enterocolitis. This may be assessed in the context of a scenario where the intensivist is called upon to assist in resuscitation and stabilisation of a newborn being delivered at or presenting to their hospital with one of these conditions.

To help prepare for the paediatric questions in the Adult ICU Fellowship examination, candidates should:

- be aware of the admission characteristics of paediatric admissions to general ICUs in Australia and New Zealand. The majority (40%) of children are referred from the emergency department with the most common diagnoses of bronchiolitis, seizures, asthma, croup, head trauma, pneumonia or pneumonitis, diabetic ketoacidosis and septic shock.
- complete an Advanced Paediatric Life Support (APLS) provider course or at least study the relevant sections of the APLS Manual.
- prepare model answers to previous short answer questions in both general and paediatric Fellowship examinations and study the abovementioned topics.
- gain clinical experience in a paediatric intensive care unit. Any time spent working in a CICM-accredited PICU can be credited towards ICU training for the general FCICM.

Training in paediatric intensive care medicine in Australasia

Training requirements

The requirements for endorsement in paediatric intensive care of the Fellowship of the CICM of Australian and New Zealand can be found on the college website: www.cicm.org.au/cmsfiles/Regulations.pdf (see Section 5.5.5 (e)). The requirements are identical to those of the General ICU Fellowship, except that the PICU trainee must complete 18 months of core training in a College-recognised PICU and must also complete a 12-month Paediatric Medicine rotation.

The candidate must successfully complete four supervised clinical examinations ('hot cases') of children in intensive care prior to registering for the final examination.

The structure of the examination for the endorsement in paediatric intensive care is identical to that of the general Fellowship examination: two written papers; each with 15 short answer questions (duration 150 minutes). Candidates who achieve a pass mark in the written examination will be invited to attend the clinical component of the examination. The clinical component of the examination consists of two 'hot cases' in PICU (20 minutes each) and eight, 10-minute structured vivas, including a 'communication' and a 'procedure' station.

The *Objectives of Training for Paediatric Intensive Care* can be found on the college website, and these essentially represent the curriculum. Candidates can expect to be examined on any of this material with an emphasis on conditions commonly encountered in a tertiary level PICU.

Strategies for success

This chapter provides a brief outline of the topics that can be assessed in the written examination, during the oral vivas or at the bedside during the clinical examination. Examples of some typical PICU hot cases are given with a suggested systematic approach to the clinical examination of these children.

'Hot cases' are selected from available children in the PICU on the day of the examination and candidates are usually asked to examine the child, with emphasis on a particular system or problem. Candidates would be well advised to consider the usual profile of children in a tertiary PICU in Australia and New Zealand and focus their examination preparation accordingly. A significant proportion of all admissions to PICUs in Australia and New Zealand are for postoperative management of children with congenital cardiac disease. The majority of non-elective admissions to a PICU are for diagnoses of bronchiolitis, seizures, asthma, head trauma, respiratory failure, pneumonia or pneumonitis, diabetic ketoacidosis, septic shock, upper airway obstruction (e.g. croup) and central apnoea. Two-thirds of the children are aged less than 5 years of age, with infants under 12 months of age making up more than half this group (approximately one-third of all PICU admissions).

Examination candidates are assessed on their ability to problem solve and think like a consultant in paediatric intensive care. Accordingly, candidates should be able to support their arguments with evidence from relevant literature. A section summarising some of the most useful papers pertaining to the speciality is therefore included.

It should be appreciated that much of adult critical care practice can be extrapolated to the management of critically ill children with some adjustments for relevant change in size and physiology. Candidates should therefore not limit their attention only to this chapter on the paediatric examination, but will benefit from much of the content of the chapters on the practice of adult intensive care medicine. In particular, Chapter 2 provides many useful tips on how to optimise performance in exams.

Blueprint for the PIC Fellowship examination

In an attempt to 'sample' from the entire curriculum, short answer and viva questions are based on a blueprint of the curriculum prepared by the examiners, an example of which is provided in Table 10.2. Candidates are advised to cover all of these topics or themes. Candidates should develop and rehearse a structured approach to possible viva questions. Similarly, it is crucial to develop a structured approach to communication, with rehearsal of typical conversations likely to be encountered in the communications station. Paediatric advanced life support algorithms should be practised in a simulated environment. It is evident on studying this table that significant amounts of this material are addressed in the preceding chapters of this book.

TABLE 10.2 Blueprint for the Paediatric Intensive Care Fellowship examination

System	Basic science	Pathophysiology	Clinical applications	Equipment and procedures
Cardiac	Physiology • Cardiac output • Changes in circulation at birth • Normal ECG • Correlation with pressure waves	Low cardiac output state Arrhythmias • SVT • JET	Postoperative management • Congenital heart disease • Arterial switch • Tetralogy of Fallot • Duct-dependent lesions • Pulmonary hypertension	Measurement • Direct and indirect blood pressure • Cardiac output • Central venous pressure Vascular access • Central venous access • Peripherally inserted central venous lines • Intra-arterial lines • Intraosseous needle insertion • Venous cutdown
		DiGeorge syndrome	Postoperative complications • Heart block • Chylothorax • Diaphragm palsy • Cardiac tamponade	Pericardiocentesis Pacemakers Defibrillation
	Pharmacology of vasoactive drugs: • Dopamine • Dobutamine • Adrenaline • Noradrenaline • Vasopressin • Phenylephrine • Phenoxybenzamine • Milrinone • Levosimendan • Nitric oxide • Amiodarone	ECG changes due to electrolyte abnormalities and temperature	Algorithms • Asystole • PVT • VF • PEA • SVT	
		Single ventricle physiology – balanced circulation	Cardiomyopathy Myocarditis Bacterial endocarditis	ECLS • ECMO • VAD
			Clinical dilemmas Tetralogy of Fallot Shunt vs early correction	ICU design – cardiac protection

Continued

TABLE 10.2 Blueprint for the Paediatric Intensive Care Fellowship examination—cont'd

System	Basic science	Pathophysiology	Clinical applications	Equipment and procedures
Respiratory	Physiology • Oxygen – haemoglobin dissociation curve • Acid–base physiology • Alveolar gas equation • Oxygen cascade • Cardiopulmonary interactions Gas laws and physical properties of gases Anatomy of bronchial tree and lungs Upper airway anatomy Difference between child and adult airway Pharmacology • Salbutamol • Atrovent • Corticosteroids	Respiratory failure V/Q mismatch Shunt (A–a) O_2 gradient Methaemoglobinaemia Acid–base disorders Ventilator-induced lung injury Barotrauma Volutrauma Congenital abnormalities Airway haemangioma Congenital cystic adenomatoid malformation Congenital lobar emphysema Chylothorax Congenital diaphragmatic hernia Gastroschisis Omphalocoele Mediastinal and thoracic tumours Jeune's thoracic dystrophy	Status asthmaticus ARDS Fat embolism Laryngotracheobronchitis (croup) Epiglottitis Bacterial tracheitis Bronchiolitis Pneumonia Pertussis Empyema management Tracheomalacia Tracheal stenosis	Oxygen therapy and delivery devices Humidification O_2 electrode CO_2 electrode Pulse oximeter Co-oximeter Capnography Oxygen analysers Flowmeters Intubation Difficult airway Cricothyroidotomy Fibre-optic laryngoscopy Bronchoscopy Bronchoalveolar lavage Mechanical ventilation Non-invasive ventilation High-frequency oscillatory ventilation Heliox High-flow nasal prong oxygen Bubble CPAP Tracheostomy V V ECMO Indications for extubation Management of failed extubation

Continued

TABLE 10.2 Blueprint for the Paediatric Intensive Care Fellowship examination—cont'd

System	Basic science	Pathophysiology	Clinical applications	Equipment and procedures
Metabolic Gastrointestinal nutrition	Physiology of swallowing	Inborn errors of metabolism Glycogen storage diseases	Management of oesophageal reflux in ICU	Management of Sengstaken-Blakemore tubes
	Energy expenditure	Refeeding syndrome Overfeeding	Pseudomembranous colitis Necrotising enterocolitis	Immunonutrition parenteral and enteral nutrition
	Liver physiology	Liver failure	Postoperative management of liver transplantation	Liver support
		Congenital gut malformations Bowel obstruction	Intra-abdominal sepsis Short gut syndromes Abdominal compartment syndrome	Bladder pressure monitoring
Neurology		Cerebral oedema Cerebral neoplasms Botulinism Tetanus Cerebral palsy Arnold-Chiari malformation	Critical illness neuropathy and myopathy Myasthenia gravis Motor neuron disease Duchenne's muscular dystrophy Spinal muscular atrophy Paraplegia Quadriplegia Peripheral and central demyelinating syndromes	Lumbar puncture – indications and risks
	Normal EEG ICP waves		Status epilepticus Intracranial haemorrhage Meningitis	Near infrared spectroscopy (NIRS)

Continued

TABLE 10.2 Blueprint for the Paediatric Intensive Care Fellowship examination—cont'd

System	Basic science	Pathophysiology	Clinical applications	Equipment and procedures
Renal fluids electrolytes	Physiology of solute transport and ultrafiltration	Renal failure Pre-renal failure Acute tubular necrosis Rhabdomyolysis	Haemolytic uraemic syndrome Nephrotic syndrome Management of renal transplant	Renal replacement therapies Peritoneal dialysis Insertion of Tenckhoff catheter CVVH(D)F Haemodialysis Insertion of dialysis catheter
	Albumin vs saline	Hyper/hyponatraemia		RRT – complications
Haematology oncology immunology	Coagulation Platelet function	Coagulation disorders Factor deficiency Platelet abnormalities	Transfusion reactions	Transfusion guidelines Thromboelastography (TEG)
	Pharmacology • Heparin • Warfarin • Tranexamic Acid • Factor VIIa	Toxic epidermal necrolysis Stevens-Johnson syndrome Anaphylaxis Allergic reactions	Febrile neutropenia – antibiotic choice Post BMT sepsis	Plasmapheresis
		Tumour lysis syndrome	Solid tumours	
	Physiology of immunity	Immunodeficient states		
Endocrine	Thyroid function	Hypo/hyperthyroidism	Sick euthyroid	
	Adrenal function		Adrenal insufficiency	
	Glucose metabolism		Diabetic ketoacidosis	

Continued

TABLE 10.2 Blueprint for the Paediatric Intensive Care Fellowship examination—cont'd

System	Basic science	Pathophysiology	Clinical applications	Equipment and procedures
Trauma Burns Poisoning Envenomation	Physiology Cerebral blood flow	Diabetes insipidus Cerebral salt wasting Inappropriate ADH secretion	Head and cervical spine trauma How to clear the C spine ICP management Management of organ donor	ICP monitoring Cooling mats Diagnosis of brain death
	Pharmacology • Tricyclic antidepressants • Valproic acid • Quinine • Beta-blockers	Burns Smoke inhalation Pathophysiology of shock	Chest trauma Abdominal trauma Conservative management of splenic trauma Drowning	Underwater sealed chest tube drainage
		Toxidromes	Management of poisoning • Organophosphates • Iron • Paracetamol	
			Envenomation • Snake bite • Spider bite • Blue-ringed octopus	Snake venom detection kit
Infectious diseases	Pharmacology Ceftriaxone Gentamicin Meropenem	Sepsis Septic shock SIRS	Purpura fulminans Meningococcal disease Tuberculosis	Universal precautions Infection control procedures Sepsis bundles Goal-directed therapy of septic shock
		Vancomycin-resistant enterococcus Healthcare-related acquired infections	Handwashing	

Continued

TABLE 10.2 Blueprint for the Paediatric Intensive Care Fellowship examination—cont'd

System	Basic science	Pathophysiology	Clinical applications	Equipment and procedures
Transport	Pressure effects of flight			Hyperbaric oxygen therapy
Anaesthesia and pain management	Pain physiology	Post-anesthesia apnoea in preterm infants	Malignant hyperthermia Propofol infusion syndrome	Patient-controlled analgesia (PCA) Patient-controlled epidural analgesia (PCEA)
	Pharmacology • Opiates – morphine fentanyl, methadone • Benzodiazepines – midazolam • Ketamine • Dexmedetomidine	Withdrawal symptoms		
Research Ethics Medical law	Statistical tests • Chi squared • Fisher's exact test • Logistic regression • Parametric and non-parametric tests Bias and confounding	Standardised mortality ratio (SMR)	Meta-analysis	Blood transfusion in Jehovah Witness child Scoring systems • PRISM • PIM 2
	Pharmacogenetics		Communication Managing adverse outcomes Withdrawal or limitation of interventions Request for organ donation Disclosure of error	Brain death testing

The clinical component of the FCICM

Candidates should be aware that 30% of the total marks for the Fellowship examination are allocated to the hot cases component of the examination. Sufficient time and effort should be invested in preparing for this. Candidates will be asked to examine a child in the PICU and to address a particular diagnostic or management issue. Approximately 10 minutes should be allocated to the actual examination of the patient and a further 10 minutes will be occupied summarising the clinical findings and discussing the relevant management issues. Candidates should adopt a systematic approach to their examination of the child in intensive care, similar to the structured approach for the clinical cases in the general Fellowship examination outlined in Chapter 8 of this book. Specific examples are provided of commonly encountered paediatric cases.

Clinical cases

1. Is this child suitable for extubation?

Common cases
- The child intubated for severe croup
- The child ventilated for severe pneumonia.

Appropriate thoughts
Establish that the child meets the criteria for successful weaning from ventilation, including:
- resolution of the pathology necessitating intubation
- the child is awake with intact airway reflexes
- ensuring adequate inspiratory effort
- adequate oxygenation in FiO_2 <40%
- minimal secretions
- evidence of leak around tube with sustained inflation pressure >30 cmH$_2$O (not an absolute requirement).

On examination
- Consider syndromes with associated craniofacial abnormalities with potential for a difficult airway (e.g. Goldenhar, Treacher Collins, Pierre Robin).
- Look for macroglossia associated with Beckwith-Wiedemann syndrome and trisomy 21.
- Look for cutaneous manifestations of haemangiomas or cystic hygroma.
- Assess the size of the endotracheal tube and ascertain whether it is cuffed or uncuffed.
- Deflate the cuff and assess for presence of a leak around the tube with sustained inflation pressure >30 mmHg.
- Assess the child's nutritional state.
- Assess neurological function.

Useful questions
- 'What was the Mallampati score on intubation?'
- 'How long has the child been intubated?'
- 'Have there been any failed extubation attempts? If so, why did the child fail?'

- 'Has the child received steroids?'
- 'Is the child still being fed? If not, for how long have they been fasted?'

Considerations
- Time of day – preference for extubating in morning
- Experienced personnel present capable of reintubating if the extubation fails
- No planned procedures.

Useful statements
'I would be cautious about extubating this child because of the following: The child is still requiring moderate ventilatory support. The child's nutritional state is poor and he looks fatigued. There is no air leak around the tube on testing and although this is not an absolute requirement, I am concerned because airway oedema may still be present …'

Topics for discussion
- Management of post-extubation stridor
- Long-term plan if child fails extubation
- Role of cricoid split in child with endotracheal tube-related subglottic stenosis
- Physical properties of heliox and its use in post-extubation airway obstructions
- Role of steroids to reduce incidence of failed extubation
- When to involve ENT surgeons
- Timing of and risks associated with tracheostomy.

2. The post-cardiac surgical paediatric case

Common cases
- Children with an uncomplicated ICU course following surgery for more complex congenital cardiac conditions, such as atrioventricular septal defect (AVSD), tetralogy of Fallot, transposition of the great vessels (TGA) or total anomalous pulmonary venous return (TAPVR).
- Children with congenital cardiac conditions not suitable for total correction undergoing palliation (e.g. hypoplastic left heart syndromes undergoing Norwood procedure, cavopulmonary shunts).
- Children requiring urgent procedures following patent ductus arteriosus closure (e.g. repair of neonatal coarctation, systemic–pulmonary shunt or re-implantation of coronary arteries in babies with anomalous coronary arteries).
- Children with complications of elective cardiac surgical procedures requiring intervention (e.g. bleeding, chylothorax or phrenic nerve palsy).

Appropriate thoughts
- Ascertain indication for surgery (e.g. duct closure, cyanotic tetralogy of Fallot, heart failure, etc).
- Determine if the postoperative course has been routine or complicated; look for evidence of complications (e.g. chyle in chest drains, elevated hemidiaphragm on chest X-ray).
- Look for evidence of low cardiac output state.

On examination
The cubicle
Multiple staff members caring for the complex child (may include nurses, medical, surgical and perfusionist).

Infusions
- Vasoactive drugs
- Blood products – packed cells, fresh frozen plasma, platelets for the management of deranged coagulation causing excessive postoperative bleeding
- Sedation and analgesia, including adjuncts such as dexmedetomidine, suggesting a patient who is difficult to sedate
- Muscle relaxant infusions, suggesting the child is critically unwell
- Maintenance fluids/glucose infusions
- Peritoneal dialysis fluid and urine/PD drainage.

Ventilation
- FiO_2, PIP, PEEP, MAP and respiratory rate; if settings outside expected normal, consider reasons
- Nitric oxide in use suggests pulmonary hypertension/right ventricular failure.

The monitor
- ECG – heart rate, rhythm, regularity, pacing spikes, obvious conduction defects
- SpO_2 – measured pre-/post-ductal
- If SpO_2 is low it suggests either right to left shunt in biventricular heart or univentricular heart
- Arterial line trace – blood pressure (BP), respiratory swing
- Invasive arterial BP; compare to non-invasive, especially post-coarctation repair
- CVP trace – note value and character, evaluate for A, C and V waves
- Near-infrared-spectroscopy (NIRS) monitor for cerebral saturations and/or renal parenchymal saturations
- Direct RA/LA line trace – value and relationship to CVP, especially in single ventricle anatomy
- Temperature – core temperature vs skin temperature.

Equipment
- Indwelling urinary catheter
- Central venous lines
- Continuous O_2 saturation catheter
- Number and position of pacing wires
- Pacemaker settings – pacing mode, rate, output (mV) and sensitivity (mA)
- Surgical drains – check patency and note the nature and amount of losses and check for presence of an air leak
- Other drains: pleural drains – note swinging, draining and bubbling with the respiratory cycle. Check if drains are under suction and occlude suction to look for air leak.
- Peritoneal dialysis (Tenckhoff) catheter/vascular catheter – suggestive of acute kidney injury
- Cooling mattress – suggests patient being cooled for management of arrhythmia (e.g. JET)
- ECMO – pump, arterial and venous catheters, inlet/outlet pressure, oxygenator flow settings/FiO_2/sweep gas flow
- EEG – suggestive of perioperative or postoperative seizures
- Train of four (TOF) measurement – muscle relaxant infusion suggests unstable patient.

The child
- Note any dysmorphic features (e.g. trisomy 21, Noonan syndrome, Williams syndrome, Marfan syndrome, Alagille syndrome).
- Note abnormal facies – velocardiofacial syndromes.

- Assess general growth parameters, looking for failure to thrive or short stature.
- Extremities – looking for finger or toe clubbing and splinter haemorrhages.
- Look for dependent pitting oedema and assess for general oedema, e.g. chest wall.
- Check the child's temperature centrally/peripherally.
- Is the fontanel tense/sunken?
- Check for ptosis and unequal pupils – suggestive of Horner's syndrome.
- Check conjunctiva for pallor and sclera for icterus (haemolysis associated with artificial valves).
- Examine the tongue and gums for cyanosis.
- Check teeth for caries as a possible risk for bacterial endocarditis.
- Check the location of any surgical incisions and drains.
- Check wounds for signs of infection.
- Sternum – open or closed; skin – open or closed?
- Check pulse character (radial, brachial and femoral) rate, volume, character – differences upper/lower limbs.
- Check skin colour and temperature gradients; capillary refill time.
- Palpate for heaves, thrills and locate point of maximal apical impulse.
- Auscultate over apex with diaphragm and bell of stethoscope, then up the parasternal border and over the pulmonary and aortic areas.
- Note intensity of S1 and S2, and whether S2 splits normally with respiration.
- Listen for added sounds and systolic and diastolic murmurs.
- Note radiation to axillae or carotids.
- Check respiratory rate.
- Assess chest movement on respiration – looking for any asymmetry or increased work of breathing (intercostal or subcostal recession); asymmetry may suggest paralysed hemidiaphragm.
- Auscultate and percuss, checking for unequal air entry and abnormal sounds.
- Seek permission to either sit patient up or, if ventilated, to roll patient in order to examine the chest posteriorly.
- Abdomen – palpate liver edge and assess volume responsiveness with liver compression.
- Check liver for pulsatility.
- Look for splenomegaly.
- Examine abdomen for ascites.

Useful questions
- 'Could I please see details of surgery and the underlying condition?'
- 'What was the duration of the cardiac bypass and cross-clamping?'
- 'Were there any problems related to coming off bypass? (e.g. arrhythmias or bleeding)
- Could I please check drain losses post-surgery?'
- 'Could I please check the position of the surgical drains?' (e.g. mediastinal, pleural, pericardial)
- 'Could I please see a recent chest radiograph?' – to check position of ETT, all central venous lines, wires and drains and to exclude other cardiac or respiratory pathology
- 'Could I please see an abdominal radiograph?' – if umbilical lines in place
- 'Could I please review a recent 12-lead ECG?' (or atrial ECG)
- 'What are the recent echocardiography findings?'
- If rhythm is paced: 'When were the sensitivity and pacing thresholds last checked?' If fully paced: 'What has the underlying rhythm and rate been?'

Useful statements

'Thirty-six hours after total correction of tetralogy of Fallot, this 10-month-old child appears to be progressing well. She is haemodynamically stable on dopamine 5 mcg/kg/min and milrinone 0.25 mcg/kg/min. She is in sinus rhythm, not requiring pacing and has warm peripheries and an adequate urine output. Her CVP is 8 cmH$_2$O and her liver edge is 1 cm below her costal margin, suggesting that there is no right ventricular diastolic dysfunction. There are no murmurs suggestive of pulmonary regurgitation. She is receiving minimal ventilatory support and is awake and comfortable on morphine 20 mcg/kg/hr. Her chest drain loss has been minimal over the last 12 hours. My plan would be to remove the pacing wires and then the chest drains after consultation with the cardiac surgeons and then proceed to extubation ...'

'This 14-day-old baby, 24 hours post switch procedure, has the following signs of low cardiac output state ...'

'I suspect that this 7-day-old baby, who remains ventilated four days after an aortic coarctation repair, has a paralysed right hemidiaphragm because ...'

Topics for discussion
- Management of post-cardiac surgical bleeding (e.g. role of activated factor VIIa)
- Causes and management of low cardiac output state
- Management of junctional ectopic tachycardia and other arrhythmias post-cardiac surgery
- Management of chylothorax
- Causes of diaphragmatic palsy
- Indications for and timing of diaphragmatic plication for phrenic nerve palsy
- Evidence for and against early correction of tetralogy of Fallot
- Management of postoperative pulmonary hypertension.

3. The child on extracorporeal life support (ECLS)

Common cases
- Child post-cardiac arrest – 'crashed' onto ECMO
- Baby post-cardiac surgery – failed to wean from cardiopulmonary bypass
- Child with cardiomyopathy – bridge to transplant
- Baby with diaphragmatic hernia – pulmonary hypoplasia
- Child with severe pneumonia/pneumonitis and respiratory failure.

Appropriate thoughts
- Underlying pathology – aetiology and progress
- Type of ECLS – duration and progress
- Suitability for weaning of ECLS
- Any complications of underlying condition and ECLS
- Evidence of multi-organ failure.

On examination
The cubicle
- Infection control procedures in place
- Family members – clues to diagnosis (genetic syndromes)
- Length of admission – family photos, balloons and toys.

Infusions
- Multiple syringe pumps – vasoactive drugs, sedation and analgesia, frusemide infusions
- Blood products – red blood cells, platelets, fresh frozen plasma, cryoprecipitate
- Total parenteral/enteral nutrition
- Maintenance fluids
- Albumin/saline fluid boluses.

Ventilation
- Conventional ventilator – settings
- High frequency oscillator – possibility of continuing air leak.

The monitor
- Heart rate – tachycardia could signify patient discomfort or seizures if intermittent
- Invasive blood pressure – MAP indicative of flow and peripheral resistance
- Look for pulsatile flow if VA-ECMO – signify return of cardiac function
- CVP/RA pressures indicative of vascular filling
- Circuit pressures – arterial and venous line pressures
- Temperature – evidence of infection.

Equipment
- ECMO pump and circuit, +/– bridge; check circuit for fibrin strands and clots
- Arterial and venous cannulae/double lumen venous cannula
- Oxygenator – check for fibrin/clots
- Oxygen/air blender and flowmeter – check FiO_2 and sweep flows
- Haemofilter: check from signs of haemolysis in ultrafiltrate
- Urinary drainage collection system – examine urine for evidence of haemolysis
- Nitric oxide – pulmonary hypertension in congenital diaphragmatic hernia or congenital cardiac disease
- Device for measuring activated clotting time (ACT) or thromboelastography (TEG).

The child
- From end of bed assess alertness and activity.
- Note the colour and presence of generalised body oedema.
- Note the nature and location of arterial/venous cannulae.
- Is the sternum open or closed?
- What is the urine colour and volume?
- Examine limbs for perfusion (temperature, colour), presence and characteristics of pulses.
- Examine the chest for air entry/added sounds.
- Examine the abdomen for hepatomegaly/ascites.
- Examine the chest wall and dependent oedema.
- Ask to review a recent chest X-ray – check position of ETT/cannulae/lines and tubes.

Useful questions
- 'Why is the child on ECLS and how long has he been on it?'
- 'Could I please see the results of any recent arterial and venous blood gases?'
- 'Is there a need for left atrial decompression?' (e.g. septectomy or cannula)
- 'What is the coagulation status?'

- 'Are there any bleeding and transfusion requirements?'
- 'What is the fluid balance?'
- 'Could I please see the results of any recent cardiac echocardiography and head ultrasound?'

Useful statements
'This 14-year-old boy with H1N1 influenza was placed on VV-ECMO 16 days ago. He is sedated with morphine and midazolam. He is enterally fed. He requires no inotropic support with stable blood pressure, inlet pressure – 5 mmHg and outlet pressure 75–85 mmHg. He is on ventilation rest settings (PEEP 10, PIP 20, rate 10, FiO_2 40%), his saturations are acceptable with ECMO flow (100 mL/kg/min) and sweep gas flow (800 mL/min) and FiO_2 = 60 mmHg. To evaluate suitability for weaning, his ventilation could be weaned to PEEP 5 cmH_2O, and the ECMO FiO_2 reduced gradually to FiO_2 21%'.

Topics for discussion
- Indications for ECLS
- Differences between VV and VA ECMO
- Complications of ECLS
- Management of anticoagulation on ECLS
- Nutrition on ECLS
- Weaning from ECLS.

4. The child post-transplant

Common cases
- Liver and kidney transplant recipients for postoperative management or management of late complications (e.g. sepsis, rejection and organ support).
- Bone marrow transplantation – for septic complications requiring ventilatory and inotropic support or graft vs host disease requiring intensive care management.

Appropriate thoughts
- Consider perioperative, early and late onset complications related to surgery
- Reperfusion injury with early poor graft function
- Specific problems related to anastomotic leaks, thromboses or late stenoses
- Early bacterial and delayed opportunistic infections (e.g. fungal)
- Rejection – hyperacute or chronic
- Graft vs host disease
- Drug side effects
- Veno-occlusive disease.

On examination
The cubicle
- Isolation room (positive or negative pressure) with infection control precautions
- Waste disposal bins for cytotoxic agents.

Infusions
- Immunosuppressant medication
- Antibiotics – may suggest likely infective agents
- Vasoactive infusions – suggesting septic shock or myocardial dysfunction.

Ventilation
- Non-invasive ventilation or mechanical ventilation via endotracheal tube
- Increased PEEP/ FiO_2/reduced lung compliance – consider ARDS/infection/fibrosis/veno-occlusive disease.

The monitor
- Temperature – fever may suggest sepsis, SIRS, rejection, drug fever
- O_2 saturation – low saturations suggest lung involvement
- Cardiovascular parameters – invasive monitoring suggests acute deterioration.

Equipment
Haemofiltration indicating acute kidney injury.

The child
- Is the child alert? – assess mental state, encephalopathy.
- Does the child have alopecia? – chemotherapy, radiation.
- Assess growth parameters – height/weight.
- Look for Cushingoid features from steroid therapy.
- Eyes – conjunctival pallor, scleral icterus. Check external ocular movements for evidence of cranial nerve palsy, neuropathy.
- Examine the mouth, teeth and tongue – mucositis, mucous membranes, dental abnormalities.
- Check thyroid – nodules.
- Examine skin – pallor, bruises, dermatitis, hyperpigmentation or desquamation.
- Look for scars and lumps.
- Look for stigmata of liver disease – spider naevi, bruising, bleeding, scratch marks, jaundice, asterixis.
- Do a precordial assessment for cardiomegaly or evidence of congestive cardiac failure (cardiomyopathy, pericarditis).
- Undertake a full respiratory examination for tachypnoea, cough or crackles due to interstitial pneumonitis or pulmonary fibrosis, respiratory infection (opportunistic viruses, bacteria/fungi if still on chemotherapy).
- Assess bony tenderness at sternum, clavicles and spine.
- Examine abdomen for scars (previous diagnostic, curative or debulking surgery), prominent veins, hepato-splenomegaly and genitals.
- Assess limbs for oedema, swelling and power – thromboses, neuropathy, venous obstruction.
- Look at the temperature chart – recurrent fevers.
- Look at the weight chart – short-term weight gain suggests fluid overload, congestive cardiac failure or veno-occlusive disease.

Useful questions
- To help assess graft viability – 'Could I please see the results of investigations?' – e.g. urea, creatinine and electrolytes, liver function tests, blood glucose and coagulation profiles
- Could I please see the results of an abdominal ultrasound?' – portal vein and hepatic/renal artery patency, kidney perfusion, exclude haematoma/abscess
- 'Could I please see the results of any recent biopsies?'

Useful statements
'This child, who is 10 days post bone marrow transplant, was intubated and ventilated for respiratory failure. It appears that the lung pathology is resolving, although I am concerned that he is now showing signs of veno-occlusive disease in that he is

jaundiced and has hepatomegaly. I would be interested in recent weight gain and the results of the liver biopsy …'

Topics for discussion
- Goal-directed therapy in paediatric septic shock
- Recent improved ICU outcome of ventilated patients with haematological malignancy and relationship of mortality to presence of multi-organ failure
- Recognition and management of graft vs host disease
- ARDS in septic shock
- Role of steroids in septic shock
- Diagnosis and management of veno-occlusive disease.

5. The child with a head injury

Common cases
- Severe traumatic brain injury
- Infant with non-accidental injury – acute on chronic subdural haemorrhages.

Appropriate thoughts
- Isolated head injury or multiple trauma – mechanism of injury
- Time since injury
- Complicating factors – secondary brain injury.

On examination
The cubicle
- Family members – age, attitude, behaviour towards each other

Infusions
- Sedation – usually morphine and midazolam
- Neuromuscular blocking agent – used to prevent shivering during cooling
- Intravenous phenytoin for seizure prophylaxis or management
- Vasoactive drugs (noradrenaline) to maintain cerebral perfusion pressure
- Osmotherapy – 3% saline or mannitol infusions.

Ventilation
- High FiO_2/PEEP may reflect associated chest injuries, aspiration, ventilator-associated pneumonia or ARDS.

The monitor
- MAP, ICP, CPP usually displayed
- Note ICP waveform character
- $ETCO_2$ monitoring – 35–40 mmHg is target range; variable if uncuffed ETT in situ
- Core temperature – may be cooled to moderate hypothermia for ICP control if refractory raised pressure or to normothermia if febrile.

Equipment
- EVD or parenchymal ICP monitor
- If EVD: note height of reservoir, note CSF pressure when drainage limb occluded, colour of CSF and volume drained
- Continuous electroencephalogram (EEG) may be used to detect seizures in a drug-paralysed patient

- Jugular venous bulb monitoring equipment
- Cooling mattress
- Nasogastric or transpyloric tube and feed pump if being fed enterally
- Urinary catheter: note the colour and ask for volume of urine in the previous 24 hours. If polyuria, consider diabetes insipidus, cerebral salt wasting or effects of osmotherapy.

The child

- Note the head position: Usually midline with 30° head-up.
- Look for head wounds: traumatic or surgical.
- Look for evidence of base of skull fracture – haemotympanum, otorrhea or rhinorrhea, bruising over the mastoid region, bilateral periorbital bruising.
- Assess the GCS: clarify that the child is not drug paralysed and speaks English.
- If child does not respond to voice, ask permission before applying painful stimuli; apply painful stimuli to each limb (brisk responses could be spinal reflexes) and both supraorbital ridges.
- Check pupil size, shape, symmetry, direct and consensual light reflexes, pupil defects (traumatic mydriasis).
- Fundoscopy: retinal haemorrhages, papilloedema.
- Examine cranial nerves if appropriate age and level of consciousness.
- If the child is unconscious, assess corneal reflexes, assess cough and gag reflexes.
- Palpate the cervical spine: ask if spinal precautions still in place.
- Perform a motor exam: peripheral tone, power if child responsive and deep tendon reflexes symmetry and briskness, plantar responses.
- Assess sensation if child responsive.
- Look for involuntary movements.

Useful questions

- 'Does the child cough and gag on suctioning?'
- 'Could I please review neuroradiology (and other radiology, such as a skeletal survey)?'
- If there is polyuria, 'Could I please see recent paired urine and serum electrolytes and osmolality?'
- 'When did sedation cease? What type of drugs were administered? For how long?'
- 'Could I please assess kidney and liver function?' – to ascertain the potential for residual drug effect to contribute to conscious level.

Useful statements

'This child, with a history of head trauma 3 days ago, is irritable and restless. His Glasgow Coma Score is 9…'

'This child, with a vague history of trauma, remains sedated, paralysed and cooled to 32.5°C, 36 hours after admission. There is an intracranial pressure monitor in place and although the current ICP is 19 mmHg, he has recently received 3% saline. The pupils are both 4 mm in size and react sluggishly to light. There are retinal haemorrhages present bilaterally. There is bruising present on the anterior chest wall suggestive of finger marks. I am concerned that this child has had a cerebral insult as a result of a shaking injury. I would like to review any recent neuroimaging.'

Topics for discussion

- Pathophysiology of traumatic brain injury
- Features of non-accidental injury in children
- Head injury – difference between adults and children
- Indications for monitoring the ICP in traumatic brain injury

- Methods of monitoring ICP – advantages and disadvantages of each
- Strategies for controlling ICP in children – evidence for, complications and risks
- Intravenous therapy – saline vs colloid
- Approaches to clearance of cervical spine (adult-specific guidelines do not provide guidance for cervical spine clearance for a child with traumatic brain injury)
- Evidence for and against decompressive craniotomy.

6. The child with acute kidney injury

Common cases
- Haemolytic uraemic syndrome
- Post-nephrotoxin kidney injury (e.g. rhabdomyolysis, tumour lysis syndrome, other nephrotoxins)
- Child with hereditary nephropathy (e.g. cystinosis)
- Child with chronic kidney disease (e.g. due to congenital renal anomalies)
- Child with chronic kidney disease resulting from glomerulonephritis.

Appropriate thoughts
- What is the underlying pathology? Acute or chronic kidney disease? Congenital or acquired kidney disease?
- Is there evidence of fluid overload or electrolyte disturbances?
- What type of RRT? (e.g. peritoneal dialysis, CVVHF or CVVHDF.)

On examination
The cubicle
- Look for features of hereditary kidney disease in family members (e.g. parent wearing a hearing aid (Alport syndrome) or siblings with growth retardation).
- Look for evidence of chronic hospitalisation (e.g. increased personal belongings in the bedspace, balloons, posters, toys).

Infusions
- Vasoactive drugs (e.g. dobutamine/noradrenaline suggests possible sepsis)
- Blood products – packed cells (e.g. anaemia of chronic kidney disease); fresh frozen plasma; platelets for the management of deranged coagulation possibly associated with HUS or sepsis
- Sedation and analgesia – especially in small children, suggests acute rather than chronic kidney injury. Children often require chemical restraint following catheter placement and for the initiation of RRT
- Peritoneal dialysis fluid and urine/PD drainage
- Enteral feeds or total parenteral nutrition (TPN).

The ventilator
- Ventilator settings – why is the patient being ventilated?
- High FiO_2 and PEEP suggest fluid overload or possibility of MOF

The monitor
- ECG – heart rate and rhythm – tachycardia may suggest hypovolaemia
- ECG morphology – prolonged PR interval, widened QRS and peaked T waves suggest hyperkalaemia; flattened or inverted T waves, a U wave and prolongation of the QT interval suggest hypokalaemia
- If SpO_2 low – consider ARDS and MOF

- Arterial line trace including respiratory swing suggesting underfilling
- Evidence of hypertension from renal insufficiency
- CVP – ask about trends
- Temperature – core temperature vs skin temperature.

Equipment
- Nasogastric tube
- Gastrostomy tube or button
- Indwelling urinary catheter
- Central venous lines
- Surgical drains – indicating recent laparotomy or abdominal compartment syndrome
- If multiple trauma, look for other drains (e.g. pleural drains – note swinging, draining and bubbling with the respiratory cycle. Check if drains are under suction and occlude suction to look for air leak)
- Peritoneal dialysis (Tenckhoff) catheter – acute peritoneal dialysis 'stick' catheter or 'chronic' surgically placed Tenckhoff catheter
- Vascular access haemofiltration catheter
- Ascertain whether CVVHF or CVVHDF is being used
- Check haemofiltration and dialysis fluid being used
- Check pump flow rate plus dialysis and haemofiltration replacement fluid flow rates
- Ascertain whether heparin or citrate is being used for anticoagulation and ask how this is being monitored – ACT, APPT or TEG
- Ask for ultrafiltrate flow rate – to calculate overall hourly balance
- Examine filter for evidence of clots.

The child
- Note the general features – does the child look sick or well?
- Note any dysmorphic features.
- Assess general growth parameters, looking for failure to thrive or short stature associated with chronic kidney disease (CKD).
- Is there any evidence of chronic steroid therapy?
- Assess the child's nutritional status – muscle bulk and subcutaneous fat stores will be reduced in CKD.
- Assess skin: colour – sallow in CKD, pallor in CKD and HUS, jaundice in hepatorenal syndrome, bruising and/or petechiae in CKD, and scratch marks from hyperuricaemia in CKD.
- Look for dependent pitting oedema and assess for general body oedema for evidence of fluid overload.
- Is the fontanel tense/sunken? Look for evidence of hydration status.
- Check conjunctiva for pallor and sclera for icterus (hepatorenal syndrome).
- Check face for hirsutism (minoxidil therapy for hypertension).
- Examine the mucous membranes to assess hydration and note uraemic breath (CKD).
- Examine the chest to exclude any bony deformities (e.g. rachitic rosary in CKD).
- Examine the praecordium for cardiomegaly (fluid overload, cardiomyopathy), murmurs (anaemia), rub (uraemic pericarditis) and signs of cardiac failure (fluid overload).
- Measure the respiratory rate – tachypnoea: respiratory compensation for metabolic acidosis.
- Auscultate and percuss the chest, looking for pleural effusions (nephrosis) and pulmonary oedema (fluid overload).

- Inspect the abdomen, looking for a peritoneal dialysis catheter and other interventions; signs of associated congenital anomalies (e.g. prune belly syndrome); scars – current or previous kidney transplants (previous kidney transplant has central abdominal scar in younger children, and scar in either iliac fossa for older children) and other surgery, including previous peritoneal dialysis scars; ascites – peritoneal dialysis fluid or nephrosis:
  - palpate musculature (absent in prune belly syndrome); kidneys (enlarged with polycystic disease, hydronephrosis); lymph nodes and genitalia (cryptorchidism in prune belly syndrome)
  - assess for signs of peritonism
  - percuss bladder and listen for bowel sounds
- Seek permission to either sit the patient up or, if ventilated, to roll patient in order to examine the back looking for sacral oedema.

Useful questions

- 'Could I please see the temperature trends over the last 24 hours?' Fever may indicate infection, transplant rejection.
- 'Could I please see details of the underlying condition and previous surgery or transplant?'
- If HUS is suspected, 'Is there a history of diarrhoea?' Especially ask for evidence of bloody diarrhoea and whether shiga-like toxin has been detected in the stool specimen or from rectal swab. Initial haemoglobin, platelet count and results of a blood smear may confirm diagnosis of HUS if there is evidence of anaemia, red cell fragmentation, and thrombocytopenia.
- 'Was Streptococcus PCR positive or was there evidence of T antigen activation in the blood?' Reduced activity of ADAMST-13 would lead to a diagnosis of thrombotic thrombocytopenia purpura (TTP).
- 'Could I please see a recent chest radiograph?' This will allow you to check the position of ETT if intubated, central venous lines, and to check cardiac silhouette (globular heart if uraemic pericarditis) and evidence of fluid overload (pulmonary oedema).
- If there are concerns about peritonitis or Tenckhoff function – 'Could I please see an abdominal radiograph?'
- 'Could I please see recent abdominal ultrasound findings?' These may elucidate the cause of kidney failure or other intra-abdominal pathology.
- Could I please see the most recent biochemistry results?'
- To exclude electrolyte disturbances, 'Could I please review a recent 12-lead ECG?'
- If the patient is not anuric, 'I would like to request a urinalysis.'

Useful statements

'This 3-year-old boy, who most likely has haemolytic uraemic syndrome, is cardiovascularly stable and is currently undergoing continuous veno-venous haemodiafiltration. He remains anuric but does not appear anaemic and there is no evidence of thrombocytopaenia. He is cardiovascularly stable. There is no evidence of fluid overload or any evidence of electrolyte disturbances such as hyperkalaemia based on the normal ECG trace. I would be interested in his pathology results on admission, particularly whether he was anaemic or thrombocytopaenic with evidence of red cell fragmentation on a peripheral blood smear …'

Topics for discussion

- Management of oliguria/anuria
- Indication for renal replacement therapy
- Benefits and risks of CRRT vs peritoneal dialysis
- CVVHF vs CVVHDF

- Management of acute electrolyte disturbances in renal failure
- Difference between HUS and TTP
- Management of HUS
- Role of plasma exchange in acute kidney injury (TTP)
- Managing nutrition in a patient with acute kidney injury
- Features of CKD.

Paediatric critical care literature

The articles in this section have been selected on the basis that they provide a foundation for the contemporary practice of paediatric ICM. Unlike the adult critical care literature, there is a paucity of large, quality trials to guide practice. Select papers are presented in this section on the grounds of their perceived importance and usefulness as a resource. In most cases each reference is accompanied simply by a comment on its significance. The subject areas have been arranged alphabetically and do not reflect the importance of one area over another. Articles within each subject have been listed in order to reflect issues such as historic and significant developments in a particular field. Inferences are frequently drawn from the adult literature and the exam candidate is therefore referred to Chapter 9.

BOX 10.2 Index of paediatric critical care literature

Brain death and organ donation
Burns
Cardiovascular medicine
Endocrine
Fluids and electrolytes
Haematology
Neurology
Nutrition
Renal medicine
Respiratory medicine
Resuscitation
Sedation and analgesia
Sepsis

Brain death and organ donation

Lutz-Dettinger N, de Jaeger A, Kerremans I. Care of the potential pediatric organ donor. Pediatric Clinics of North America. 2001; 48: 715–49.

Significance: This paper highlights the importance of early recognition of brain death and the consequent 'radical switch of the treatment goal from preservation of the patient's brain and life to preservation of organs' and considers the thyroid hormone controversy and the differential applicability of inotropic, vasoactive, or fluid-centred strategies to optimise post-transplant function.

Burns

Ansermino M. ABC of burns: intensive care management and control of infection. BMJ. 2004; 329: 220–3.

Significance: 'The goal in management of an acute burn is to limit the extent of the systemic insult. Intensive care management should not be seen as rescue for failed initial treatment but as a preventive measure in patients at high risk of organ failure. Intensive care units have the resources for improved monitoring and expertise in managing acute physiological changes. Intensive care management should not, however, become an obstacle to early aggressive surgical excision of the burn wound, which is associated with improved outcome.'

Cardiovascular medicine

Andreasen JB, Johnsen SP, Ravn HB. Junctional ectopic tachycardia after surgery for congenital heart disease in children. Intensive Care Medicine. 2008; 34: 895–902.

Significance: 'JET occurred in approximately 10% of children following cardiac surgery in this observational study and was associated with higher mortality and longer ICU stay. Risk factors included high inotropic requirements after surgery and extensive myocardial injury in terms of high CK-MB values and longer CPB duration.'

Bronicki RA, Anas NG. Cardiopulmonary interaction. Pediatric Critical Care Medicine. 2009; 10: 313–22.

Significance: A useful review of 'the physiology and pathophysiology of cardiopulmonary interaction in the critically ill paediatric patient'.

Carotti A, Digilio MC, Piacentini G, et al. Cardiac defects and results of cardiac surgery in 22q11.2 deletion syndrome. Developmental Disabilities Research Reviews. 2008; 14(1): 35–42.

Significance: 'The conotruncal heart defects occurring in patients with 22q11.2 deletion syndrome include tetralogy of Fallot, pulmonary atresia with ventricular septal defect, truncus arteriosus, interrupted aortic arch, isolated anomalies of the aortic arch and ventricular septal defect. A range of associated problems should be anticipated, including intellectual delay, hypocalcaemia (hypoparathyroidism), immune deficiency (thymic aplasia), vasomotor instability, bronchospasm and laryngeal webs.'

Conway J, Dipchand AI. Heart transplantation in children. Paediatric Clinics of North America. 2010; 57: 353–73.

Significance: 'In the last 40 years orthotopic heart transplantation has been established as a realistic treatment strategy for infants and children with severe forms of congenital heart disease and cardiomyopathy. The evaluation, management, and outcomes of these patients have continued to improve. These achievements have advanced pediatric cardiac transplantation and allowed more attention to be focused on improving quality of life after transplantation and reducing the long-term complications.'

Deal BJ, Mavroudis C, Jacobs JP, et al. Arrhythmic complications associated with the treatment of patients with congenital cardiac disease: consensus definitions from the Multi-Societal Database Committee for Pediatric and Congenital Heart Disease. Cardiology in the Young. 2008; Dec; 18 Suppl 2: 202–5.

Significance: 'Arrhythmias (defined as any cardiac rhythm other than normal sinus rhythm) can not only result from perturbations of other organ systems, such as renal failure, but can also produce dysfunction in other organ systems due to haemodynamic compromise or embolic phenomena. They are classified by location, mechanism, aetiology, timing of onset, duration and frequency.'

Dimmick S, Badawi N, Randell T. Thyroid hormone supplementation for the prevention of morbidity and mortality in infants undergoing cardiac surgery. Cochrane Database Systematic Reviews 2004; 3: CD004220.

Significance: 'Paediatric studies have demonstrated that cardiopulmonary bypass is associated with a decline in thyroid hormone levels. Adult patients who undergo open-heart surgery and receive tri-iodothyronine supplementation have demonstrated a dose-dependent increase in cardiac output, which has been associated with an improved clinical outcome. At present, there is a lack of evidence concerning the effects of tri-iodothyronine supplementation in infants undergoing cardiac surgery. Further randomised, controlled trials that include sufficiently large subject numbers in a variety of different age strata (neonates, infants and older children) need to be undertaken.'

Frommelt PC. Update on pediatric echocardiography. Current Opinion in Pediatrics. 2005; Oct; 17(5): 579–85.

> Significance: 'Paediatric echocardiography has clearly expanded from a diagnostic tool used to describe anatomic abnormalities associated with congenital heart disease to a non-invasive myocardial monitoring tool that allows serial assessment of the pathological effects of both cardiac and non-cardiac disease. Tissue Doppler imaging is used for regional assessment of myocardial velocities and to assess diastolic function. Myocardial performance index assesses myocardial function. Integrated backscatter analysis evaluates abnormal ventricles. 3-D echo assists determination of flow rates and volumes including shunt and regurgitant volumes. Fetal echo has enabled early clarification of abnormalities.'

Hoffman TM, Wernovsky G, Atz AM, et al. Efficacy and safety of milrinone in preventing low cardiac output syndrome in infants and children after corrective surgery for congenital heart disease. Circulation 2003; 107: 996–1002.

> Significance: Because LCOS occurs frequently in paediatric patients after congenital heart surgery, the prophylactic use of a positive inotropic and vasodilatory agent, such as milrinone, may improve cardiac function and lower the risk of morbidity and mortality. The purpose of the PRIMACORP trial (PRophylactic Intravenous use of Milrinone After Cardiac OpeRation in Pediatrics) was to evaluate the efficacy and safety of the prophylactic use of milrinone in paediatric patients at high risk of developing LCOS after cardiac surgery. The prophylactic use of high-dose milrinone (75 mcg/kg bolus followed by a 0.75 mcg/kg/min infusion) reduced the risk of LCOS after paediatric congenital heart surgery. Although hypotension, thrombocytopenia, and arrhythmias have been reported in adult patients, they occurred infrequently in paediatric patients and were not associated with milrinone use.

Jaquiss RD, Imamura M. Single ventricle physiology: surgical options, indications and outcomes. Current Opinion in Cardiology. 2009; Mar; 24(2): 113–18.

> Significance: 'The development of a number of inventive operations, combined with a greater understanding of the physiologic requirements for success after single ventricle reconstruction, has resulted in dramatic improvements in outcomes. The identification and modification of risk factors, as well as the recent development of catheter-based intervention, offer the real prospect of significant continued improvement.'

Jones B, Hayden M, Fraser JF, Janes E. Low cardiac output syndrome in children. Current Anaesthesia and Critical Care. 2005; 16: 347–58.

> Significance: Management of LCOS in children aims to achieve the optimal balance between oxygen delivery and consumption. Preload and afterload should be optimised prior to escalation of inotropic support. Specifically remediable causes should be excluded (e.g. airway and ventilation problems, pericardial tamponade, residual anatomic defects, pulmonary hypertensive crises, arrhythmias, electrolyte abnormalities) Positive-pressure ventilation and non-pharmacological strategies (e.g. sternal reopening, hypothermia, mechanical support) are also useful.

Kantor PF, Mertens LL. Clinical practice: heart failure in children. Part I: clinical evaluation, diagnostic testing, and initial medical management. European Journal of Pediatrics. 2010; 169: 269–79.

> Significance: 'Current evidence suggests that almost half of all children with cardiomyopathy and symptomatic heart failure will die or require a cardiac transplant within 5 years of diagnosis. This review provides a framework for this diagnostic assessment and gives an overview of the treatment options available for children with heart failure (e.g. diuretics, vasoactive drugs especially inodilators, ACE inhibitors, cardioselective beta-blockers, oral anticoagulants, non-invasive ventilation, mechanical support and transplantation). Common causes of heart failure in infancy and childhood include rheumatic heat disease, acute myocarditis, incessant SVT, antineoplastic drugs, myopathies, metabolic disorders and cardiomyopathies.'

Kantor PF, Mertens LL. Clinical practice: heart failure in children. Part II: current maintenance therapy and new therapeutic approaches. European Journal of Pediatrics. 2010; 169: 403–10.

Significance: 'The goals of therapy are to maintain circulatory and end-organ function and to allow for recovery and reverse remodelling to occur. When maintenance therapy fails, the alternative of device therapy must be considered. Patients with electromechanical dysynchrony of ventricular systolic function have demonstrated a benefit from biventricular pacing devices (cardiac resynchronisation therapy), with improved functional capacity and quality of life and, in some patients, avoidance of the need for transplantation.'

Lawrenson J, Eyskens B, Vlasselaers D, Gewillig M. Manipulating parallel circuits: the perioperative management of patients with complex congenital cardiac disease. Cardiology in the Young. 2003; 13: 316–22.

Significance: 'In patients undergoing complex palliations, the pulmonary and systemic circulations can be compared to two circuits in parallel. Manipulations of variables, such as resistance or flow, in one circuit, can profoundly affect the performance of the other circuit. A large pulmonary flow might result in a large increase in the saturation of haemoglobin with oxygen returning to the heart via the pulmonary veins at the expense of a decreased systemic flow. Accurate balancing of these parallel circulations requires an appreciation of all interventions that can affect individual components of both circulations.'

Mendeloff EN, Glenn GF, Tavakolian P, et al. The role of thromboelastography in directing blood product usage in infant open-heart surgery. Innovations. 2009; 4: 282–90.

Significance: 'Thromboelastography allows for proactive, goal-directed blood component therapy with improved postoperative hemostasis in infants undergoing cardiopulmonary bypass.'

Morris MC, Wernovsky G, Nadkarni VM. Survival outcomes after extracorporeal cardiopulmonary resuscitation instituted during active chest compressions following refractory in-hospital pediatric cardiac arrest. Pediatric Critical Care Medicine. 2005; 5: 440–6.

Significance: 'Extracorporeal cardiopulmonary resuscitation can be used to successfully resuscitate selected children following refractory in-hospital cardiac arrest, and can be implemented during active cardiopulmonary resuscitation. Intact neurologic survival can sometimes be achieved, even when the duration of in-hospital cardiopulmonary resuscitation is prolonged. In this series, children with isolated heart disease were more likely to survive following extracorporeal cardiopulmonary resuscitation than were children with other medical conditions. Survival rates of 33% to hospital discharge are described (10% if non-cardiac condition).'

Ohye RG, Sleeper LA, Mahony L, et al. Comparison of shunt types in the Norwood procedure for single-ventricle lesions. New England Journal of Medicine. 2010; 362: 1980–92.

Significance: 'Twelve-month transplantation-free survival was higher with the use of a right ventricle-pulmonary artery shunt than with the use of a modified Blalock Taussig shunt. However, the RVPA shunt was associated with a higher rate of unintended cardiovascular interventions and complications during the first 12 months. There was no significant difference between the two groups with respect to transplantation-free survival beyond 12 months.'

Pinsky WW, Arciniegas E. Tetralogy of Fallot. Pediatrics Clinics of North America. 1990; 37: 179–92.

Significance: 'Tetralogy of Fallot is the most common malformation of children born with cyanotic heart disease, with an incidence of approximately 10 per cent of congenital heart disease. There can be a wide spectrum as to the severity of the anatomic defects, which include ventricular septal defect, aortic override, right ventricular outflow tract obstruction, and right ventricular hypertrophy. Cyanosis may vary from mild to severe, and patients may present as newborns or, more commonly, young infants. This review suggests that infants with classic tetralogy of Fallot and stable anatomy should undergo primary complete intracardiac repair.'

Plumpton K, Justo R, Haas N. Amiodarone for post-operative junctional ectopic tachycardia. Cardiology in the Young. 2005; 15: 13–18.

> Significance: Junctional ectopic tachycardia is defined as HR >180, with a QRS complex the same as prior to the arrhythmia, AV discordance and warm-up. It usually resolves spontaneously and worsens cardiac output via AV dysynchrony, loss of ventricular filling and increased myocardial oxygen demand. Amiodarone controls rate effectively. Not uncommon after TOF and VSD repairs.

Rossi AF, Khan DM, Hannan R, et al. Goal-directed medical therapy and point-of-care testing improve outcomes after congenital heart surgery. Intensive Care Medicine. 2005; 31: 98–104.

> Significance: 'The combination of goal-directed therapy and point-of-care testing was associated with a marked decrease in mortality for patients undergoing congenital heart surgery. Improvement was greatest in the highest risk patients.'

Seear MD, Scarfe JC, Leblanc JG. Predicting major adverse events after cardiac surgery in children. Pediatric Critical Care Medicine. 2008; 9: 606–11.

> Significance: 'Lactate and SVO$_2$ are the only postoperative measurements with predictive power for major adverse events. Forming a ratio of the two (SVO$_2$/lactate), seems to improve predictive power, presumably by combining their individual predictive strengths. Both measures have excellent specificities but lower sensitivities. Predictive power of single measures is only fair but can be improved, in high-risk patients, by monitoring repeated measures over time.'

Shekerdemian L. Perioperative manipulation of the circulation in children with congenital heart disease. Heart. 2009; 95: 1286–96.

> Significance: 'All patients undergoing surgery on cardiopulmonary bypass are at risk of developing low cardiac output state, especially younger patients undergoing more complex surgery.' 'Strategies for management of low cardiac output state focus on manipulating the circulation to optimise systemic oxygen delivery.'

Stocker CF, Shekerdemian LS. Recent developments in the perioperative management of the paediatric cardiac patient. Current Opinion in Anaesthesiology. 2006; 19: 375–81.

> Significance: 'Survival of infants born with complex cardiac anomalies has dramatically improved, and the growing population of patients with congenital heart disease reaching adulthood has resulted in an increased incidence of long-term complications related to the perioperative period. This review focuses on recent advances in strategies to prevent, detect, treat, or predict early and late complications arising from open-heart surgery for congenital heart disease.' The evidence basis for a range of interventions, including medications to manage post-operative bleeding, mechanical support and cardiac and cerebral protective strategies, are discussed.

Theilen U, Shekerdemian L. The intensive care of infants with hypoplastic left heart syndrome. Archives of Disease in Childhood. 2005; 90: F97–F102.

> Significance: 'Hypoplastic left heart syndrome (HLHS) is a continuum that can affect all left-sided cardiac structures, from the mitral valve to the aortic arch. Since Norwood's first description of surgical palliation in 1981, HLHS has been managed either by staged palliation in the majority of cases, or, in a minority, by primary cardiac transplantation. This article reviews the early medical and surgical management of the neonate with HLHS, focusing on the evolution of new surgical strategies, and on the changing emphasis of perioperative circulatory management on the intensive care unit.'

Tissot C, Beghetti M. Advances in therapies for pediatric pulmonary arterial hypertension. Expert Reviews of Respiratory Medicine. 2009; 3: 265–82.

> Significance: 'Pulmonary arterial hypertension (PAH) is a life-threatening disease characterised by progressive obliteration of the pulmonary vasculature, leading to right heart failure and death if left untreated.' It is defined as PAP >25 mmHg at rest with PAWP less than or equal to 15 mmHg and increased PVRI greater or equal to 3 Wood units. 'Prior to the current treatment era, pulmonary hypertension carried a poor prognosis with a high mortality rate, but its prognosis has changed over the past decades in relation to new therapeutic agents. Nevertheless, pulmonary hypertension continues to be a

serious condition, which is extremely challenging to manage. The data in children is often limited owing to the small number of patients, and extrapolation from adults to children is not straightforward. While none of these new therapeutic agents have been specifically approved for children, there is evidence that each can appropriately benefit the PAH child. This is a useful review the current understanding of paediatric pulmonary hypertension, classification, diagnostic evaluation and available treatment. A description of targeted pharmacological therapy and new treatments in children is outlined.'

Wernovsky G, Ghanayem N, Ohye RG, et al. Hypoplastic left heart syndrome: consensus and controversies in 2007. Cardiology in the Young. 2007; Sep; 17 Suppl 2: 75–86.

Significance: 'This review assesses the variability in practice at a large number of centres that manage neonates with hypoplastic left heart syndrome, with an emphasis on practice before, during, and after the first stage of the Norwood sequence of operations.' There have been no randomised trials of the different approaches.

Endocrine

Yung M, Wilkins B, Norton L, Slater A, for the Paediatric Study Group; Australian and New Zealand Intensive Care Society. Glucose control, organ failure, and mortality in pediatric intensive care. Pediatric Critical Care Medicine. 2008; 9: 147–52.

Significance: 'Hyperglycemia is common in PICUs, occurs early, and is independently associated with organ failure and death. However, early hyperglycemia is not associated with later or worsening organ failure.' Australasian PICUs seldom use insulin for glycaemic control. Possible mechanisms of harm are discussed.

Vlasselaers D, Milants I, Desmet L, et al. Intensive insulin therapy for patients in paediatric intensive care: a prospective, randomised controlled study. Lancet 2009; 373: 547–56.

Significance: Randomised controlled trial of intensive insulin targeting a BSL of 2.8–4.4 mmol/L in infants and 2.9–5.6 mmol/L in children compared with a liberal policy of tolerating levels up to 12 mmol/L. Improved outcomes were found with intensive therapy (e.g. reduced mortality, length of stay and secondary infections). Of note, the feeding regimens were quite aggressive and thus of questionable generalisability. For example, only 5% children require insulin in Australasia (see above study) compared to the 50% and almost 100% of patients in the study arms. It may be possible that the beneficial effects are purely related to managing the ill-effects of overfeeding and hyperglycaemia. The long-term effects of hypoglycaemia are also unclear from this paper. A previous study found that the extremes of blood glucose are associated with increased mortality and length of stay (Wintergerst, K. Association of hypoglycaemia, hyperglycaemia, and glucose variability with morbidity and death in the PICU. Pediatrics. 2006; 118: 173–9).

Glaser N, Barnett P, McCaslin I, et al. Risk factors for cerebral edema in children with diabetic ketoacidosis. New England Journal of Medicine. 2001; 344: 264–9.

Significance: Children are at increased risk of cerebral oedema if they have a low partial pressure of CO_2 and high urea nitrogen at presentation and are treated with bicarbonate.

Hoorn EJ, Carlotti AP, Costa LA, et al. Preventing a drop in effective plasma osmolality to minimise the likelihood of cerebral oedema during treatment of children with diabetic ketoacidosis, Journal of Pediatrics 2007; 150: 467–73.

Significance: Cerebral oedema is associated with a drop in the effective osmolarity over the first 8 hours, related to either to drop in glucose or sodium. Such patients are more likely to have received insulin boluses and have a more positive fluid and sodium balance. Strategies to prevent this complication are discussed that may include hypertonic saline administration is the sodium is suddenly dropping as hypernatraemia is well tolerated.

Fluids and electrolytes

Hoorn EJ, Geary D, Robb M, et al. Acute hyponatremia related to intravenous fluid administration in hospitalized children: an observational study. Pediatrics. 2004; 113: 1279–84.

Significance: 'The most important factor for hospital-acquired hyponatremia is the administration of hypotonic fluid. Hypotonic fluid should not be given to children unless P_{Na} >138 mmol/L.'

Montañana PA, Alapont VM, Ocón AP, et al. The use of isotonic fluid as maintenance therapy prevents iatrogenic hyponatremia in pediatrics: a randomized, controlled open study. Pediatric Critical Care Medicine. 2008; 9: 589–97.

Significance: 'Hypotonic fluids are widely used in pediatrics. The use of hypotonic fluids increases the risk of hyponatremia when compared with isotonic fluids at 24 hrs following infusion.' This study demonstrates that 'the use of isotonic fluids does not increase the incidence of adverse events compared with hypotonic fluids'.

Haematology

Lacroix J, Hebert PC, Hutchison, et al. Transfusion strategies for patients in pediatric intensive care units. New England Journal of Medicine. 2007; 356: 1609–19.

Significance: 'In stable, critically ill children a hemoglobin threshold of 7 g per dL for red-cell transfusion can decrease transfusion requirements without increasing adverse outcomes.'

Kache S, Weiss IK, Moore TB. Changing outcomes for children requiring intensive care following hematopoietic stem cell transplantation. Pediatric Transplant. 2006; 10: 299–303.

Significance: 'Past literature has shown that respiratory failure following hematopoietic stem cell transplant is associated with a universally poor outcome, with mortality rates approaching 100%. More recent studies have suggested that patient survival is improving.' This is a retrospective review of 183 post-BMT patients. Over the course of the study, the ICU survival increased from 18% to 59%. In the latter period, 54% of the patients discharged from the ICU were alive at 100 days post-transplant. 'Factors that were significant predictors of poor outcome were malignancy as the reason for transplant, dialysis during the ICU stay, or extreme respiratory failure with a ratio of arterial oxygen tension (PaO_2)/inspired oxygen concentration (FiO_2) <300. Analysis of patients who required a high positive end-expiratory pressure or who were ventilated with permissive hypercapnia showed that they also had a higher mortality. The impact on survival of factors, such as age at time of transplant, graft vs. host disease, pneumonia, bacteraemia, sepsis, post-transplant days, Pediatric Risk of Mortality III score, engraftment status, or veno-occlusive disease, did not reach statistical significance in this cohort. Survival has improved for children who require intensive care following a bone marrow transplant; even for those who require mechanical ventilation. Patients with extreme respiratory failure and those requiring dialysis continue to have poor outcome. Because of an overall improvement in survival, children whose condition following transplant requires intensive care should be treated aggressively.'

Neurology

Banwell BL, Mildner RJ, Hassall AC, et al. Muscle weakness in critically ill children. Neurology 2003; 61: 1779–82.

Significance: The paper describes an incidence of 1.7% (0.7% in <3 yo; 5.4% >10 yo), which is much lower than in adults. It may be higher in post-pubertal children and the pick-up in infants lower than the true incidence. All have evidence of myopathy and some also have neuropathy. Most recovered, albeit slowly (over up to 2 yrs). One died from it. All affected children were ventilated >5 days and most received steroids, neuromuscular blocking agents and/or aminoglycosides. BMT patients were disproportionately represented.

Hughes RA, Swan AV, Raphael JC, et al. Immunotherapy for Guillain-Barré syndrome: a systematic review. Brain 2007; 130: 2245–57.

Significance: The authors found that plasma exchange improves recovery compared with placebo, but no significant difference between plasma exchange and intravenous immunoglobulin (IVIG). Four plasma exchanges appear optimal. No benefit was found of administering IVIG after plasma exchange. Oral steroids appeared to worsen recovery and intravenous methylprednisolone had no effect.

Riordan FAI, Cant AJ. When to do a lumbar puncture. Archives of Disease in Children 2002; 87: 35–7.

Significance: The authors conclude that a lumbar puncture is appropriate if meningitis is suspected and there are no contraindications. Contraindications are signs of cerebral herniation, GCS <8, abnormal papillary responses, absent doll's eye movements, tonic posturing, respiratory abnormalities, papilloedema, focal neurological signs, prolonged seizure, shock, local infection in the area the needle will transverse and bleeding disorders. It must be appreciated that a normal CT does not rule out raised ICP (Shetty AK, Dessell BC, Craver RD, Steele RW. Fatal cerebral herniation after lumbar puncture in a patient with a normal computed tomography scan. Pediatrics 1999; 103: 1284–7).

Andrews PJ, Citerio G. Intracranial pressure. Part one: historical overview and basic concepts. Intensive Care Medicine. 2004; 30: 1730–3.

Significance: Useful revision of basic concepts; ICP physiology and waveforms.

Citerio G, Andrews PJ. Intracranial pressure. Part two: clinical applications and technology. Intensive Care Medicine. 2004; 30: 1882–5.

Significance: Current management strategies for acute brain injury patients encompass the principle of physiological stability. Although there is debate about which precise thresholds should be striven for, without monitoring intracranial pressure (ICP) considerable information is missing and objective management of the patient is difficult. ICP monitors have an acceptably low complication rate; offer a high yield in information gained and should be the cornerstone of all critical care management of acute brain injury.

Carney NA, Chesnut R, Kochanek PM. Guidelines for the acute medical management of severe traumatic brain injury in infants, children, and adolescents. Pediatric Critical Care Medicine. 2003; 4: S1.

Significance: This article summarises the evidence-based recommendations that guide the principal management strategies for head-injured children. They are also available at the Brain Trauma Foundation Guidelines (www.braintrauma.org). The optimal cerebral perfusion pressure in children remains unclear. Key issues to consider are contemplated in another key article (Chambers IR, Kirkham FJ. What is the optimal cerebral perfusion pressure in children suffering from traumatic coma? Neurosurgical Focus. 2003; 15: E3).

Giza CC, Mink RB, Medikians A. Pediatric traumatic brain injury: not just little adults. Current Opinion in Critical Care. 2007; 12: 143–52.

Significance: 'The developing brain is not simply a smaller version of the mature brain. Studies have uncovered important distinctions of the younger brain after traumatic brain injury, including an increased propensity for apoptosis, age-dependent parameters for cerebral blood flow and metabolism, development-specific biomarkers, increased likelihood of early post-traumatic seizures, differential sensitivity to commonly used neuroactive medications and altered neuroplasticity during recovery from injury. Specifically, there is strong preclinical evidence for increased neuronal apoptosis in the developing brain being triggered by anesthetics and anticonvulsants, making it paramount that future studies more clearly delineate preferred agents and specific indications for use, incorporating long-term functional outcomes, as well as short-term benefits. In addition, the young brain may actually benefit from therapeutic interventions that have been less effective following adult traumatic brain injury, such as decompressive craniectomy and hypothermia.' Importantly, the mechanisms of injury vary, with non-accidental injury being an important cause in young children, and older children having injury patterns more like adults.

Hutchison JS, Ward RE, Lacroix J, et al. Hypothermia therapy after traumatic brain injury in children. New England Journal of Medicine. 2008; 358: 2447–56.

Significance: A meta-analysis that suggests that while iatrogenic hypothermia may confer a marginal benefit in neurological outcome, there does not appear to be clear evidence of lower mortality rates in unselected traumatic brain injury patients. Prolonged hypothermia may confer a benefit, particularly in patients with elevated

ICP refractory to conventional manipulations. Conclusions regarding the use of hypothermia are controversial and not strongly supported by the available evidence.

Jagannathan J, Okonkwo DO, Dumont AS et al. Outcomes following decompressive craniectomy in children with severe traumatic brain injury: a 10 year single-center experience with long-term follow up. Journal of Neurosurgery. 2007; 106 (4 Suppl): 268–75.

Significance: Retrospective review of 23 patients undergoing decompressive craniectomy for severe head trauma with 69% survival rate and 82% of survivors having a good outcome.

Klimo P, Ware ML, Gupta N, Brockmeyer D. Cervical spine trauma in the pediatric patient. Neurosurgery Clinics of North America. 2008; 599–620.

Significance: Injuries to the paediatric cervical spine are uncommon. Although children can sustain similar injuries to those observed in adults, there are several unique features characteristic of paediatric cervical spine injuries (e.g. SCIWORA). These are attributable to differences in the anatomy of the immature spine and its response to deformational forces. In this article, the authors review epidemiological data, biomechanics, and classification of paediatric cervical spine injuries and discuss in detail the injuries that are more common or unique to the paediatric spine.

Taylor A, Butt W, Rosenfeld J, et al. A randomized trial of very early decompressive craniectomy in children with traumatic brain injury and sustained intracranial hypertension. Child's Nervous System. 2001; 17: 154–62.

Significance: This pilot study suggests that 'when children with traumatic brain injury and sustained intracranial hypertension are treated with a combination of very early decompressive craniectomy and conventional medical management, it is more likely that ICP will be reduced, fewer episodes of intracranial hypertension will occur, and functional outcome and quality of life may be better than in children treated with medical management alone.'

Fortune PM, Shann F. The motor response to stimulation predicts outcome as well as the full Glasgow Coma Scale in children with severe head injury. Paediatric Critical Care Medicine. 2010; 11: 339–42.

Significance: 'Both the full Glasgow Coma Scale score and the motor response provide a useful indication of long-term outcome, although neither score is sufficiently accurate to be used to limit treatment. The full Glasgow Coma Scale does not have a linear relationship with mortality, and there is poor interobserver agreement. The motor response should be used in children in preference to the full Glasgow Coma Scale; the predictive power is equivalent to the full Glasgow Coma Scale, there is a linear relationship to mortality, and it is easier to collect accurately.'

Van de Beek D, de Gans J, et al. Corticosteroids for acute bacterial meningitis. Cochrane Database Systematic Reviews. 2007: CD004405.

Significance: The study evaluated the effect of steroids when given with the first dose of antibiotics, in both adults and children. An overall decrease in hearing loss and adverse long-term neurologic sequelae and mortality was found. In children the benefits were greatest in *Haemophilus influenzae* type b in terms of reducing hearing loss. There was also a trend to improved survival in those with meningococcal disease.

Geddes JF, Plunkett J. The evidence base for shaken baby syndrome. BMJ 2004; 328: 719–20.

Significance: Retinal haemorrhage is not pathognomonic for shaken baby. Shaken baby is usually diagnosed based on subdural and retinal haemorrhages with brain damage in infants/young child in the context of inappropriate or inconsistent history and commonly accompanied by other inflicted injuries.

Nutrition

del Castillo SL, McCulley ME, Khemani RG, et al. Reducing the incidence of necrotizing enterocolitis in neonates with hypoplastic left heart syndrome with the introduction of an enteral feed protocol. Pediatric Critical Care Medicine. 2010; 11: 373–7.

Significance: 'Measures directed at reducing the incidence of necrotising enterocolitis may reduce morbidity in neonates with hypoplastic left heart syndrome and reduce cost by decreasing hospital length of stay. A standardised feeding protocol contributed to reducing the incidence of necrotising enterocolitis in this high-risk population.'

Jaksic T, Hull MA, Modi BP, et al. ASPEN Clinical Guidelines: nutrition support of neonates supported with extracorporeal membrane oxygenation. Journal of Parenteral and Enteral Nutrition. 2010; 34: 247–53.

Significance: 'ECMO does not provide a 'metabolic rest', rather, neonates on ECMO have demonstrated some of the highest rates of protein catabolism reported. Appropriate provision of nutrition support in ECMO patients is predicated upon a clear understanding of the changes in their metabolism, metabolic reserves, and nutrition requirement. This clinical guideline addresses the nutritional support of neonatal patients on ECMO.'

Natarajan G, Reddy AS, Aggarwal S. Enteral feeding of neonates with congenital heart disease. Neonatology. 2010; 4: 330–6.

Significance: 'The majority of infants with CHD achieve moderate enteral intake prior to surgery, even while on prostaglandins. Despite this and the early initiation of postoperative enteral feeds, many infants need gavage feeds at discharge.'

Willis L, Thureen P, Kaufman J, et al. Enteral feeding in prostaglandin-dependent neonates: is it a safe practice? Journal of Pediatrics. 2008; 153: 867–9.

Significance: In a retrospective study of 67 children, 34 infants were found to have been enterally fed while receiving PGE1 therapy. No patient developed necrotising enterocolitis; one patient had feed intolerance, suggesting that enteral feeding in PGE1-dependent neonates can be done safely.

Renal medicine

Flynn JT. Choice of dialysis modality for management of pediatric acute renal failure. Pediatric Nephrology. 2002; 1: 61–9.

Significance: 'Acute renal failure in children requiring dialysis can be managed with a variety of modalities, including peritoneal dialysis, intermittent haemodialysis and continuous haemodiafiltration. The choice of dialysis modality to be used in managing a specific patient is influenced by several factors, including the goals of dialysis, the unique advantages and disadvantages of each modality, and institutional resources.' This paper serves aspects of acute renal failure management and provides practical guidance regarding modality selection of appropriate renal replacement therapy. There is no clear evidence of benefit of one modality over another in all situations.

Foland JA, Fortenberry JD, Warshaw BL, et al. Fluid overload before continuous hemofiltration and survival in critically ill children: a retrospective analysis. Critical Care Medicine. 2004; 32: 1771–6.

Significance: 'Improved survival in critically ill children receiving CVVH may be associated with less fluid overload in patients with ≥ 3-organ MODS. Prospective studies are necessary to determine whether earlier use of CVVH to control fluid overload in critically ill children can improve survival.'

Schneider J, Khemani R, Grushkin C, Bart R. Serum creatinine as stratified in the RIFLE score for acute kidney injury is associated with mortality and length of stay for children in the pediatric intensive care unit. Critical Care Medicine. 2010; 38: 933–9.

Significance: Retrospective analysis of prospectively collected clinical data in 533 children concludes that RIFLE criteria serves well to describe acute kidney injury in critically ill pediatric patients.

Resuscitation

The International Liaison Committee on Resuscitation. Circulation 2010; 122; 16: Suppl 2.

Significance: Evidence-based international expert consensus on issues relating to basic and advanced life support. The entire supplement is devoted to updating the ILCOR 2005 guidelines. This is a continuing recommendation for a 3:1 chest compression-ventilation ratio for newborns at delivery when a cardiac problem is unlikely, but 15:2 for non-delivery room neonates/infants/child CPR with two rescuers. A ratio of 30:1 is recommended for all lone lay rescuers of non-newborn paediatric patients. Neonatal assessment now focuses on three parameters (heart rate, respiratory rate and oximetry rather than colour). Initial resuscitation with air rather than 100%

oxygen is advised for term babies; a 1-minute delay in cord clamping in babies not requiring resuscitation. There is a new recommendation for an initial dose of 2–4 J/kg in the shockable pathway with continued recommendation, like the adult algorithm for single rather than stacked shocks. There is considerable discussion regarding the role of therapeutic hypothermia, concluding that for newborns with birth asphyxia it appears safe and may improve survival and neurological outcome, but in children further quality trial evidence is needed as retrospective studies have failed to show a benefit. Resuscitation councils in different countries have produced ratified versions of these recommendations (e.g. British, European and Australian Resuscitation Councils). These vary slightly according to local practices and needs.

Abend NS. Licht DJ. Predicting outcome in children with hypoxic ischemic encephalopathy. Pediatric Critical Care Medicine. 2008; 9: 32–9.

Significance: 'Hypoxic ischemic encephalopathy (HIE) is common in children, and providing accurate and timely prognostic information is important in determining the appropriate level of care.' 'When performed at least 24 hrs after the inciting event, abnormal clinical signs (pupil reactivity and motor response), absent N20 waves bilaterally on somatosensory evoked potentials, electrocerebral silence or burst suppression patterns on electroencephalogram (not due to metabolic or medication etiology), and abnormal magnetic resonance imaging with diffusion restriction in the cortex and basal ganglia are each highly predictive of poor outcome.' 'Combining these modalities improves the overall predictive value several days after hypoxic-ischemic injury, and often multiple tests are required to improve prognostic ability and rule out potentially confounding conditions.'

Nadkarni VM, Larkin GL, Peberdy MA, et al. First documented rhythm and clinical outcome from in hospital cardiac arrest among children and adults. JAMA. 2006; 295: 50–7.

Significance: 'In this multicentre registry of in-hospital cardiac arrest, the first documented pulseless arrest rhythm was typically asystole or PEA in both children and adults. Because of better survival after asystole and PEA, children had better outcomes than adults despite fewer cardiac arrests due to VF or pulseless VT.'

Atkins DL, Everson-Stewart, S, Sears, G, et al. Epidemiology and outcome from out of hospital cardiac arrest in children. Circulation 2009; 119: 1484–91.

Significance: This epidemiological observational study demonstrates that 'the incidence of out-of-hospital cardiac arrest in infants approaches that observed in adults'. Remarkably, pediatric patients were more likely to survive to discharge than adults, and children and adolescents were twice as likely to survive compared with infants or adults. Patients with an initial rhythm of VT/VF have better survival than those with asystole/pulseless electric activity.

Respiratory medicine

Werner HA. Status asthmaticus in children: a review. Chest 2001; 119: 1913–29.

Significance: The article reviews the pathophysiology of asthma and the various strategies for managing critically ill children with asthma, including pharmacological and non-pharmacological therapies. Both conventional and non-established therapies are described. Various guidelines exist in different regions that are useful adjuncts to enable recent developments to be appreciated (e.g. UK British Thoracic Society at www.brit-thoracic.org.uk; National Asthma Council Australia at www.nationalasthma.org.au).

Gozal D, Colin AA, Jaffe M, Hochberg Z. Water, electrolyte and endocrine homeostasis in infants with bronchiolitis. Pediatric Research. 1990; 27: 204–9.

Significance: 'Bronchiolitis of infancy is characterised by both increased antidiuretic hormone secretion and hyper-reninaemia with secondary hyperaldosteronism, which induce water retention but counterbalance each other with respect to serum sodium. Increased ADH secretion, as well as increased plasma renin activity, are not 'inappropriate' but rather suggest a response to the perception of hypovolaemia by intrathoracic receptors.'

Kellner JD, Ohlsson A, Gadomski AM, Wang EE. Bronchodilators for bronchiolitis. Cochrane Database Systematic Reviews. 2000; (2): CD001266.

Significance: Bronchodilators produce small, short-term improvements in clinical scores among infants with bronchiolitis and may slightly improve oxygenation in those treated as outpatients. However, given the high costs, incidence of adverse effects and uncertain efficacy based on the findings of this meta-analysis, bronchodilators cannot be recommended for routine management of first-time wheezers who present with the clinical findings of bronchiolitis. Bronchodilators should not be used routinely in patients who are hospitalised with bronchiolitis.

Hanna S, Tibby SM, Durward A, Murdoch IA. Incidence of hyponatraemic seizures in severe respiratory syncytial virus bronchiolitis. Acta Paediatrica. 2003; 92: 430–4.

Significance: 'Hyponatraemia is common among infants with RSV bronchiolitis presenting to intensive care. Neurological complications may occur and fluid therapy in vulnerable infants should be tailored to reduce this risk.'

Hartling L, Russell K, Patel H, et al. Epinephrine for bronchiolitis. Cochrane Database Systematic Reviews. 2004; 1: CD003123.

Significance: There is no evidence to support adrenaline in this condition in inpatients. There is some evidence favouring adrenaline over salbutamol and placebo in outpatients.

Russell KF, Wiebe N, Saenz A, et al. Glucocorticoids for croup. Cochrane Database Systematic Reviews. 2004 CD001955.

Significance: Although various regimens have been studied, in a range of studies, it can be concluded that dexamethasone and budesonide are effective at reducing symptom severity, representation and readmission and length of stay during admissions. Steroids are beneficial for croup of all severities. In contrast, a Cochrane Review found no benefit of steroids in bronchiolitis (Patel H, Platt R, Lozano J, Wang E. 2004; 3: CD004878).

McCaffrey J, Farrell C, Whiting P, et al. Corticosteroids to prevent extubation failure: a systematic review and meta-analysis. Intensive Care Medicine. 2009; 35: 977–86.

Significance: 'Corticosteroids reduce laryngeal oedema and importantly reduce the incidence of extubation failure in critically ill patients of all ages. The effect of corticosteroids tended to be more pronounced in studies when used at least 12 h prior to attempted extubation.'

Kornecki A, Frndova H, Coates AL, Shemie SD. A randomized trial of prolonged prone positioning in children with acute respiratory failure. Chest. 2001; 119: 211–18.

Significance: 'In children with acute respiratory failure, oxygenation is significantly superior in the PP than in the SP. This improvement occurs early, remains sustained for a 12-h period, and is independent of changes in lung mechanics.'

Sokol J, Jacobs SE, Bohn D. Inhaled nitric oxide for acute hypoxemic respiratory failure in children and adults. Cochrane Database Systematic Reviews. 2000; 4: CD002787.

Significance: Only a transient improvement in oxygenation was found to be significant, but no improvements in mortality were identified. This is an expensive therapy and the role remains unclear, but it is of possible benefit to the sickest group of children where further randomised studies are needed.

Keckler SJ, Laituri CA, Ostlie DJ, St Peter SD. A review of venovenous and venoarterial extracorporeal membrane oxygenation in neonates and children. European Journal of Pediatric Surgery. 2010; 1: 1–4.

Significance: 'The use of extracorporeal membrane oxygenation (ECMO) has increased since its inception. As this modality gained wider acceptance, its application in a variety of disease states has increased. The initial use of ECMO required cannulation of both the carotid artery and internal jugular vein (VA ECMO). Ligation of the carotid artery and concern regarding potential long-term sequelae prompted the development of the single cannula venous only (VV ECMO) technique. Various reports in the literature have compared VV ECMO and VA ECMO. This is a useful review of the literature with regard to both physiology and clinical application.'

Wratney AT, Benjamin DK Jr, Slonim AD, et al. The endotracheal tube air leak test does not predict extubation outcome in critically ill pediatric patients. Pediatric Critical Care Medicine. 2008; 9: 490–6.

Significance: 'An endotracheal tube air leak pressure $\geq$30 cmH$_2$O measured in the non-paralysed patient before extubation or for the duration of mechanical ventilation was common and did not predict an increased risk for extubation failure. Pediatric patients who are clinically identified as candidates for an extubation trial but do not have an endotracheal tube air leak may successfully tolerate removal of the endotracheal tube.'

Markovitz BP, Randolph AG. Corticosteroids for the prevention of reintubation and postextubation stridor in pediatric patients: a meta-analysis. Pediatric Critical Care Medicine 2002; 3: 223–6.

Significance: The quality of studies was not high but it concluded that there was a trend to reduced need for re-intubation when used prophylacticaly and an improvement in post-extubation stridor especially in neonates. A trend to reduced need for re-intubation was also found in patients receiving steroids to treat airway existing obstruction.

Sedation and analgesia

Berens RJ, Meyer MT, Mikhailov TA, et al. A prospective evaluation of opioid weaning in opioid-dependent pediatric critical care patients. Anesthesia and Analgesia. 2006; 102: 1045–50.

Significance: 'Critically ill children are treated with opioid medication in an attempt to decrease stress and alleviate pain during prolonged pediatric intensive care. This treatment plan places children at risk for opioid dependency.' Once dependent, children can be weaned using oral methadone or risk development of a withdrawal syndrome on abrupt cessation of medication.

Hosokawa K, Shime N, Kato Y, et al. Dexmedetomidine sedation in children after cardiac surgery. Pediatric Critical Care Medicine. 2010; 11: 39–43.

Significance: Continuous sedation with a 0.4–0.6 mcg/kg/hr infusion of dexmedetomidine is a useful adjunct to postoperative sedation analgesia regimens and enables early extubation of paediatric patients after cardiac surgery. Because of its potential adverse haemodynamic effects, the risks of haemodynamic complications must be weighed carefully against the respiratory benefits, particularly in haemodynamically unstable, cardiac patients.

Sepsis

Butt W. Septic shock. Pediatric Clinics of North America. 2001; 48: 601–25.

Significance: Of children admitted to PICU 82% develop SIRS, 23% sepsis, 4% severe sepsis and 2% septic shock, with a mortality of 6% (higher if sepsis develops later in the admission). Responsible organisms, monitoring, resuscitation, organ support and specific therapies are discussed. The Surviving Sepsis Guidelines also includes a section on evidence-based recommendations for sepsis management (Dellinger RP, Carlet JM, Masur H, et al. Surviving Sepsis Campaign guidelines for management of severe sepsis and septic shock. Critical Care Medicine. 2004; 32: 858–73).

Booy R, Habibi P, Nadel S, et al. Meningococcal Research Group. Reduction in case fatality rate from meningococcal disease associated with improved healthcare delivery. Archives of Disease in Childhood. 2001; 85: 386–90.

Significance: 'A significant improvement in outcome for children admitted with meningocoal disease to a PICU has occurred in association with improvements in initial management of patients with meningocoal disease at referring hospitals, use of a mobile intensive care service, and centralisation of care in a specialist unit.'

De Kleijn ED, Joosten KF, Van Rijn B, et al. Low serum cortisol in combination with high adrenocorticotrophic hormone concentrations are associated with poor outcome in children with severe meningococcal disease. Pediatric Infectious Disease Journal. 2002; 21: 330–6.

Significance: Cortisol levels were significantly lower and ACTH significantly higher in non-survivors than survivors. Non-survivors had a higher level of IL6 (stimulates ACTH release) and TNF alpha (inhibits ACTH release centrally). The paper raises interesting ideas about a potential mechanism of steroids influencing survival. The pathophysiology of meningococcal meningitis and septicaemia is addressed comprehensively in another paper (Pathan N, Faust S, Levin M. Pathophysiology of meningococcal meningitis and septicaemia. Archives of Disease in Children. 2003; 88: 601–7).

Carcillo JA. Role of early fluid resuscitation in pediatric septic shock. JAMA. 1991; 266: 1242–5.

Significance: 'Rapid fluid resuscitation in excess of 40 mL/kg in the first hour following emergency department presentation was associated with improved survival, decreased occurrence of persistent hypovolaemia, and no increase in the risk of cardiogenic pulmonary oedema or adult respiratory distress syndrome in this group of pediatric patients with septic shock.'

Casartelli CH, Garcia PC, Branco RG, et al. Adrenal response in children with septic shock. Intensive Care Medicine. 2007; 33: 1609–13.

Significance: 'Adrenal insufficiency is a frequent finding in children with septic shock. The low-dose corticotrophin stimulation test seems to be an important tool to distinguish between a normal cortisol response to stress and evidence of adrenal failure. Mortality was significantly higher in children that failed to respond to a corticotrophin stimulation test.' All children who died had a high baseline cortisol. It is hypothesised that a progression is seen with a good initial response above a low baseline, then a parabola of maximal response ending in a high, then low baseline that is unable to respond. It is possible that the last two groups may benefit from exogenous steroids.

de Oliveira CF, de Oliveira DS, Gottschald AF, et al. ACCM/PALS haemodynamic support guidelines for paediatric septic shock: an outcomes comparison with and without monitoring central venous oxygen saturation. Intensive Care Medicine. 2008; 34: 1065–75.

Significance: Goal-directed therapy using the endpoint of a $ScvO_2$ ≥70% in addition to conventional measures has a significant and additive impact on the outcome of children and adolescents with septic shock. Other authors also postulate that the central venous arterial carbon dioxide difference may be an additionally useful marker. Using a a–$cvCO_2$ difference >6 mmHg identified a group with lower CO and lactate clearance over subsequent 12 hours despite $ScvO_2$ >70%, suggesting $ScvO_2$ >70% may miss some under resuscitated patients. Higher mortality was found in these children (Vallee F, Vallet B, Mathe O, et al. Central venous-to-arterial carbon dioxide difference: an additional target for goal-directed therapy in septic shock? Intensive Care Medicine. 2008; 34: 2218–25).

McMaster P, Shann F. The use of extracorporeal techniques to remove humoral factors in sepsis. Pediatric Critical Care Medicine. 2003; 4: 2–7.

Significance: A useful literature review of the evidence for the use of haemofiltration or plasmapheresis in the management of sepsis in children. The balance of data supports an improvement in haemodynamic parameters but there is less convincing evidence in terms of survival. Plasmafiltration appears more effective than haemofiltration. Large multicentre trials are needed.

Nadel S, Goldstein B, Williams MD, et al. REsearching severe Sepsis and Organ dysfunction in children: a gLobal perspective (RESOLVE) study group. Drotrecogin alfa (activated) in children with severe sepsis: a multicentre phase III randomised controlled trial. Lancet. 2007; 369: 836–43.

Significance: The study was not able to show a significant decrease in complete organ failure recovery time or mortality with the use of drotrecogin alfa activated (DrotAA). Although not statistically significant, there was an increased risk of bleeding and CNS bleeding associated with the use of DrotAA, especially in children less than 60 days old and 4 kg, which makes the risk-benefit ratio too high to use. Current sepsis management guidelines, based upon this study, specifically recommend NOT using DrotAA for paediatric severe sepsis. It should be appreciated, however, that the trial was underpowered, as it was stopped early due to adverse interim analysis results.

Pollard AJ, Britto J, Nadel S, et al. Emergency management of meningococcal disease. Archives of Disease in Children. 2001; 85: 386–90.

Significance: Careful assessment of all children with abnormal vital signs may lead to earlier recognition of meningococcal sepsis and application of the meningococcal treatment algorithm described here may help in the early management of critically ill patients with meningococcal disease.

References

The following sources have been used as reference material in the preparation of this chapter.

Harris W. Examination Paediatrics. Churchill Livingstone; 3rd edn: 2006.

Mackway-Jones K, et al. Advanced Paediatric Life Support. The Practical Approach. Blackwell Publishing; 4th edn: 2005.

Murphy P, Marriage SC, Davis PJ. Case Studies in Pediatric Critical Care. Cambridge University Press; 1st edn: 2009.

Stack C, Dobbs P. Essentials of Paediatric Intensive Care. Greenwich Medical Media limited; 1st edn: 2004.

List of abbreviations

A–a gradient	Alveolar–arterial oxygen gradient
AA	Amino acid
ABG	Arterial blood gas
AC	Alternating current
ACA	Anterior cerebral artery
ACE-I	Angiotensin converting enzyme inhibitor
ACEM	Australasian College for Emergency Medicine
ACh	Acetylcholine
ACLS	Advanced cardiac life support
ACS	Acute coronary syndrome
ACT	Activated clotting time
AD	Autosomal dominant
ADP	Adenosine diphosphate
ADRs	Adverse drug reactions
AF	Atrial fibrillation
AFB	Acid-fast bacilli
AG	Anion gap
AHA	American Heart Association
AICD	Automated implantable cardioverter defibrilator
AIHA	Autoimmune haemolytic anaemia
AIkT	Alkaline phosphatase
ALI	Acute lung injury
AMI	Acute myocardial infarct
ANZCA	Australian and New Zealand College of Anaesthetists
APO	Acute pulmonary oedema
APRV	Airway pressure release ventilation
aPTT	Activated partial thromboplastin time
AR	Autosomal recessive/aortic regurgitation
ARDS	Acute respiratory distress syndrome
ARF	Acute renal failure
AS	Aortic stenosis
ASA	American Society of Anesthesiologists
ATLS	Advanced trauma life support
ATRA	All-trans-retinoic acid syndrome
ATN	Acute tubular necrosis
AVR	Aortic valve replacement
BBB	Blood–brain barrier/bundle branch block
BCAA	Branched chain amino acid
BDZ	Benzodiazepine
BFR	Blood flow rate
β-hCG	Beta human chorionic gonadotrophin
BMI	Body mass index
BMR	Basal metabolic rate
BP	Blood pressure
BSL	Blood sugar level

C&S	Culture and sensitivity
CABG	Coronary artery bypass graft
CAPS	Catastrophic Antiphospholipid Syndrome
CBF	Cerebral blood flow
CCC	Cholecystokinin
CCF	Congestive cardiac failure
CCU	Coronary care unit
cfu	Colony-forming units
cGMP	Cyclic glyceryl monophosphate
CHI	Closed head injury
CHO	Carbohydrate
CI	Cardiac index
CICM	College of Intensive Care Medicine of Australia and New Zealand
CK	Creatine kinase
CLD	Chronic liver disease
CME	Continuing medical education
CMP	Calcium, magnesium and phosphate
Cn	Cyanide
CNS	Central nervous system
CO	Cardiac output
CO_2	Carbon dioxide
COAD	Chronic Obstructive Airways Disease
COMT	Catechol-O-methyltransferase
COPD	Chronic obstructive pulmonary disease
COPD	Chronic obstructive pulmonary disease
CPB	Cardiopulmonary bypass
CPP	Cerebral perfusion pressure
CPR	Cardiopulmonary resuscitation
CREST	Form of systemic scleroderma characterised by Calcinosis, Raynaud's syndrome, oEsophageal dysmotility, Sclerodactyly, Telangiectasia
CRF	Chronic renal failure
CRRT	Continuous renal replacement therapy
CRT	Capillary refill time
CSF	Cerebrospinal fluid
CSWS	Cerebral salt wasting syndrome
CT	Computed tomography
CT KUB	Computed tomography of kidneys, ureter and bladder
CTA	Computed tomography angiogram
CTD	Connective tissue disease
CTG	Cardiotocograph
CVA	Cerebrovascular accident
CVC	Central venous catheter
CVL	Central venous line
CVP	Central venous pressure
CVS	Cardiovascular system
CVVHD	Continuous veno-venous haemodialysis
CVVHDF	Continuous veno-venous haemodiafiltration
CVVHF	see CVVHDF
CXR	Chest X-ray

dBP	Diastolic blood pressure
DC	Direct current
DCD	Donation after cardiac death
DDVAP	Desmopressin or 1-deamino-8-D-arginine vasopressin
DIC	Disseminated intravascular coagulation
DLCO	Carbon monoxide diffusing capacity
DM	Diabetes mellitus
DO_2	Oxygen delivery
DSA	Digital subtraction angiography
DVT	Deep venous thrombosis
ECG	Electrocardiogram
ECMO	Extracorporeal membrane oxygenation (vv = venovenous ⇒ oxygenation; va = venoarterial ⇒ myocardial pump inadequacy)
EDH	Extradural haemorrhage
EMG	Electromyogram
EMST	Emergency management of severe trauma
EN	Enteral nutrition
ENT	Ear, nose and throat
ESBL	Extended spectrum β-lactamase
$EtCO_2$	End tidal carbon dioxide concentration
ETT	Endotracheal tube
EUC	Urea, creatinine and electrolytes
EVD	Extraventricular drain
EVLWI	Extra vascular lung water index
f	Frequency (set ventilator respiratory rate)
FRC	Functional residual capacity
FVC	Forced vital capacity
G-6-PD	Glucose-6-phosphate dehydrogenase
G&H	Group and hold
GCS	Glasgow Coma Scale
GM-CSF	Granulocyte macrophage colony stimulating factor
GTN	Glyceryl trinitrate
GXM	Group and cross-match
HAP	Hospital-acquired pneumonia
Hb	Haemoglobin
HBO_2	Hyperbaric oxygen
HBOC	Haemoglobin-like oxygen carrier
HDU	High dependency unit
HE	Hepatic encephalopathy
HELLP	Haemolytic anaemia, elevated liver enzymes and low platelets
HES	Hydroxyethylstarch
HFOV	High frequency oscillatory ventilation
HFV	High frequency ventilation
HHH	Hypervolaemia, hypertension and haemodilution therapy for cerebral vasospasm after SAH therapy for cerebral vasospasm after SAH
HITTS	Heparin-induced thrombocytopaenia and thrombotic syndrome

HIV	Human immunodeficiency virus
HMWK	High molecular weight kininogen
HOCM	Hypertrophic obstructive cardiomyopathy
HR	Heart rate
HRCT	High-resolution CT scan
HRS	Hepatorenal syndrome
HT	Hypertension
HUS	Haemolytic uraemic syndrome
I&V	Intubate and ventilate
IABP	Intra-aortic balloon pump
ICC	Intercostal catheter
ICH	Intracranial haemorrhage/intracranial hypertension
ICM	Intensive care medicine
ICP	Intracranial pressure
ICU	Intensive care unit
IDC	Indwelling urinary catheter
IDDM	Insulin-dependent diabetes mellitus
IHD	Ischaemic heart disease/intermittent haemodialysis
IJ	Internal jugular
ILCOR	International Liaison Committee On Resuscitation
INR	International normalised ratio
iPEEP	Intrinsic pulmonary end-expiratory pressure
ITBUI	Intrathoracic blood volume index
ITP	Idiopathic thrombocytopenic purpura
IUGR	Intrauterine growth retardation
IV	Intravenous
IVDU	Intravenous drug use
IVI	Intravenous infusion
IVIG	Intravenous immunoglobulin
IVP	Intravenous pyelogram
JVP	Jugular venous pressure
K+	Potassium
LA	Left atrium
LAD	Left axis deviation
LAP	Left atrial pressure
LDH	Lactate dehydrogenase
LFTs	Liver function tests
LHF	Left heart failure
LOA	Loss of appetite
LOC	Loss of conciousness
LOW	Loss of weight
LQTS	Long QT syndrome
LV	Left ventricle
LVAD	Left ventricular assist device
LVEDP	Left ventricular end-diastolic pressure
LVEDV	Left ventricular end-diastolic volume
LVEF	Left ventricular ejection fraction

M-FAST-HUGS	Mobilisation; feeding; analgesia; sedation; thromboprophylaxis; head up minimum 30°; ulcer prophylaxis; glycaemic control; skin care
MAHA	Microangiopathic haemolytic anaemia
MAO	Monoamine oxidase
MAP	Mean arterial pressure
MBT	Massive blood transfusion
MCA	Middle cerebral artery
MCD	Minimal change disease
Met-Hb	Methaemoglobin
MHPG	3-methoxy-4-hydroxyphenylglycol
MI	Myocardial infarction
MMSE	Mini Mental State Examination
MOF	multi-organ failure
MOPS	Maintenance of professional standards
MR	Mitral regurgitation
MSk	Musculoskeletal
MVC	Motor vehicle collision
MvO_2	Myocardial oxygen demand
MVP	Mitral valve prolapse
MVR	Mitral valve replacement
MWt	Molecular weight
N/V	Nausea or vomiting
Na	Sodium
NAdr	Noradrenaline
NAPQI	N-acetyl-p-benzoquinonimine
NIV	Non-invasive ventilation
NPV	Negative predictive value
NUM	Nurse unit manager
nvCJD	New variant Creutzfelt-Jakob disease
O_2	Oxygen
OCP	Oral contraceptive pill
OPD	Outpatients department
OT	Operating theatre/occupational therapy
PA	Pulmonary artery
PAC	Pulmonary artery catheter
PAOP	Pulmonary artery occlusion pressure
PAP	Positive airway pressure/pulmonary artery pressure
PCA	Patient-controlled analgesia/posterior cerebral artery
PCKD	Polycystic kidney disease
PCP	*Pneumocystis carinii* pneumonia (now *Pneumocystis jiroveci* pneumonia)
PCV	Packed cell volume
PCWP	Pulmonary capillary wedge pressure
PE	Pulmonary embolism
PEEP	Pulmonary end-expiratory pressure
PEG	Percutaneous entero-gastrostomy tube
PEJ	Percutaneous entero-jejunostomy tube
PICC	Peripherally inserted central catheter

PIFR	Peak inspiratory flow rate
PLT	Platelet
PMHx	Past medical history
PMNs	Polymorphonuclear cells (neutrophils)
PPM	Permanent pacemaker
PPV	Positive-pressure ventilation/positive predictive value
PR	Pulse rate or per rectum
PRBC	Packed red blood cells
PT	Prothrombin time
PUO	Pyrexia of unknown origin
PVR	Pulmonary vascular resistance
Px	Prevention
q6h	Every 6 hours
QALY	Quality adjusted life year
QI	Quality improvement
RACP	Royal Australian College of Physicians
RACS	Royal Australian College of Surgeons
RAD	Right axis deviation
RAS	Reticular activating system
RhF	Rheumatoid factor
RHF	Right heart failure
RN	Registered nurse
ROC	Receiver operator characteristic
RRT	Renal replacement therapy
RSI	Rapid sequence induction
RTI	Respiratory tract infection
RV	Residual volume
RVCPP	Right ventricular coronary perfusion pressure
S1, S2	First heart sound, second heart sound
SAAG	Serum to ascitic fluid albumen gradient
SAH	Subarachnoid haemorrhage
SAM	Systolic anterior motion of the mitral valve
SBP	Spontaneous bacterial peritonitis
sBP	Systolic blood pressure
SC	Subclavian
SCD	Sudden cardiac death
SCUF	Slow continuous ultrafiltration
SDH	Subdural haemorrhage
SES	Socioeconomic status
SIADH	Syndrome of inappropriate ADH secretion
SIRS	Systemic inflammatory response syndrome
SLE	Systemic lupus erythematosis
SLED	Slow low efficiency dialysis
SMR	Standardised mortality rate
SNP	Sodium nitroprusside
SpO_2	Pulse oximeter oxygen saturation
SSRI	Serotonin specific reuptake inhibitor
STD	Sexually transmitted disease

SV	Stroke volume
SVR	Systemic vascular resistance
T	Temperature
T1DM	Type I diabetes mellitus
T2DM	Type II diabetes mellitus
TB	Tuberculosis
TBI	Traumatic brain injury
TBSA	Total body surface area
TCAD	Tricyclic antidepressant
TG	Triglyceride
TIA	Transient ischaemic attack
TIPPS	Transjugular intra-hepatic portosystemic shunt
TL-CVC	Triple lumen central venous catheter
TLC	Total lung capacity
TOE	Transoesophageal echocardiography
TPN	Total parenteral nutrition
TR	Tricuspid regurgitation
TRALI	Transfusion-related lung injury
TT	Thrombin time
TTE	Transthoracic echocardiography
TTP	Thrombotic thrombocytopenic purpura
U/A	Urine analysis
U/O	Urine output
U&E	Urea and electrolytes
UTI	Urinary tract infection
VAP	Ventilator-associated pneumonia
VATS	Video assisted thoracoscopy
VDK	Venom detection kit
VF	Ventricular fibrillation
VISA	Vancomycin intermediate resistant *staphylococcus aureus*
VMA	Vanillylmandelic acid
VO_2	Oxygen consumption rate
VRE	Vancomycin-resistant enterococcus
VSD	Ventricular septal defect
Vt	Tidal volume
VT	Ventricular tachycardia
vWF	Von Willebrand factor
WFNS	World Federation of Neurosurgeons
ZN	Ziel-Nielsen stain

Index

A

abdominal aortic aneurysm repair, 253–4
  appropriate thoughts, 253
  discussion topics, 254
  examination, 253–4
    cubicle, 253
    equipment, 253
    infusions, 253–4
    monitor, 253
    physical, 253–4
    ventilation, 253
  possible cases, 253
  useful questions, 254
  useful statements, 254
abdominal ultrasound, 126
  abnormalities seen on, 126t
  specific types of, 126t
abdominal X-rays, 121
  abnormalities seen on, 121–2t
  air in biliary tree, 123f
  small bowel obstruction, 124–5f
actor stations, 77
  communication, 81b
  role-play communication, 82t
  scenario examples, 80–1
acute kidney injury, child with, 301–4
  appropriate thoughts, 301
  common case, 301
  discussion topics, 303–4
  examination, 301–3
    cubicle, 301
    equipment, 302
    infusion, 301
    monitor, 301–2
    physical, 302–3
    ventilator, 301
  useful questions, 303
  useful statements, 303
acute myocardial infarction, 165
ADAPT *see* Australian Donor Awareness Program
  Training
Advanced Paediatric Life Support (APLS), 13–14, 283
airway management
  critical care literature, 1
  as viva topic, 204
airway obstruction
  fixed upper, 169f
  lower, 168f
  variable extrathoracic upper, 169f
  variable intrathoracic upper, 169f

airway resistance
  lung volume compared to, 29f
  respiratory system, 26
alveolar gas equation, 179b
alveolar opacification, 112f
anagelsia, 316
anatomy
  bronchial, 88f
  chest, 87f
  cubital fossa, 89f
  femoral triangle, 90f
  foot arterial, 90f
  head, 132f
  neck, 85–6f
  practical and procedural skills, 85
  wrist, 89f
ankylosing spondylitis, 140f
ANZICS *see* Australian and New Zealand Intensive
  Care Society
aortic dissection, 161
  CT scan of, 120f
aortic regurgitation, 162, 163f
aortic stenosis, 162
APLS *see* Advanced Paediatric Life Support
apnoea test examination, 94f
ARDS
  lung physiology, 26
arterial blood gas analysis, 175–7
  alevolar gas equation, 179b
  important gaps, 178t
  interpretation rules, 176t
  major acid-base abnormality differential diagnosis,
    177t
arterial waveforms, 152, 152f, 153t
ascitic fluid analysis, 198t
assessment classification, 77–8
  actor stations, 77
  full body manikins, 78, 91, 91t, 96f
  hybrids, 78, 99–100t
  part task trainers, 78
atrioventricular septal defect (AVSD), 292
Australasia paediatric intensive care medicine training,
  283–4
  PIC Fellowship examination blueprint, 284, 285–90t
  success strategies, 284
  training requirements, 283–4
Australian Donor Awareness Program Training
  (ADAPT), 13
The Australian Intensive Care Medicine clinical
  refresher course, 14

Page references followed by *f*, indicate figure, by *b*, indicate box, and by *t* indicate table.

Australian and New Zealand Intensive Care Society
     (ANZICS), 13
Australian Short Course in Intensive Care
     Medicine, 14
autoimmune markers, 184, 184–5t
AVSD *see* atrioventricular septal defect

B
back anatomy, 91f
bariatric patients, 265–7
    appropriate thoughts, 265
    discussion topics, 266–7
    examination, 266
        equipment, 266
        infusions, 266
        monitor, 266
        physical, 266
        ventilation, 266
    possible cases, 265
    respiratory system, 33
    useful questions, 266
    useful statements, 266
    as viva topic, 204
BBB *see* blood brain barrier
bile, 47
bile salts, 47
biliary tree, air in, 123f
bilirubin, 47
biochemistry data sets
    electrolytes disorders, 181–2t
    urea-to-creatinine ratio, 179, 184f
        classic exam, 179–80t
        liver function, 183t
biochemistry tests, 175–87
    arterial blood gas analysis, 175–7, 176–8t, 179b
    autoimmune markers, 184, 184–5t
    data sets, 179, 179–80t, 183t, 184f
    iron studies, 186
    miscellaneous other tests, 186–7
    short Synacthen test, 184–5, 185f
    thyroid function tests, 186
    tumour markers, 186
blood brain barrier (BBB), 44
blood clotting platelets, 50
blood counts, 187–90
blood cross-matching, 49–50
body fluid analysis, 195
    ascitic fluid, 198t
    cerebrospinal fluid, 198t
    joint fluid, 199t
    pleural fluid, 197t
    urine, 195–7t
box and whisker plot, 273f
brain death, 231–3
    appropriate thoughts, 231
    discussion topics, 233
    examination, 231–2
        apnoea test, 94f
        coma, 93f

corneal reflex, 93f
cough reflex, 94f
cubicle, 231
demonstration of, 92, 92f
equipment, 232
equipment for, 92f
gag reflex, 94f
infusions, 232
monitor, 232
physical, 232
pupillary light reflex, 93f
sample marking grid, 95, 95t
ventilation, 232
vestibular-ocular test, 94f
    paediatric intensive care literature on, 304
    possible cases, 231
    useful questions, 233
    useful statements, 233
bronchial anatomy, 88f
bronchiectasis, 119f
burns, 261–3
    appropriate thoughts, 261
    discussion topics, 263
    examination, 261–3
        cubicle, 261–2
        equipment, 262
        infusions, 261–2
        monitor, 261
        physical, 262–3
        ventilation, 262–3
    inflammatory/infective phase of, 261
    paediatric intensive care literature on, 304
    possible scenarios, 261
    post-resuscitation phase of, 261
    resuscitation phase of, 261
    useful questions, 263
    useful statements, 263
    as viva topic, 204–5

C
C2 fracture, 138f
calorimetry, indirect, 174
The Canberra ICU course, 14
capnography, 174
    normal waveform, 174f
    traces, 175t
CAPPS *see* catastrophic antiphospholipid
     syndrome
carbon dioxide dissociation curve, 30, 32f
cardiac arrest survivor, 240–2
    appropriate thoughts, 240
    discussion topics, 241–2
    examination, 240–1
        cubicle, 240
        equipment, 241
        infusions, 240
        monitor, 240
        physical, 241
        ventilation, 240

possible cases, 240
  useful questions, 241
  useful statements, 241
cardiogenic shock, 19f
cardiomyopathy
  dilated, 164
  hypertrophic obstructive, 164–5
  restrictive, 164
  Takotsubo, 165, 165f
cardiovascular medicine
  paediatric intensive care literature on, 305
cardiovascular system, 33–9
  central venous pressure and, 38
  coronary circulation, 34–5, 35f
  ECG electrochemical basis, 33
  haemorrhage response, 36–8
  problems of, 205
  ventricular pressure-volume relationships, 35, 37–8f
catastrophic antiphospholipid syndrome (CAPPS), 195
central venous pressure (CVP) waveforms, 151
  analysis, 151t
  normal, 151f
cerebral artery territory infarct, 135f
cerebral blood flow, 44–5, 45f
cerebrospinal fluid analysis, 198t
cervical spine X-rays, 137f
chest anatomy, 87f
chest trauma, 115f
chest X-rays, 103–11
  abnormalities seen on, 107–10t
  alveolar opacification, 112f
  chest trauma, 115f
  fissure location, 106f
  hemithorax white-out, 114f
  interstitial infiltration, 113f
  lung lobes, 106f
  multiple medical devices, 111f
  ruptured hemidiaphragm, 116f
  systematic assessment of, 104–5b
chronic obstructive pulmonary disease, 238–40
  appropriate thoughts, 239
  discussion topics, 239–40
  examination, 239
  possible cases, 238–9
  useful questions, 239
  useful statements, 239
chronic subdural haematoma, 134f
CICM see College of Intensive Care Medicine
clinical and oral examination, of EDIC, 3–4
  minimum criteria for, 3
  pass marks for, 4
coagulation studies, 190–3
  disorders, 192–3t
  thromboelastograph, 193
CoBaTrICE see Competency-Based Training in Intensive Care Medicine in Europe
collagen vascular diseases, 205

College of Intensive Care Medicine (CICM), 7
  pass marks of, 9t
  primary examination for, 7–9
    format of, 8
    oral section of, 8
    viva for, 208
    written section of, 8
coma examination, 93f
Competency-Based Training in Intensive Care Medicine in Europe (CoBaTrICE), 1
compliance, respiratory system, 29
computed tomography (CT) scans
  abdomen, 127
    abnormalities seen on, 127t
    impaired renal perfusion, 130f
    metastatic lymphoma, 129f
    traumatic liver injury, 128f
    traumatic renal injury, 128f
    traumatic spleen rupture, 129f
  chest and neck, 117
    abnormalities seen on, 117t
    aortic dissection, 120f
    bronchiectasis, 119f
    interstitial lung disease, severe, 119f
    pneumothorax, 118f
    saddle pulmonary embolism, 118f
  head, 131
    abnormalities seen on, 131t
    basic neuroanatomy seen on, 132f
    cerebral artery territory infarct, 135f
    chronic subdural haematoma, 134f
    diffuse axonal injury, 134f
    diffuse cerebral oedema, 133f
    extradural haematoma, 133f
    subarachnoid haemorrhage, 135f
consolidate learning concepts, 60
corneal reflex examination, 93f
coronary circulation, 34–5, 35f
cough reflex examination, 94f
creatinine, 41–2
  GFR compared to, 41f
  urea ratio, 179, 184f
Critical Care and Resuscitation, 7
critical care literature, 269
  airway management, 1
  overview of, 269–70
  topics covered by, 270–1b
CT see computed tomography scans
cubital fossa anatomy, 89f
CVP see central venous pressure waveforms

D
data, 272
  box and whisker plot for, 273f
  normal distribution curve, 273f
  summarising of, 272
  types of, 102b
data interpretation
  DICM, 101

data interpretation (*Continued*)
  EDIC, 101
  FCICM, 101
  for intensive care medicine, 101
  overview of, 101–2
  see also imaging studies
dead space
  Fowler's estimation method, 31f
  respiratory system and, 30
defibrillator, 73f, 74–5t
diagnostic tests, 276–7, 276f, 277f
diagrams and graphs, 52–3
  on drug response mechanisms, 53f, 54t
  non-linear receptor binding, 53
  occupational theory anomalies, 52–3
  receptor reserve, 53
  transducer molecules, 53
DICM *see* Diploma in Intensive Care Medicine
diffuse axonal injury, 134f
diffuse cerebral oedema, 133f
diffusing capacity of carbon monoxide (DLCO),
    167, 168t
Diploma in Intensive Care Medicine (DICM), UK
    intercollegiate, 4–6
  data interpretation of, 101
  dissertation for, 5–6
  entry criteria for, 5
  exam format of, 6
  examiner presentation, 217
  expanded case summaries for, 6
  modules of, 5
  pass marks for, 6
  preparation courses for, 12–13
  viva for, 203–8
Diploma of the Irish Board of Intensive Care Medicine
    preparatory course, 13
dissertation
  for DICM, 5–6
  domains of, 5–6
DLCO *see* diffusing capacity of carbon monoxide

E
ECG *see* electrocardiograph
echocardiography
  abnormalities, 161–7
  acute myocardial infarction, 165
  aortic dissection, 161
  aortic regurgitation, 162, 163f
  aortic stenosis, 162
  apical four-chamber window, 160f
  cardiomyopathy, dilated, 164
  cardiomyopathy, hypertrophic obstructive, 164–5
  cardiomyopathy, restrictive, 164
  cardiomyopathy, Takotsubo, 165, 165f
  endocarditis, 164, 164f
  hardware, 167
  intracardiac masses, 166–7
  left ventricular diastolic dysfunction, 161
  left ventricular systolic dysfunction, 161

  left ventricular wall thickness, 161
  mitral regurgitation, 163, 163f
  mitral stenosis, 162
  parasternal long-axis window, 160f
  pericardial effusion and tamponade, 161
  pulmonary hypertension, 165–6
  right ventricular dysfunction, 165
  shunts, 165f, 166
ECLS *see* extracorporeal life support
EDIC *see* European Diploma of Intensive Care
    Medicine
electrocardiograph (ECG), 36f, 147, 147f
  electrochemical basis, 33
  patterns and abnormalities of, 148–50t
electrolyte disorders, 181–2t
  see also fluids and electrolytes
Emergency Management of Severe Trauma
    (EMST), 14
endocarditis, 164, 164f
endocrine
  paediatric intensive care literature on, 309
  physiology, 52
endocrine disease, 205
environmental clues, in ICU, 211–13
  cubicle, 211
  equipment, 212–59
  infusions, 211
  monitor, 212
  ventilator, 212
epiglottitis, 139f
equipment, 68
  abdominal aortic aneurysm repair examination, 253
  acute kidney injury examination, 302
  bariatric patient examination, 266
  brain dead examination, 92f, 232
  burns examination, 262
  cardiac arrest survivor examination, 241
  ECLS examination, 264, 296
  febrile examination, 234–5
  head injury examination, 247–8, 299–300
  ICU environmental clues, 212–59
  intra-abdominal catastrophe examination, 252
  jaundice examination, 227
  library arrangement of, 70–5
  long-stay patient examination, 267
  obstetric patient examination, 255
  oncology patient examination, 259
  overview of, 68–76
  physics and clinical measurement and, 75–6
  post-cardiac surgical paediatric case examination, 293
  post-cardiac surgical patient examination, 243
  post-transplant examination, 298
  renal failure examination, 225
  SAH examination, 245–6
  sample question for, 68–70
  sedation examination, 228
  severe respiratory failure examination, 218
  shock examination, 223–4
  spinal injury examination, 249–50

trauma injury examination, 236
ventilation weaning examination, 220
weakness examination, 230
ESICM *see* European Society of Intensive Care
    Medicine
European Diploma of Intensive Care Medicine
    (EDIC), 1–4
    clinical and oral examination of, 3–4
    data interpretation of, 101
    examiner presentation, 216
    MCQ paper of, 2–3
    preparation courses for, 12–13
    short cases of, 216–17t
    viva for, 203–8
European Society of Intensive Care Medicine
    (ESICM), 1
exam templates, 66
examiner presentation, 214–17
    common questions regarding, 215
    for DICM candidates, 217
    for EDIC candidates, 216
    for FCICM candidates, 215–16
extracorporeal life support (ECLS), 263–5
    appropriate thoughts, 263–4
    discussion topics, 265
    examination, 264–5
        cubicle, 264
        equipment, 264
        infusions, 264
        monitor, 264
        physical, 264–5
        ventilation, 264
    possible cases of, 263
    useful questions, 265
    useful statements, 265
extracorporeal life support (ECLS), of child, 295–7
    appropriate thoughts, 295
    common cases, 295
    discussion topics, 297
    examination, 295–6
        cubicle, 295
        equipment, 296
        infusion, 296
        monitor, 296
        physical, 296
        ventilation, 296
    useful questions, 296–7
    useful statements, 297
extradural haematoma, 133f
extubation, 221–2
    appropriate thoughts, 221–2
    child suitable for, 291–2
        appropriate thoughts, 291
        common cases, 291
        considerations, 292
        discussion topics, 292
        examination, 291
        useful questions, 291–2
        useful statements, 292

    considerations, 222
    discussion topics, 222
    examination, 222
    possible cases, 221–2
    useful questions, 222
    useful statements, 222

F
fact cards, 61
Faculty Intensive Care Medicine (FICM), 4–5
FCICM *see* Fellowship of the College of Intensive Care
    Medicine
febrile, 233–5
    appropriate thoughts, 233
    discussion topics, 235
    examination
        cubicle, 234
        equipment, 234–5
        infusions, 234
        monitor, 234
        physical, 234–5
        ventilation, 234
    possible cases, 233
    useful questions, 235
    useful statements, 235
Fellowship of the College of Intensive Care Medicine
    (FCICM)
    admittance to, 6
    completion of, 7
    data interpretation of, 101
    examination for, 9–11
        clinical, 11
        cross-table viva, 10
        format for, 10–11
        oral, 10
        pass marks for, 11, 11t
        results, 11
        written, 10
    examiner presentation, 215–16
    preparation courses for, 13–14
    training requirements of, 6–11
        core knowledge and resources, 6–7
    viva for, 203–8
femoral triangle anatomy, 90f
FICM *see* Faculty Intensive Care Medicine
flow-volume loops, 168
    fixed upper airway obstruction, 169f
    lower airway obstruction, 168f
    restrictive lung disease, 170f
    variable extrathoracic upper airway obstruction,
        169f
    variable intrathoracic upper airway obstruction,
        169f
fluid infusion, 42, 43f
fluid management
    as viva topic, 205
fluids and electrolytes
    paediatric intensive care literature on, 309
foot arterial anatomy, 90f

forest plot, 275
Fowler's method, for dead space estimation, 31f
Frank-Starling mechanism, 37f, 38
full body manikins, 78, 91
   scenarios using, 91t
   set-up, 96f

G
gag reflex examination, 94f
gastric emptying factors, 48
gastric secretion, 47–8
gastrointestinal system, 46–8
   bile, bilirubin and bile salts, 47
   gastric emptying factors, 48
   gastric secretion, 47–8
   liver blood flow, 46–7
   problems of, 205
   urea cycle, 47, 184
glomerular filtration rate (GFR), 40–1, 41f

H
haematologic data sets, 193
   CAPPS, 195
   normal values, 194t
   pre-eclampsia, 193–5
   thromboelastogram, 194f
   thrombotic thrombocytopenic purpura, 193
haematological system, 49–50
   blood clotting platelets, 50
   blood cross-matching, 49–50
   haemostasis, 50, 51f
haematology, 187–95
   blood counts, 187–90
   body fluid analysis, 195, 195–9t
   coagulation studies, 190–3, 192–3t
   data sets, 193, 194f, 194t
   HIT pre-test, 191t
   paediatric intensive care literature on, 310
   platelet disorders, 190f
   red and white blood cell disorders, 188–9t
haemodynamic monitoring, 151–67
   arterial waveforms, 152, 152f, 153t
   CVP waveforms, 151, 151f, 151t
   echocardiography, 159–67
   intra-aortic balloon pump waveforms, 153, 153–5f
   mixed venous oxygen saturation and central venous
      oxygen saturation, 152, 152f
   newer measurement devices, 158
   oesophageal Doppler, 158, 159f
   pulmonary artery catheters, 155, 156–7f, 156t
haemorrhage response, cardiovascular system and,
     36–8
haemostasis, 50, 51f
head injury, 246–9
   appropriate thoughts, 246
   child with, 299–301
      appropriate thoughts, 299
      common cases, 299
      discussion topics, 300–1

      examination, 299–300
      useful questions, 300
      useful statements, 300
   discussion topics, 248–9
   examination, 247–8
   possible cases, 246
   useful questions, 248
   useful statements, 248
heart
   Frank-Starling mechanism of, 37f, 38
hemidiaphragm, ruptured, 116f
hemithorax white-out, 114f
heparin infusion, 211
heparin-induced thrombocytopenia (HIT)
      pre-test, 191t
high frequency oscillatory ventilator
   answer on, 70
   sample question on, 70
HIT *see* heparin-induced thrombocytopenia pre-test
host defence, 49
hybrids, 78, 99–100t
hypersensitivity reactions, 49

I
ICU *see* intensive care unit
imaging studies, 102–46
   abdominal ultrasound, 126, 126t
   abdominal X-rays, 121, 121–2t, 123–5f
   of anatomical structures, 103f
   chest X-rays, 103–11, 104–5b, 106–7f, 107–10t
   CT scans
      abdomen, 127, 127t, 128–30f
      chest and neck, 117, 117t
      head, 131, 131t, 132–5f
   modalities for, 146
   MRI, 147t
   skeletal and soft tissue, 136, 136–43f,
      144–5t, 146f
immunology, 49
impaired renal perfusion, 130f
infection control, as viva topic, 205–6
inferential statistics, 272–4
intensive care medicine, 101
   basic sciences for, 24
      diagrams and graphs, 52–3
      exam templates, 66
      fact cards, 61
      introduction to, 24–5
      learning consolidate concepts, 60
      lists, 58–60
      mind maps, 60, 61f
      past papers, 61
      pharmacology, 25, 52–67
      physics/clinical measurement, 25
      physiology, 24–52
      question creation, 64
      quizzes, 66–7
      research methods/statistics, 25
      sample questions, 62–6

statistics, 271–7
tables, 55
training, 1
EDIC, 1–4
FCICM, 6–11
UK intercollegiate DICM, 4–6
intensive care unit (ICU)
clinical cases in, 209, 209–10b
environmental clues, 211–13
examiner presentation, 214–17
generic approach to, 210–17
introduction to, 209
systemic clinical examination, 213–14
diagnostic problems, 217–38
brain dead, 231–3
extubation, 221–2
febrile, 233–5
jaundice, 226–8
multi-organ failure, 238
renal failure, 225–6
sedation, 228–9
severe respiratory failure, 217–19
shock, 223–5
trauma injuries, 235–7
ventilation weaning, 219–21
weakness, 229–31
intravenous fluids used in, 55t
scoring systems in, 207
specific patient groups, 238–68
abdominal aortic aneurysm repair, 253–4
bariatric, 265–7
burns, 261–3
cardiac arrest survivor, 240–2
chronic obstructive pulmonary disease, 238–40
ECLS, 263–5
head injury, 246–9
intra-abdominal catastrophe, 251–2
long-stay patient, 267–8
obstetric patient, 254–6
oncology patient, 258
post-cardiac surgical patient, 242–5
spinal injury, 249–51
subarachnoid haemorrhage, 245–6
transplant patient, 256–8
interstitial infiltration, 113f
interstitial lung disease, severe, 119f
intra-abdominal catastrophe, 251–2
appropriate thoughts, 251
discussion topics, 252
examination, 251–2
cubicle, 251
equipment, 252
infusions, 251
monitor, 251–2
physical, 252
ventilation, 251
possible cases, 251
useful questions, 252
useful statements, 252

intra-aortic balloon pump, 83f
insertion of, 83t–5t
waveforms, 153
early deflation, 154f
early inflation, 154f
late deflation, 155f
late inflation, 155f
normal, 153f
intracardiac mass, 166–7
invasive blood pressure monitoring, 68–70, 69f
invasive positive pressure ventilation (IPPV), 33
iron studies, 186
isomerism, 62b

J
jaundice, 226–8
appropriate thoughts, 227
discussion topics, 228
examination, 227
possible cases, 226
useful questions, 227
useful statements, 227
Joint Faculty of Intensive Care Medicine (JFICM), 7
joint fluid analysis, 199t

L
Le Fort facial fracture classification, 136f
left ventricular diastolic dysfunction, 161
left ventricular systolic dysfunction, 161
left ventricular wall thickness, 161
literature see critical care literature
liver blood flow, 46–7
liver function tests, 183t
liver injury, traumatic, 128f
long-stay patient, 267–8
appropriate thoughts, 267
discussion topics, 268
examination, 267–8
possible cases, 267
useful questions, 268
useful statements, 268
lung
ARDS physiology, 26
normal
airway resistance compared to, 29f
fissure location, 106f
lobes of, 106–7f
physiology, 25–6
PVR compared to, 30f

M
magnetic resonance imaging (MRI), 147t
manikins see full body manikins
MCQ see multiple choice question
medical crises, 206
meta-analysis, 275–6
metastatic lymphoma, 129f
mind maps, 60, 61f
mitral regurgitation, 163, 163f

mitral stenosis, 162
mixed venous oxygen saturation and central venous
        oxygen saturation, 152, 152f
MRI *see* magnetic resonance imaging
multi-organ failure, 19f, 238
multiple choice question (MCQ), 1
    of EDIC, 2–3
        blueprint topic question distribution for, 3t
        minimum criteria for, 2
        pass mark for, 3
        type A question, 2, 2t
        type K question, 2, 2t
multiple medical devices, 111f
musculoskeletal system, 48–9

N
National Intensive Care exam revision course, 13
neck anatomy, 85–6f
nerve axon conduction, 45
nerve fibre classification, 46t
neurological system, 44–6
    BBB, 44
    cerebral blood flow, 44–5, 45f
    nerve axon conduction, 45
    nerve fibre classification, 46t
    pain pathways and mediators, 45–6
neurology
    paediatric intensive care literature on, 310
    as viva topic, 206
normal distribution curve, 273f
nutrition
    paediatric intensive care literature on, 312
    physiology, 52
    as viva topic, 206

O
obesity *see* bariatric patients
objective structured clinical examinations (OSCEs), 8
*Objectives of Training for Paediatric Intensive
        Care*, 284
obstetrics and gynaecology, 50–2, 254–6
    appropriate thoughts, 254
    discussion topics, 256
    examination, 254–5
    placenta gas exchange, 52
    possible cases, 254
    useful questions, 255–6
    useful statements, 256
    as viva topic, 206
occupational theory anomalies, 52–3
oesophageal Doppler, 158, 159f
oncology patient, 258
    appropriate thoughts, 259
    discussion topics, 260
    examination, 259–60
        cubicle, 259
        equipment, 259
        infusions, 259
        monitor, 259

physical, 259–60
    ventilation, 259
    possible cases, 258
    useful questions, 260
    useful statements, 260
    as viva topic, 206–7
organ donation, 304
OSCEs *see* objective structured clinical examinations
osmolality, 39f
oxygen cascade, 27f
oxygen flux, 33
oxygen-haemoglobin dissociation curve, 27f

P
PACT *see* Patient-centered Acute Care Training
paediatric intensive care, 279
    Australasia training for, 283–4
    chapter content of, 279–80b
    clinical cases of, 291–304
        acute kidney injury, 301–4
        ECLS child, 295–7
        extubation, 291–2
        head injury, 299–301
        post-cardiac surgical, 292–5
        post-transplant, 297–9
    FCICM component of, 283
    introduction to, 279
    key facts for, 280–2t
    literature on, 304, 304b
Paediatric Intensive Care Fellowship
    clinical component of, 291
    examination blueprint, 284, 285–90t
paediatric intensive care literature, 304, 304b
    brain death and organ donation, 304
    burns, 304
    cardiovascular medicine, 305
    endocrine, 309
    fluids and electrolytes, 309
    haematology, 310
    neurology, 310
    nutrition, 312
    renal medicine, 313
    respiratory medicine, 314
    resuscitation, 313
    sedation and analgesia, 316
    sepsis, 316
pain medicine
    as viva topic, 207
pain pathways, 45–6
part task trainers, 78, 82–3
past papers, 61
Patient-centered Acute Care Training (PACT), 1–2
PEEP *see* positive and expiratory pressure
pelvis, 142f
    fractures, 143f
pericardial effusion and tamponade, 161
pharmacokinetic terms, 59–60
pharmacology
    diagrams and graphs for, 52–3

drug interaction mechanisms and, 59
exam templates, 66
fact cards, 61
learning consolidate concepts, 60
lists, 58–60
mind maps, 60, 61f
past papers, 61
question creation, 64
quizzes, 66–7
sample questions, 62–6, 66f
as science for intensive care medicine, 25, 52–67
tables, 55, 55–8t
terms for, 59–60
vancomycin, 60b
physics/clinical measurement, 25
physiology
   in ARDS lung, 26
   cardiovascular system, 33–9
   endocrine and nutrition, 52
   gastrointestinal system, 46–8
   haematological system, 49–50
   immunology and host defence, 49
   musculoskeletal system, 48–9
   neurological system, 44–6
   in normal lung, 25–6
   obstetrics, 50–2
   renal system, 39–44
   respiratory system, 26–33
   sample question, 25–6
   as science for intensive care medicine, 24–5
   thermoregulation, 48
PiCCO data, 158, 158t
platelet disorders, 190f
pleural fluid analysis, 197t
pneumothorax, 118f
positive and expiratory pressure (PEEP)
   flow-time waveform with, 173f
   pressure support with, 173f
   respiratory system, 32
post-cardiac surgical paediatric case, 292–5
   appropriate thoughts, 292
   common cases, 292
   discussion topics, 295
   examination, 292–3
      cubicle, 292
      equipment, 293
      infusion, 293
      monitor, 293
      physical, 293–4
      ventilation, 293
   useful questions, 294
   useful statements, 295
post-cardiac surgical patient, 242–5
   appropriate thoughts, 242
   discussion topics, 244–5
   examination, 242–4
      equipment, 243
      infusions, 242
      monitor, 242

      physical, 243–4
      ventilation, 242–3
   possible cases, 242
   useful questions, 244
   useful statements, 244
post-transplant, child, 297–9
   appropriate thoughts, 297
   common cases, 297
   discussion topics, 299
   examination, 297–8
      cubicle, 297
      equipment, 298
      infusion, 297
      monitor, 298
      physical, 298
      ventilation, 298
   useful questions, 298
   useful statements, 298–9
posture changes
   cardiovascular system and, 39
   respiratory system, 32
potassium handling, by kidney, 40
practical and procedural skills, 77
   advice for, 78–80, 79t
   anatomy, 85
   assessment classification, 77–8
   overview of, 77
   role-play communication approach, 82t
   scenario examples for, 80–91
pre-eclampsia, 193–5
preparation courses
   for EDIC and DICM, 12–13
   exam courses for, 14
   for FCICM, 13–14
   scientific meetings as, 12–13
   for success strategies, 12–14
pressure transducer, 71f, 72–3t
pressure-volume loops, 170, 170f
pulmonary artery catheters, 155
   interpretation, 157f
   parameters, 156t
   waveforms, 156f
pulmonary blood flow, 33
pulmonary hypertension, 165–6
pulmonary vascular resistance (PVR), 26–9, 30f
pupillary light reflex examination, 93f
PVR see pulmonary vascular resistance

Q
quizzes, 66–7

R
receiver operator characteristic (ROC) curve, 272
red and white blood cell disorders, 188–9t
renal disease, 207
renal failure, 225–6
   appropriate thoughts, 225
   discussion topics, 226
   examination, 225–6

renal failure (*Continued*)
   cubicle, 225
   equipment, 225
   infusion, 225
   monitor, 225
   physical, 226
   ventilation, 225
  possible cases, 225
  useful questions, 226
  useful statements, 226
renal medicine
  paediatric intensive care literature on, 313
renal system, 39–44
  acid-base balance control, 42–4
  blood flow features, 39
  buffer system, 44
  counter-current mechanisms, 40
  creatinine, 41–2
  fluid infusion, 42, 43f
  GFR factors, 40–1
  potassium handling, 40
  sodium handling, 40
  TBW, 42
  traumatic injury, 128f
research methods/statistics
  data, 272
  diagnostic tests, 276–7, 276f
  factors involved in, 275
  forest plot, 275
  inferential statistics, 272–4
  meta-analysis, 275–6
  paper reports, 277
  ROC curve, 277f
  sample question for, 271
  as science for intensive care medicine, 25, 271–7
  trials, 274–5
  as viva topic, 207
respiratory failure, severe, 217–19
  appropriate thoughts, 217
  discussion topics, 219
  examination, 217–19
   cubicle, 217–18
   equipment, 218
   infusions, 218
   monitor, 218
   physical, 218–19
   ventilation, 218
  possible cases, 217
  useful questions, 219
  useful statements, 219
respiratory function tests
  DLCO, 167, 168t
  flow-volume loops, 168, 168–70f
  pressure-volume loops, 170, 170f
  spirometry, 167, 167f
respiratory medicine
  paediatric intensive care literature on, 314
  as viva topic, 207
respiratory system, 26–33
  airway resistance, 26

  arterial and end-tidal pCO$_2$ difference, 32
  carbon dioxide dissociation curve, 30, 32f
  compliance, 29
  control, 33
  dead space, 30, 31f
  IPPV, 33
  lung volume compared to airway
   resistance, 29f
  obesity, 33
  oxygen flux, 33
  PEEP effects, 32
  posture changes effects, 32
  pulmonary blood flow features, 33
  PVR, 26–9, 30f
  spirometry, 28f
  venous admixture, 26
restrictive lung disease, 170f
resuscitation
  paediatric intensive care literature on, 313
right ventricular dysfunction, 165
ROC *see* receiver operator characteristic curve

S
saddle pulmonary embolism, 118f
SAH *see* subarachnoid haemorrhage
sample marking grid
  for brain dead examination, 95
  for ventilation high peak airway pressures scenario,
   98, 98t
SAQs *see* short-answer questions
scoliosis, 146f
sedation, 228–9
  appropriate thoughts, 228
  discussion topics, 229
  examination, 228–9
   cubicle, 228
   equipment, 228
   infusions, 228
   monitor, 228
   physical, 229
   ventilation, 228
  paediatric intensive care literature on, 316
  possible cases, 228
  useful questions, 229
  useful statements, 229
  as viva topic, 207
sepsis
  paediatric intensive care literature on, 316
SFQs *see* short-fact questions
shock, 223–5
  appropriate thoughts, 223
  discussion topics, 224–5
  examination, 223–4
   cubicle, 223
   equipment, 223–4
   infusions, 223
   monitor, 223
  possible cases, 223
  useful questions, 224
  useful statements, 224

short Synacthen test, 184–5, 185f
short-answer questions (SAQs), 8
short-fact questions (SFQs), 8
shunts, 165f, 166
skeletal and soft tissue imaging, 136
    abnormalities seen on, 144–5t
    ankylosing spondylitis, 140f
    C2 fracture, 138f
    cervical spine X-rays, 137f
    epiglottitis, 139f
    Le Fort facial fracture classification, 136f
    pelvic fractures, 143f
    pelvis, 142f
    scoliosis, 146f
    spinal fracture, 141f
    subcutaneous emphysema, 139f
    swimmer's view with dislocation, 138f
small bowel obstruction, 103f, 124f
sodium handling, by kidney, 40
spinal fracture, 141f
spinal injury, 249–51
    appropriate thoughts, 249
    discussion topics, 250–51
    examination, 249–50
        cubicle, 249
        equipment, 249–50
        infusions, 249
        monitor, 249
        physical, 250
        ventilation, 249
    possible cases, 249
    useful questions, 250
    useful statements, 250
spirometry, 28f, 167, 167f
spleen rupture, traumatic, 129f
statistics see inferential statistics; research methods/
    statistics
study notes, 15–16
subarachnoid haemorrhage (SAH), 245–6
    appropriate thoughts, 245
    CT scan of, 135f
    discussion topics, 246
    examination, 245–6
        equipment, 245–6
        infusions, 245
        monitor, 245
        physical, 245–6
        ventilation, 245
    possible cases, 245
    useful questions, 246
    useful statements, 246
subcutaneous emphysema, 139f
success strategies, 12
    clinical cases and, 20
    exam day and, 21
    failure coping and, 22
    generic clinical assessment and, 18f
    personal care as, 17–18
    preparation courses for, 12–14
        EDIC and DICM, 12–13

right impression creation and, 21
study groups for, 18–20
study notes for, 15–16
textbooks, journals and online resources as, 14–15
timing for, 12
travel considerations, 21
viva and, 20
Sydney Intensive Care Equipment course, 14
The Sydney Short Course in Intensive Care Medicine, 14
systemic clinical examination, 213–14
    EDIC short cases of, 216–17t
    patient positioning, 213

T
tables, pharmacology, 55, 55–8t
TAPVR see total anomalous pulmonary
    venous return
TBW see total body water
textbooks, journals and online resources, 14–15
TGA see transposition of great vessels
thermoregulation, 48
thromboelastograph, 193
thyroid function tests, 186
total anomalous pulmonary venous return
    (TAPVR), 292
total body water (TBW), 42
toxicology
    specific investigations, 16–17t
    study notes for, 16, 16f
    as viva topic, 207
transfusion medicine, 205
transplant patient, 256–8
    appropriate thoughts, 256–7
    discussion topics, 258
    examination, 257–8
        cubicle, 257
        infusions, 257
        monitor, 257
        physical, 258
        ventilation, 257
    possible cases, 256
    useful questions, 258
    useful statements, 258
    as viva topic, 207–8
transposition of great vessels (TGA), 292
trauma
    as viva topic, 208
trauma injuries, 235–7
    appropriate thoughts, 235–6
    chest, 115f
    discussion topics, 237
    examination, 236–7
        equipment, 236
        infusions, 236
        monitor, 236
        physical, 236–7
        ventilation, 236
    liver, 128f
    possible cases, 235
    renal, 128f

trauma injuries (*Continued*)
   spleen rupture, 129f
   useful questions, 237
   useful statements, 237
trials, 274–5
tumour markers, 186
type A question, 2, 2t
type K question, 2, 2t

U
urea cycle, 47, 184f
urea-to-creatinine ratio, 179, 184f
   classic exam, 179–80t
   liver function, 183t
urine analysis, 195–7t

V
Valsalva manoeuvre, 34f
vancomycin pharmacokinetics, 60b
venous admixture, 26
ventilation, high peak airway pressures scenario, 96–8
   equipment set-up, 96
   manikin set-up, 96f
   procedure, 97f
   sample making grid for, 98, 98t
   setting review, 96f
   vital sign readings and, 97f
ventilation weaning, 219–21
   appropriate thoughts, 219–20
   discussion topics, 221
   examination, 220–1
      cubicle, 220
      equipment, 220
      infusion, 220
      monitor, 220
      physical, 220–1
      ventilation, 220
   possible cases, 219
   useful questions, 221
   useful statements, 221
ventilator waveform, 171–2
   autoflow and pressure support, 172f
   flow-time waveform with PEEP, 173f
   pressure support with PEEP, 173f
   volume control with pressure support, 170f

ventricular pressure-volume relationships, 35
vertebral levels, 103f
vestibular-ocular test examination, 94f
viva, 201
   for CICM primary examination, 208
   for EDIC, DICM and FCICM examinations, 203–8
   format of, 203
   generic advice on, 201–3
   success strategies and, 20
   topics of, 204–8
      airway management, 204
      bariatric patients, 204
      burns, 204–5
      cardiovascular problems, 205
      collagen vascular diseases, 205
      endocrine disease, 205
      fluid replacement and transfusion medicine, 205
      gastrointestinal problems, 205
      ICU scoring systems, 207
      infection control, 205–6
      medical crises, 206
      neurology, 206
      nutrition, 206
      obstetric patients, 206
      oncology, 206–7
      pain and sedation management, 207
      renal disease, 207
      respiratory medicine, 207
      statistics and research, 207
      toxicology, 207
      transplantation medicine, 207–8
      trauma, 208
      welfare issues, 208

W
weakness, 229–31
   appropriate thoughts, 230
   discussion topics, 231
   examination, 230
   possible cases, 229
   useful questions, 231
   useful statements, 231
welfare issues, 208
wrist anatomy, 89f